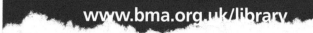
Diabetic Cardiology

Diabetes

dp

in Practice

Other titles in the Wiley Diabetes in Practice Series

Exercise and Sport in Diabetes Second Edition
Edited by Dinesh Nagi
978 0470 022061

Complementary Therapies and the Management of Diabetes and Vascular Disease
Edited by Patricia Dunning
978 0470 014585

Diabetes in Clinical Practice: Questions and Answers from Case Studies
Edited by N. Katsilambros, E. Diakoumopoulou, I. Ioannidis, S. Liatis, K. Makrilakis, N. Tentolouris and P. Tsapogas 978 0470 035221

Obesity and Diabetes
Edited by Anthony Barnett and Sudhesh Kumar
978 0470 848982

Prevention of Type 2 Diabetes
Edited by Manfred Ganz
978 0470 857335

Diabetes – Chronic Complications Second Edition
Edited by Kenneth Shaw and Michael Cummings
978 0470 865798

The Metabolic Syndrome
Edited by Christopher Byrne and Sarah Wild
978 0470 025116

Psychology in Diabetes Care Second Edition
Edited by Frank J. Snoek and T. Chas Skinner
978 0470 023846

The Foot in Diabetes Fourth Edition
Edited by Andrew J. M. Boulton, Peter R. Cavanagh and Gerry Rayman
978 0470 015049

Gastrointestinal Function in Diabetes Mellitus
Edited by Michael Horowitz and Melvin Samson
978 0471 899167

Diabetic Nephropathy
Edited by Christoph Hasslacher
978 0471 489924

Nutritional Management of Diabetes Mellitus
Edited by Gary Frost, Anne Dornhorst and Robert Moses
978 0471 497516

Diabetes in Pregnancy: An International Approach to Diagnosis and Management
Edited by Anne Dornhorst and David R. Hadden
978 0471 962045

Hypoglycaemia in Clinical Diabetes Second edition
Edited by Brian M. Frier and Miles Fisher
978 0470 018446

Diabetic Cardiology

Editors

Miles Fisher

Glasgow Royal Infirmary, Glasgow, UK

John J. McMurray

*Clinical Research Initiative in Heart Failure and Department of Medicine,
University of Glasgow, Glasgow, UK*

BICENTENNIAL
1807
WILEY
2007
BICENTENNIAL

John Wiley & Sons, Ltd

Other Wiley Editorial Offices

John Wiley & Sons Inc., 111 River Street, Hoboken, NJ 07030, USA

Jossey-Bass, 989 Market Street, San Francisco, CA 94103-1741, USA

Wiley-VCH Verlag GmbH, Boschstr. 12, D-69469 Weinheim, Germany

John Wiley & Sons Australia Ltd, 33 Park Road, Milton, Queensland 4064, Australia

John Wiley & Sons (Asia) Pte Ltd, 2 Clementi Loop #02-01, Jin Xing Distripark, Singapore 129809

John Wiley & Sons Canada Ltd, 6045 Freemont Blvd, Mississauga, Ontario, L5R 4J3, Canada

Wiley also publishes its books in a variety of electronic formats. Some content that appears in print may
not be available in electronic books.

Anniversary Logo Design: Richard J. Pacifico

Library of Congress Cataloging in Publication Data

Diabetic cardiology / edited by Miles Fisher, John J. McMurray.
      p.   ;   cm.
Includes bibliographical references and index.
ISBN 978-0-470-86204-9 (alk. paper)
1. Heart—Diseases. 2. Cardiovascular system—Diseases.   3. Diabetes—Complications.
I. Fisher, Miles.   II. McMurray, John J., MD. [DNLM: 1. Cardiovascular Diseases—etiology.
2. Diabetes Complications.   3. Cardiovascular Diseases—therapy.   4. Diabetes
Mellitus—therapy. WG 120 D536 2008]
RC682.D52 2008
616.6'1—dc22
                                                                              2007024231

British Library Cataloguing in Publication Data

A catalogue record for this book is available from the British Library

ISBN 978-0-470-86204-9

Typeset in 10/12pt Times by Integra Software Services Pvt. Ltd, Pondicherry, India
Printed and bound in Great Britain by Antony Rowe Ltd, Chippenham, Wiltshire
This book is printed on acid-free paper responsibly manufactured from sustainable forestry in which at
least two trees are planted for each one used for paper production.

Contents

List of Contributors ix

Introduction xi

1 Epidemiology of Vascular Disease in Diabetes 1
Susan Laing

    1.1   Introduction 1
    1.2   The Role of Epidemiological Studies 1
    1.3   Cohort Studies of People with Diabetes 2
    1.4   Cardiovascular Disease and Diabetes 4
    1.5   Mortality from Coronary Heart Disease 6
    1.6   Mortality from Cerebrovascular Disease 8
    1.7   Discussion 10
    References 12

2 Pathogenesis of Atherosclerosis and Vascular Disease in Type 2 Diabetes 16
Naveed Sattar and Alistair Cormack

    2.1   Introduction 16
    2.2   What is Insulin Resistance? 17
    2.3   Dyslipidaemia and Type 2 Diabetes 19
    2.4   Hypertension 22
    2.5   Endothelial Dysfunction and Type 2 Diabetes 23
    2.6   Inflammation 25
    2.7   Adipokines – Adiponectin 26
    2.8   Haemostatic Changes in Type 2 Diabetes 27
    2.9   Hyperinsulinaemia 28
    2.10   Role of Hyperglycaemia 29
    2.11   Metabolic Syndrome as a Link between Insulin Resistance and CVD? 30
    2.12   Effects of Anti-diabetic Drugs on Risk Factor Pathways 31
    2.13   Conclusions 32
    References 32

3 Coronary Heart Disease and Diabetes 37
Colin Berry, Miles Fisher and John J. McMurray

    3.1   Nature of Coronary Heart Disease in Diabetes 37
    3.2   Presentation of CHD in Diabetes 38

3.3   Non-invasive Investigation   39
3.4   Pharmacological Treatment of CHD in People
       with Diabetes   40
3.5   Coronary Revascularisation in Diabetes   42
3.6   Stents for Coronary Artery Disease in Diabetes   50
3.7   Drug-eluting Stents   53
3.8   Drug Therapy and PCI in Diabetic Patients   56
3.9   Conclusions   59
       References   59

4 Diabetes and Acute Coronary Syndromes   **69**
   Colin Berry, Miles Fisher and John J. McMurray

4.1   Introduction   69
4.2   Antiplatelet Agents   69
4.3   Thrombolysis   71
4.4   Beta-blockers   73
4.5   ACE Inhibitors   74
4.6   Angiotensin Receptor Blockers   74
4.7   Heparin   76
4.8   Glycoprotein IIb/IIIa Inhibitors   76
4.9   Revascularisation for Acute Coronary Syndromes   79
4.10   Device Therapy Post-MI   84
4.11   Management of Glycaemia   84
4.12   Conclusions   87
       References   87

**5 Diabetes, Left Ventricular Systolic Dysfunction and Chronic
   Heart Failure**   **93**
   Michael R. MacDonald, Mark C. Petrie,
   Nathaniel M. Hawkins and John J. McMurray

5.1   Introduction   93
5.2   Prevalence   93
5.3   Incidence   98
5.4   Risks of Developing CHF and Diabetes   99
5.5   Diabetes and Mortality in Patients with CHF   100
5.6   Morbidity   102
5.7   Chronic Heart Failure and Abnormalities of Insulin and
       Glucose Metabolism   103
5.8   Why do Patients with Diabetes develop CHF?   105
5.9   Reducing the Risk of Diabetes in Patients with CHF   109
5.10   Reducing the Development of CHF in Patients with
       Diabetes   109
5.11   Treatment of Diabetes in Patients with CHF   110
5.12   Treatment of CHF in Patients with Diabetes   117
5.13   Conclusions   121
       References   121

6   Diabetes and Hypertension   **135**
Gordon T. McInnes

    6.1   Introduction   135
    6.2   Metabolic Syndrome   137
    6.3   Risk Stratification   139
    6.4   Strategies to Reduce Cardiovascular Risk   140
    6.5   Strategies to Reduce Kidney Disease Risk   149
    6.6   Risk of Diabetes Mellitus with Antihypertensive Drugs   156
    6.7   Conclusions   160
    References   162

7   Diabetes and Stroke / Transient Ischaemic Attacks   **175**
Christopher S. Gray and Janice E. O'Connell

    7.1   Introduction   175
    7.2   Diabetes as a Risk Factor for Stroke   176
    7.3   Diabetes, Post-stroke Hyperglycaemia and Outcome from Stroke   178
    7.4   Hyperglycaemia and Ischaemic Cerebral Damage   181
    7.5   Management of Diabetes and Hyperglycaemia following Stroke 182
    7.6   Prevention of Stroke in Diabetic Patients   185
    7.7   Diabetes, Cognitive Impairment and Dementia   191
    7.8   Conclusions   192
    References   193

8   Diabetes and Peripheral Arterial Disease   **199**
Iskandar Idris and Richard Donnelly

    8.1   Introduction   199
    8.2   Pathogenesis   200
    8.3   Clinical Features of PAD in Patients with Diabetes   205
    8.4   Lower Extremity Revascularisation in Patients with Diabetes   209
    8.5   Medical Therapy of PAD in Diabetes   210
    8.6   Future Therapy for PAD   217
    8.7   Conclusions   217
    References   218

9   Prevention of Cardiovascular Events in Diabetic Patients   **223**
Markku Laakso

    9.1   Introduction   223
    9.2   Coronary Artery Disease in Type 2 Diabetes   223
    9.3   Potential and Proven Risk Factors for Atherothrombosis in Patients
          with Type 2 Diabetes   227
    9.4   Treatment Effects of Cardiovascular Risk Factors on the Risk of
          CAD in Type 2 Diabetes   230
    9.5   Summary   234
    Acknowledgements   235
    References   235

**10   Prevention of Diabetes as a Means of Preventing
      Cardiovascular Disease   240**
Stephen J. Cleland and Jonathan Shaw

    10.1   Hyperglycaemia as a Risk Factor for Cardiovascular Disease   240
    10.2   Risk of Cardiovascular Disease in Pre-diabetes   243
    10.3   Intervention Trials in Pre-diabetes   245
    10.4   Screening for Pre-diabetes   252
    10.5   Summary and Conclusions   253
    References   254

11   Diabetes for Cardiologists   258
David Macfarlane, Colin Perry and Miles Fisher

    11.1   Introduction   258
    11.2   Epidemiology of Diabetes Mellitus   258
    11.3   New Diagnostic Criteria for Diabetes Mellitus   260
    11.4   Metabolic Syndrome   261
    11.5   Treatment of Diabetes Mellitus   264
    11.6   Hypoglycaemia   266
    11.7   Treatment of Type 2 Diabetes   268
    11.8   Conclusions   274
    References   275

Study Acronyms   280

Index   287

List of Contributors

Colin Berry   Department of Cardiology, Western Infirmary, Glasgow G11 6NT, UK

Stephen J. Cleland   Department of Medicine, Stobhill Hospital, 133 Balornock Rd, Glasgow G21 3UT, UK

Alistair Cormack   Department of Cardiology, Glasgow Royal Infirmary, 10 Alexandra Parade, Glasgow G31 2ER, UK

Richard Donnelly   The Medical School, Derby City General Hospital, Uttoxeter Road, Derby DE22 3DT, UK

Miles Fisher   Glasgow Royal Infirmary, 84 Castle Street, Glasgow G4 0SF, UK

Christopher S. Gray   Department of Geriatrics, Sunderland Royal Hospital, Kayll Road, Sunderland SR4 7TP, UK

Nathaniel M. Hawkins   Department of Cardiology, Stobhill Hospital, Balornock Road, Springburn, Glasgow G21 3UW, UK

Iskandar Idris   Department of Diabetes and Endocrinology, Sherwood Forest Hospitals NHS Trust, Kings Mill Hospital NHS Trust, Mansfield Road, Nottinghamshire, NG17 4JL, UK

Markku Laakso   Department of Internal Medicine, University of Kuopio, PO Box 1627, FIN-70211, Kuopio, Finland

Susan Laing   Institute of Cancer Research, Section of Epidemiology Block D, Cotswold Road, Sutton, Surrey SM2 5NG, UK

Michael R. MacDonald   Department of Cardiology, Glasgow Royal Infirmary, 10 Alexandra Parade, Glasgow G31 2ER, UK

David Macfarlane   Diabetes Centre, Glasgow Royal Infirmary, University NHS Trust, Glasgow G31 2ER, UK

Gordon T. McInnes   University of Glasgow, Division of Cardiovascular and Medical Sciences, Western Infirmary, Glasgow G11 6NT, UK

John J. McMurray   Clinical Research Initiative in Heart Failure and Department of Medicine, West Medical Building, University of Glasgow, Glasgow G12 8QQ, UK

Janice E. O'Connell   Department of Geriatrics, Sunderland Royal Hospital, Kayll Road, Sunderland SR4 7TP, UK

Colin Perry   Diabetes Centre, Glasgow Royal Infirmary, University NHS Trust, Glasgow G31 2ER, UK

Mark C. Petrie   Department of Cardiology, Glasgow Royal Infirmary, 10 Alexandra Parade, Glasgow G31 2ER, UK

Naveed Sattar   Department of Pathological Biochemistry, Glasgow Royal Infirmary, 10 Alexandra Parade, Glasgow, G31 2ER, UK

Jonathan Shaw   International Diabetes Institute, 260 Kooyong Road, Caufield, Victoria 3162, Australia

Introduction

Until recently there was little overlap between diabetes and cardiology. Epidemiological studies identified an increase risk of cardiovascular morbidity and mortality in people with diabetes, but there were no proven interventions to reduce that risk. Control of glycaemia did not seem to reduce the risk, and there was even the suggestion that certain treatments for diabetes might further increase the risk. There was a perception that the vascular disease of diabetes would not respond to treatment of conventional cardiovascular risk factors such as hypertension and hypercholesterolaemia, and as a consequence people with diabetes were excluded from large cardiovascular trials, or were included in such small numbers that meaningful analysis of diabetes-subgroups was difficult or impossible. From a cardiovascular perspective the survival of people with diabetes following myocardial infarction was reduced compared to people without diabetes, and when surgical or percutaneous interventions were performed in patients with coronary heart disease the short term results and long term survival were inferior in patients with diabetes compared to non-diabetes patients.

This has changed in the last ten years for two major reasons. Firstly, evidence from large, multi-centre studies has demonstrated that for many interventions the relative risk reduction has been the same in both diabetic and non-diabetic subjects, but because of the increased event-rate in people with diabetes the absolute risk reduction in people with diabetes is greater, so they have more to gain from these interventions. Secondly, the changes in society with reductions in physical activity and increases in overweight and obesity, coupled with detailed scrutiny of glycaemia status in patients with cardiovascular disease, has revealed that around one third of cardiac patients have diabetes and one third other degrees of dysglycaemia, and that the numbers of people with any degree of dysglycaemia are increasing rapidly.

There are now several books that examine the clinical and scientific overlap of cardiovascular disease in diabetes, and these often seem to either tackle issues from a general medical perspective, or focus more on a diabetes and metabolic perspective. In this book we have deliberately chosen to examine the area from a cardiological perspective, hence the title 'Diabetic Cardiology'. Following chapters on the epidemiology and patho-physiology of cardiovascular disease in diabetes there are detailed chapters on the way that diabetes will be viewed by those running a cardiovascular service, covering stable coronary disease, acute coronary syndromes, cardiac failure, hypertension, strokes, and peripheral vascular disease. That is not to say that diabetes and metabolic factors are not important, and the final three chapters demonstrate how a more metabolically oriented approach, including glycaemia and dyslipidaemia interventions, can reduce risk in diabetes and pre-diabetic states, and some of the other treatment considerations in diabetes that may impinge upon cardiovascular practice.

Neither is this to say that the book will not be of interest to a diabetes readership who require further information on cardiovascular aspects of diabetes, and as many diabetes physicians are also specialists in general medicine or acute medicine much of the material in the early part of the book will be of interest beyond their diabetes practice.

It takes considerable time and dedication to write a chapter for a book, and we are extremely grateful to our local, national and international colleagues who have given their precious time to write contributions to this book. Chapters arrive at different times, and there is an inevitable delay between the submission of the final manuscripts and the appearance on the shelf of the finished book. If the reader wonders why a recent large, novel or controversial study has not been included it is because the study was not published when the book was completed! Nevertheless, each chapter provides a secure foundation on which can be added future research in the area of diabetic cardiology.

1 Epidemiology of Vascular Disease in Diabetes

Susan Laing

1.1 Introduction

Mortality rates in people with diabetes exceed those in the general population despite many recent improvements in care. Diabetes is one of the most common chronic diseases in the young, and is a substantial cause of morbidity as well as mortality at all ages. After the introduction of insulin in 1922 it was hoped that adverse consequences of diabetes might become a thing of the past, but mortality rates are still higher than those in the general population and, in addition, the late complications of diabetes, in particular cardiovascular disease (CVD), have been unmasked (Kessler, 1971; Dorman *et al.*, 1984; Orchard *et al.*, 1990). The St Vincent declaration of 1989, pledged by representatives of European government health departments, patient organizations and diabetes experts, set targets for improving the outlook for people with diabetes. It urged health departments throughout Europe to work towards a reduction in the heavy burden of disease in these patients by better recognition and treatment in the early stages and reduction of long-term complications. Determining the success of these health initiatives requires accurate measurement of morbidity and mortality rates, country by country.

1.2 The Role of Epidemiological Studies

Epidemiological studies are the best means by which these outcomes, and changes in these outcomes, can be measured. Epidemiology is concerned with events that occur in populations rather than separate individuals, and it is this that differentiates epidemiology from clinical medicine. Epidemiological studies are concerned not only with people who get a disease, or in this case those people with diabetes who develop cardiovascular complications, but also with those who do not, and in particular how

Diabetic Cardiology   Editors Miles Fisher and John J. McMurray
© 2007 John Wiley & Sons, Ltd.

the two groups differ. Initially epidemiological studies can be used to measure and describe the occurrence of CVD in patients with diabetes and how it differs between males and females, between different age- or socio-economic groups or between geographical regions. Secondly, epidemiological studies are concerned with how these measurements vary over time, or following the introduction of a new treatment. Finally, by measuring cardiovascular risk factors as well as the disease itself, these studies can be used to address the question 'why?'. Why do some people with diabetes develop serious cardiovascular complications while others do not? Is it possible to identify factors (biological, environmental or lifestyle) that are associated with an increased likelihood of developing cardiovascular complications?

Epidemiological studies may measure mortality, morbidity or both, but the studies measuring mortality tend to be larger. Smaller studies are ideal for tracking morbidity as it is possible to do frequent out-patient assessments of each patient and note the development of complications of diabetes, or any changes in symptoms, as they occur. Regular measurements of possible risk factors can also be made.

Patients with diabetes cannot always be identified from routine death certificates as diabetes is frequently not recorded on the death certificate, and therefore death certificates alone cannot be used to pick out the diabetic study group. Thus national mortality statistics will underestimate the true death rates (Andresen *et al.*, 1993), and instead a cohort study is the method of choice for assessing mortality. A group or 'cohort' of people with diabetes is gathered together, often from a number of different sources, and registered centrally. When the patient dies the research group is notified and receives a copy of the death certificate. The death certificate can then be used to indicate the fact and cause of death, independent of whether or not diabetes is mentioned. This chapter will be mainly confined to mortality studies because it was as a consequence of studies of this type that CVD was first recognised as the principal complication of people with diabetes.

1.3 Cohort Studies of People with Diabetes

The Framingham study, which has provided the foundation for so much of cardiovascular epidemiology over the past five decades, was one of the first to follow people with diabetes over time. From 1948 onwards over 5000 residents from the town of Framingham in Massachusetts were followed-up for mortality and morbidity. A cohort of people with diabetes was a subgroup of this population (Garcia *et al.*, 1974; Kannel and McGee, 1979). About the same time a cohort of over 21 000 people with diabetes was also being followed-up from the Joslin Clinic in Boston (Kessler, 1971). Both of these cohort studies began within a decade or so of the introduction of insulin, and both studies reported a significant excess risk of death from CVD in patients with diabetes.

Early studies rarely distinguished between patients with type 1 and type 2 diabetes. A recent meta-analysis (Kanters *et al.*, 1999) was conducted to determine an estimate of mortality and the incidence of CVD events. Of the 27 studies that allowed calculations of at least one of the outcomes, only two were restricted solely to patients with type 1 diabetes, eleven to patients with type 2 diabetes and of the remainder only one distinguished between type 1 and type 2. It is not surprising that the majority of the studies concern patients with type 2 diabetes (Barret-Connor *et al.*, 1991; Manson *et al.*, 1991; Stamler *et al.*, 1993; Muggeo *et al.*, 1995) as this condition is the most prevalent type of diabetes and accounts for 90% of all diagnoses (Nathan *et al.*, 1997). In addition, as it is primarily a condition of older people and is often associated with, or preceded by, the detection of CVD risk factors, it is comparatively straightforward to follow this group for subsequent CVD events. Type 1 diabetes is less frequent, occurs at an earlier age and is rarely accompanied by any co-existent CVD risk factors at the time of diagnosis.

Type 1 diabetes

Cohort studies of patients with type 1 diabetes are rarely large unless they are compiled from more than one centre. The earliest report of patients with type 1 diabetes alone was from Pittsburgh in 1972 (Sultz *et al.*, 1972) and since then there have been a number of further studies published from Pittsburgh, including a cohort study of 1966 patients with type 1 diabetes in 1984 (Dorman *et al.*, 1984; Krolewski *et al.*, 1987; Lloyd *et al.*, 1996a). There have also been a number of studies of a similar size from Scandinavian countries (Deckert *et al.*, 1979; Borch-Johnsen *et al.*, 1986; Lounamaa *et al.*,1991; Laakso and Kuusisto, 1996).

To date, the largest study of patients with type 1 diabetes has come from the UK (Laing *et al.*, 1999a, 1999b). The Diabetes UK Cohort Study (formerly British Diabetic Association Cohort Study) has followed over 23 000 patients with insulin-treated diabetes, recruited from separate registers across the UK. Both prevalent and incident cases were recruited. All had been diagnosed under the age of 30 years and were treated with insulin, and were therefore presumed to have type 1 diabetes. The first patients were recruited into the study in 1972, and recruitment continued until 1993. Although insulin treatment rather than evidence of absolute insulin deficiency was the criterion for inclusion, this cohort was considered to be essentially one of patients with type 1 diabetes. From the age-specific percentages of diabetic patients with type 1 diabetes (Laakso and Pyorala, 1985) it was estimated that at least 94% will have had type 1 diabetes.

A few international studies have compared complications and outcomes between countries. A four-country comparative study run by the Diabetes Epidemiology Research International Study Group has followed patients with type 1 diabetes from the USA, Finland, Israel and Japan (Diabetes Epidemiology Research International Study Group, 1995), and the WHO Multinational Study of Vascular Disease in Diabetes (which follows patients with both type 1 and type 2 diabetes) continues to report from 10 centres worldwide (Fuller *et al.*, 2001; Morrish *et al.*, 2001).

As it is more usual nowadays to distinguish between the two types of diabetes rather than group them together, it is tempting to draw comparisons. However, there are a number of difficulties in comparing studies of patients with type 1 and type 2 diabetes. Factors that must be taken into consideration include the relative ages of the two groups, the calendar period during which the data were collected, the endpoint chosen, together with the measurement used, and the population from which the cohort was selected.

As the patients with type 2 diabetes are diagnosed at an older age, usually over 45 years, there are very few age-specific studies of these patients and the patients are generally grouped together. As mortality is known to vary with age a comparison of type 1 and type 2 patients without any reference to age group would be flawed. To complicate things further, in a number of the type 1 studies there may be insufficient numbers to subdivide by age. Mortality is also known to vary with calendar period as lifestyles change or medical treatments improve and it would be difficult to draw any comparisons between results from two studies conducted 20 or 30 years apart. Studies may also differ in the type of endpoint that is measured, for example some may report mortality, others morbidity or a combination of the two. In addition these may be reported as a rate, a proportion, or a ratio relative to the underlying general population. The variation in mortality between countries further complicates international comparisons.

Despite these difficulties, it is only by drawing comparisons that the similarities and differences in CVD risk between type 1 and type 2 diabetes can be understood, which in turn might lead to a better understanding of the mechanisms by which CVD complications develop.

1.4 Cardiovascular Disease and Diabetes

Diabetes, both type 1 and type 2, is increasing in prevalence and it is estimated that three million individuals in the UK will have type 2 disease by 2010 (Gale, 2002; Fisher, 2003). Overall the numbers of people with type 2 far exceed those with type 1 and, in addition, they are usually middle aged or elderly and often present with concomitant CVD risk factors. However, comments such as 'Diabetes mellitus, *and particularly non-insulin dependent diabetes mellitus* increases the risk for all manifestations of vascular disease' (Laakso, 1998) and 'CVD complications occur more often in patients with NIDDM than in patients with IDDM' (Laakso and Lehto, 1997) can easily be misconstrued. Epidemiological studies measure outcome in a number of different ways. While absolute numbers can be counted, other measurements, adjusted for the size of the group, are more commonly used. For example, a rate (of an event) can be calculated as the number of such events per 100 000 people per year. Another commonly used epidemiological measure is the standardised mortality ratio (SMR), which is calculated as the number of observed deaths in the study population compared with the number of deaths that would be expected if general population rates, allowing for the size and age distribution of the study group, were applied. Once the smaller numbers and younger age distribution of people with type 1 diabetes have been taken into account, comparisons can be made.

A direct comparison of all-cause mortality, matched for age, calendar period and country, was made in the WHO Multinational Study (Head and Fuller, 1990). They studied mortality among 4740 diabetic men and women, aged 35–55 years, from 10 centres around the world and they calculated age-adjusted death rates, by centre, separately for type 1 and type 2 diabetes. Death rates for patients with type 1 diabetes were almost always higher than for the corresponding type 2 group.

Standardised mortality ratios, which take into account the underlying mortality in the general population, can also be compared. All-cause mortality in middle-aged and elderly patients with type 2 diabetes is generally 2–4 times higher than the mortality in the general population (Manson *et al.*, 1991; Moss *et al.*, 1991; Muggeo *et al.*, 1995).

The Diabetes UK Cohort Study (Laing *et al.*, 1999a), of patients with type 1 diabetes, reported an overall SMR of 2.7 for men and 4.0 for women. However, at younger ages in type 1 studies the SMRs for all cause mortality are higher, partly reflecting the much lower mortality in the general population in this age group, with SMRs for the under 40s from Pittsburgh being 5.0 for men and 9.3 for women (Dorman *et al.*, 1984). The Diabetes UK Cohort Study reported all-cause SMRs of 3.7 for men and 4.9 for women in the 30–39 age group. In both studies the relative risk of death was higher in the women than men.

Causes of death

All-cause mortality statistics give no clue as to why mortality might be raised. As well as the acute complications of diabetes, such as hypoglycaemia and ketoacidosis, a number of chronic complications are well recognised. Almost all of these relate in some way to micro- or macrovascular disease, and include CVD, nephropathy, neuropathy and retinopathy. Some may feature largely in studies of morbidity but not be a major cause of mortality, for example peripheral arterial disease is a common condition among diabetic patients but is rarely the primary cause of death (Chapter 8). Studies of patients with type 2 diabetes, although not usually subdivided by age, indicate that CVD is the major cause of death in these patients, accounting for as much as 80% of the excess deaths (Blendea *et al.*, 2003). In younger patients the chronic complications of diabetes develop some time after the initial diagnosis.

Data from the Diabetes UK Cohort Study illustrates how the predominant cause of death in people with type 1 diabetes changes with age (Table 1.1). Under the age of 20 the greatest single cause of death was acute complications of diabetes, which accounted for 38% of the deaths in men and 54% of the deaths in women. In males, between the ages of 20 and 39 years, acute complications remained the greatest single cause of death but in females CVD was the cause of the greatest number of deaths even at this young age. By the 40–59 age groups CVD accounted for at least half of all the deaths in patients with type 1 diabetes. This same pattern has been seen in other studies of young people with diabetes (Lounamaa *et al.*, 1991; Moss *et al.*, 1991), acute complications initially being responsible for the greatest number of deaths but CVD complications becoming the predominant cause of death at fairly young ages.

Table 1.1 Cause of death, expressed as a percentage of the total, by age group. Data from the Diabetes UK Cohort Study.

	Males			Females		
	1–19 years	20–39 years	40–59 years	1–19 years	20–39 years	40–59 years
Diabetes	38	26	7	54	17	10
Renal disease	0	8	9	0	16	11
Cardiovascular disease	6	17	61	10	26	50
Other	56	49	23	36	41	29

Renal disease has previously been identified as a major cause of death in patients with type 1 diabetes. From Pittsburgh (Dorman *et al.*, 1984) it was reported that renal disease was responsible for the majority of deaths in the 20–29 age group of the Pittsburgh morbidity and mortality study, and studies from Denmark suggested that the high relative mortality after 20–30 years' duration of diabetes was due to the development of proteinuria (Borch-Johnsen *et al.*, 1986). In the Diabetes UK Cohort Study the proportion of deaths due to renal disease was lower than the proportion due to CVD at all ages.

Clearly if mortality and morbidity are to be reduced then the prevention and treatment of CVD must be addressed. Cardiovascular disease itself is a generic term, encompassing many specific components, and can be further divided into peripheral arterial disease, cerebrovascular disease and heart disease as well as other types of vascular disease such as venous disease and aneurysms. Even within these groups further divisions can be made, for example the term 'heart disease' includes not only ischaemic heart disease, but also valve disorders, hypertensive heart disease, cardiomyopathy, dysrrhythmias and heart failure. Large cohort studies are necessary if separate statistics are to be calculated for the individual components of CVD. A number of studies of patients with type 2 diabetes have calculated these separate statistics, although the results are rarely reported by specific age group, but among the studies of patients with type 1 diabetes the Diabetes UK Cohort Study is alone in being of sufficient size and having sufficient follow-up to examine some of the CVD outcomes separately by age (Laing *et al.*, 2003a, 2003b).

1.5 Mortality from Coronary Heart Disease

Heart disease is well recognised as a chronic complication of diabetes, and is the major cause of morbidity and mortality in patients from middle-age onwards. Type 2 diabetes is associated at the onset with risk factors for heart disease such as hypertension and obesity, raising the question of whether diabetes *per se* is an independent risk factor for heart disease. Type 1 diabetes is not associated with risk factors for heart disease at the time of diagnosis although these develop later. Both types of diabetes are also characterised by hyperglycaemia and abnormal protein and lipid metabolism (Chapter 2).

The majority of cardiovascular deaths are specifically due to heart disease (Morrish *et al.*, 2001) and it is becoming apparent that heart disease is the major cause of morbidity and mortality at young as well as older ages. Heart disease, however, is such a broad term that unless the conditions included are made clear it is difficult to interpret the results. A number of studies have now specifically reported mortality from coronary heart disease (CHD) using codes according to the International Classification of Diseases.

There is a paucity of age- and sex-specific data for mortality from CHD in patients with type 1 diabetes as most studies are too small for such subdivisions. The Diabetes UK Cohort Study has recently published rates and SMRs for mortality from ischaemic heart disease (IHD) in 10-year age groups and the results are shown for the age groups between 20 and 59 years (Table 1.2). Within each age group the mortality rates for the patients with type 1 diabetes were higher than the corresponding rates for subjects in the general population. The mortality rates in the females were not only higher than

Table 1.2 Mortality from ischaemic heart disease in patients with type 1 diabetes. Data from the Diabetes UK Cohort Study.

Age at death (years)	Males		Females	
	Rate (per 100 000 person-years)	SMR (95% CI)	Rate (per 100 000 person-years)	SMR (95% CI)
20–29	12	11.8 (5.4–22.4)	14	44.8 (20.5–85.0)
30–39	69	8.0 (5.1–11.9)	84	41.6 (26.7–61.9)
40–49	537	7.5 (5.6–9.7)	282	18.3 (11.4–27.6)
50–59	1273	4.4 (3.4–5.7)	551	7.2 (4.5–10.9)
1–84	107	4.5 (3.9–5.1)	73	8.8 (7.4–10.3)

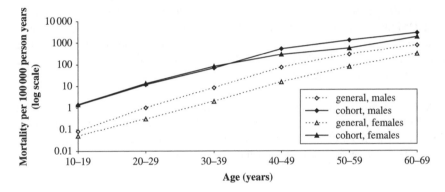

Figure 1.1 Ischaemic heart disease mortality in patients with type 1 diabetes. Data from the Diabetes UK Cohort Study.

for women without diabetes but were also considerably higher than for men without diabetes (Figure 1.1). In the general population mortality from CHD is higher for men than women at all ages but in the patients with type 1 diabetes there was no difference in mortality under the age of 40 years. The increased vulnerability of the young women is shown by the SMRs. At all ages the SMRs were higher for women than men, and under the age of 40 years the risk of mortality from CHD in women was increased 40-fold. This reflects both the mortality from CHD in these women and the low mortality rates, at younger ages, among women in the general population.

Although there are no age-specific results to compare with the findings reported here, a few studies of patients with type 1 diabetes have reported overall morbidity or mortality from CHD (Manson *et al.*, 1991). The most direct comparison can be made with the results from the population-based study from Wisconsin that recorded SMRs for CHD mortality in a group of 1200 patients diagnosed with diabetes under the age of 30 years, but the results were not subdivided by age (Moss *et al.*, 1991). They reported SMRs for IHD mortality at ages under 60 years of 9.1 for men and 15.4 for women. The exceptionally high SMRs for women in the Diabetes UK Cohort Study were only apparent after finer stratification by age.

In all reports of patients with type 2 diabetes, mortality from CHD was raised compared to the general population, and the relative risks were generally higher in women than men (Manson *et al.*, 1991; Stamler *et al.*, 1993). The data were not usually stratified by age, but there was one study from Scotland that enabled a comparison with the Diabetes UK data (Wong *et al.*, 1991). Not only was this a geographical area covered by the Diabetes UK Cohort Study, but it also specified the age at which the patients died. The SMRs for CHD mortality in the 45–64 age group were 3.7 for men and 5.4 for women. Values for the same age group from the Diabetes UK Cohort Study were 4.7 for men and 7.9 for women. In the absence of epidemiological studies of CHD in young patients with type 2 diabetes, direct comparisons cannot be made for the younger age groups, but it is of interest to note that the relative risk of death from CHD in the type 1 group was much higher at younger ages than at older ages, although the absolute risk remains low at this age.

In some cases it is possible that the high cardiovascular risk is mediated by renal disease, and in the Pittsburgh study there were more deaths certified to renal disease than to CVD among the young patients (Dorman *et al.*, 1984). It has been suggested that 'in IDDM macrovascular disease usually occurs in the presence of renal complications' (Laakso, 1998) and data from the American Diabetes Association (1989) suggest that the risk of overall CVD is much higher in type 1 patients with renal disease than in those without. Clearly the interrelationship between nephropathy and CVD is complicated.

As has already been discussed there are many more cases of CVD in patients with type 2 diabetes as it is the most prevalent type of disease and develops at an older age. However, it seems probable from the results shown above that type 1 diabetes confers the greater relative risk of a CVD event in an individual.

1.6 Mortality from Cerebrovascular Disease

Type 1 diabetes

Clinical aspects of stroke disease in people with diabetes are described in Chapter 7. Mortality from cerebrovascular disease is barely mentioned in epidemiological studies of patients with type 1 disease and usually only gets a passing mention in studies of patients with type 2 diabetes (Barrett-Connor and Khaw, 1988; Manson *et al.*, 1991; Moss *et al.*, 1991; Lehto *et al.*, 1996). Cerebrovascular disease is generally manifest in later years and most cohort studies of younger patients do not continue follow-up beyond their 40s. Further, cerebrovascular disease complications are not as frequent as heart disease and many studies will therefore be too small, with too few events, to draw any conclusions. This lack of data has led some to suggest that 'in the patient with insulin-dependent diabetes mellitus the frequency of stroke and death from stroke is less than in the patient with non-insulin dependent diabetes mellitus' (Bell, 1994). None the less it is a significant cause of mortality in patients with both types of diabetes, and in the Diabetes UK Cohort Study accounts for 6% of all deaths overall, and 8% of deaths under the age of 40 years (Laing *et al.*, 2003a). A similar proportion, 7% of the total mortality, was reported in a much smaller study of patients with type 1 diabetes by Deckert *et al.* (1979).

Table 1.3 Mortality from cerebrovascular disease in patients with type 1 diabetes. Data from the Diabetes UK Cohort Study.

Age at death (years)	Males		Females	
	Rate (per 100 000 person-years)	SMR (95% CI)	Rate (per 100 000 person-years)	SMR (95% CI)
1–19	2.3	4.6 (0.6–16.5)	2.5	6.1 (0.7–21.9)
20–30	10.2	5.2 (2.6–9.2)*	13.8	7.6 (4.0–12.9)*
40–59	100.3	4.6 (2.6–7.5)*	101.7	5.1 (2.6–8.9)*
60–84	458.7	1.7 (0.9–3.0)	548.4	2.8 (1.5–4.7)*
1–84	18.7	3.1 (2.2–4.3)*	21.1	4.4 (3.1–6.0)*

*$P < 0.05$.

The Diabetes UK Cohort Study of type 1 diabetes has recently published rates and SMRs for mortality from cerebrovascular disease and these are shown in Table 1.3. During the follow-up (an average of 17 years per person) there was a total of 1437 deaths, 80 of which were from cerebrovascular disease. The rates were comparable for men and women at all ages. Overall the rates were raised compared with the general population, though not significantly so at ages 1–19, or in the men aged 60–84 years. In the 20–39 age group the risk of cerebrovascular mortality was increased more than fivefold in men and more than sevenfold in women. There are no other studies of cerebrovascular mortality rates by age and sex in patients with type 1 diabetes, probably because available studies have not been large enough or had sufficient follow-up. Other studies have either calculated risks of combined fatal and non-fatal cerebrovascular events (Manson *et al.*, 1991) or calculated risks of cerebrovascular mortality based on only a few deaths (Moss *et al.*, 1991).

Type 2 diabetes

One of the earlier reports of the increased risk of stroke in patients with type 2 diabetes was from Framingham (Garcia *et al.*, 1974), which indicated an increased risk for stroke of 2.4 in both men and women. Other studies, of mortality, have reported SMRs similar to those in the 60–84 age group of the Diabetes UK Cohort Study and it is interesting to note that these studies have also failed to demonstrate a significantly raised risk for men, although they have demonstrated a raised risk for women. Results from the Joslin Clinic (Kessler, 1971) reported SMRs for cerebrovascular mortality of 1.1 in men and 1.2 in women, with equivalent SMRs of 1.8 and 2.2 from the Wisconsin Study (Moss *et al.*, 1991) and 1.7 and 2.6 from the Rancho Bernardo Study (Barrett-Connor and Khaw, 1988). Those studies that have included younger patients with type 2 diabetes have indicated higher risks, with a significant increase in risk for both men and women. The MRFIT study (Neaton *et al.*, 1993) of men aged predominantly under 60 reported an SMR of 2.7 and the Nurses Health Study (Manson *et al.*, 1991) of similarly aged women reported an SMR of 5.0.

Table 1.4 Risk of mortality from haemorrhagic and non-haemorrhagic stroke. Data from the Diabetes UK Cohort Study.

Age at death	Haemorrhagic		Non-haemorrhagic	
	No. of deaths	SMR (95%CI)	No. of deaths	SMR (95%CI)
Males				
1–39	5	2.3 (0.7–5.3)	6	18.6 (6.8–40.6)*
40–84	3	1.1 (0.2–3.2)	20	3.1 (1.9–4.7)*
Females				
1–39	4	2.4 (0.6–6.0)	11	37.0 (18.5–66.3)*
40–84	6	2.5 (0.9–5.4)	15	3.6 (2.0–6.0)*

*$P < 0.05$.

The risk of mortality from cerebrovascular disease has been shown in the MRFIT study to be only associated with ischaemic, non-haemorrhagic stroke, but there was no increased risk of death from subarachnoid or intracranial haemorrhage (Neaton *et al.*, 1993). Similar findings have now been shown for type 1 diabetes. The death certificates for those people who had died from cerebrovascular disease in the Diabetes UK Cohort Study were examined further to determine whether the death had occurred as a result of a haemorrhagic or non-haemorrhagic incident. Of the 80 deaths, 50 could be classified as non-haemorrhagic, 18 as haemorrhagic and the remaining 10 were excluded as there was not sufficient information on the death certificate for classification. These groups were analysed separately (Table 1.4). The risk of death from non-haemorrhagic stroke was high, especially in the under 40 age group where it was increased 18-fold in men and 35-fold in women. The risk of mortality from haemorrhagic stroke, whilst higher than for the general population, was not significantly increased but the numbers were too small to draw any firm conclusions. Although it was not possible to be certain about the exact nature of the non-haemorrhagic deaths from the death certificates, it seems probable that many of these deaths were ischaemic in origin.

As we have already noted for CVD in general, the absolute number of people with diabetes dying from cerebrovascular disease will always be higher in type 2 diabetes because this is the predominant form of diabetes among older people and cerebrovascular disease is related to age. However, at younger ages the Diabetes UK Cohort Study has demonstrated that risks of cerebrovascular mortality, relative to the general population, are raised, especially for those deaths likely to be ischaemic in origin, and although the risks are not so high in the older age groups they remain very comparable to the risks seen in patients with type 2 diabetes.

1.7 Discussion

Appraisal of epidemiological studies

Since the early days of Framingham, epidemiological studies have played an essential role in the recognition of cardiovascular complications in diabetes. Not long after the introduction of insulin, just as it was hoped that diabetes could be 'cured', the first epidemiological studies indicated that a significant excess mortality was still a feature of these patients. Subsequently, specific pathologies accounting for this raised mortality have been identified, although for the less frequent outcomes these can only be identified by very large studies – even in the Diabetes UK cohort there were still only 80 deaths from cerebrovascular disease from a cohort of over 23 000 patients with type 1 diabetes during a lengthy follow-up.

Epidemiological studies have provided quantification of these deaths, expressing mortality as an absolute number, but also expressing mortality as a rate or a rate ratio (such as an SMR) using a different, usually non-diabetic, group as the denominator. Once mortality is described and quantified, changes over time or between populations can be measured. The larger studies have also been able to report these measures according to specific age groups and gender, and measurements of mortality have been shown to vary with age and sex as well as the type of disease.

The large studies have highlighted not only the increased risk of death from CVD, but more specifically indicated that these deaths are usually atherosclerotic in origin. For example, while it was noted that there was an association between diabetes and mortality from ischaemic, non-haemorrhagic stroke it was also noted that there was no such association with subarachnoid or intracranial haemorrhage in patients with type 2 diabetes, and this has subsequently been shown to be the case in patients with type 1 diabetes as well. Similarly, for heart disease the mortality rates and SMRs are much higher for death from IHD alone than from all types of heart disease grouped together. These observations are relevant because they indicate where treatment and early detection might help reduce mortality.

Gender and cardiovascular risk in diabetes

One of the features of CVD complications in patients with diabetes that has been highlighted by epidemiological studies, and is of particular interest, is the relationship between CVD risk and gender. Mortality from cerebrovascular disease in the general population does not vary between the sexes. Although the rates are higher in the patients with type 1 diabetes these also do not differ between men and women except in the oldest age group where mortality from stroke appears to be a bit higher in women. Similar studies of patients with type 2 diabetes have also suggested that the stroke rate or the increased risk of stroke might be slightly higher for women at older ages.

In contrast mortality from heart disease in the general population is higher in men than women at all ages, and premenopausal women have a degree of cardioprotection as CHD rates remain low at this age. This premenopausal protection appears to be completely lost in young women with type 1 diabetes and CHD mortality rates are the same as for men. This accords with incidence data from Pittsburgh (Lloyd *et al.*, 1996b), in which similar rates of new coronary artery disease events were found in males and females under 40 years, and from the WHO study (Morrish *et al.*, 2001), which showed similar incidence rates for new myocardial infarctions in men and women. Even though the rates fall behind those of men in the older age groups, at all ages the rates in women with type 1 diabetes are higher than those for men in the general population. Women with type 2 diabetes appear to fare only slightly better and studies suggest that some of this survival advantage may also be lost. Data from the Rancho Bernardo Study show that survival rates in females with type 2 diabetes are similar to those in men without diabetes, and considerably worse than those for women without diabetes (Barrett-Connor *et al.*, 1991).

Clearly, although it may be convenient to do so, in reality it is impossible to generalise about the effects of diabetes on CVD risk. Not only do the rates and risks differ between the two types of diabetes but there are also considerable differences in mortality according to pathology, age group and sex. Unless the cohort is a particularly large one, it may not be possible to subdivide the deaths by age group or specific cause, but without some subdivision important differences may be overlooked and high-risk groups fail to be identified.

Although this chapter has largely concentrated on mortality, epidemiological studies that have been able to provide more detailed information, although on a smaller population, have also proved invaluable. An example of this type of study is the DARTS/MEMO Study, an electronic record linkage of multiple data sources to create a diabetes register from Tayside in Scotland (Morris *et al.*, 1997). The advantages of these studies can be illustrated by considering peripheral arterial disease. Intermittent claudication, an early symptom, is very common in patients with diabetes and is highlighted as a major problem in morbidity studies but hardly features in studies of mortality, and the incidence of below knee amputations, a more serious consequence of peripheral arterial disease, can only be determined by local audit (Morris *et al.*, 1998) (Chapter 8). A further advantage of smaller studies is that it is possible to measure cardiovascular risk factors in individuals (EURODIAB IDDM Complications Study Group, 1994; Fuller *et al.*, 2001) and it turn establish which risk factors appear to be relevant to which outcomes.

Following on from the epidemiological studies that measure risk factors come clinical trials. These trials are intervention studies that assess the best method of treatment in order to reduce the complications of diabetes. Some of these concentrate on achieving tight control of diabetes in order to reduce the adverse consequences (Diabetes Control and Complications Trial Research Group, 1995; UK Prospective Diabetes Study (UKPDS) Group, 1998) whereas others put more emphasis on treating the CVD risk factors directly (Colhoun *et al.*, 2004) (Chapter 9). These and other methods of treatment to prevent or alleviate the consequences of CVD in patients with diabetes are discussed in the subsequent chapters in this book.

References

American Diabetes Association (1989). Role of cardiovascular risk factors in prevention and treatment of macrovascular disease in diabetes. *Diabetes Care* **12**: 573–9.

Andresen EM, Lee JA, Pecoraro RE, Koepsell TD, Hallstrom AP, Siscovick DS (1993). Underreporting of diabetes on death certificates, King Country, Washington. *American Journal of Public Health* **83**: 1021–4.

Barrett-Connor EL, Khaw K (1988). Diabetes mellitus: An independent risk factor for stroke. *American Journal of Epidemiology* **128**: 116–23.

Barrett-Connor EL, Cohn BA, Wingard DA, Edelstein SLE (1991). Why is diabetes mellitus a stronger risk factor for fatal ischaemic heart disease in women than in men? The Rancho Bernardo Study. *Journal of the American Medical Association* **265**: 627–31.

Bell DSH (1994). Stroke in the diabetic patient. *Diabetes Care* **17**: 213–19.

Blendea MC, McFarlane SI, Isenovic ER, Gick G, Sowers JR (2003). Heart disease in diabetic patients. *Current Diabetic Report* **3**: 223–9.

Borch-Johnsen K, Kreiner S, Deckert T (1986). Mortality of Type I (insulin-dependent) diabetes mellitus in Denmark: a study of relative mortality in 2930 Danish Type I diabetic patients diagnosed from 1933 to 1972. *Diabetologia* **29**: 767–72.

Colhoun HM, Betteridge DJ, Durrington PN, Hitman GA, Neil HAW, Livingstone SJ, Thomson MJ, Mackness MI, Charlton-Menys V, Fuller JH, on behalf of the CARDS investigators (2004). Primary prevention of cardiovascular disease with atrovastatin in type 2 diabetes in the Collaborative Atorvastatin Diabetes Study (CARDS): multicentre randomised placebo-controlled trial. *Lancet* **364**: 685–96.

Deckert T, Poulsen JE, Larsen M (1979). The prognosis of insulin dependent diabetes mellitus and the importance of supervision. *Acta Medica Scandinavica Supplementum* **624**: 48–53.

Diabetes Control and Complications Trial Research Group (1995). Effect of intensive diabetes management on macrovascular events and risk factors in the diabetes control and complications trial. *American Journal of Cardiology* **75**: 894–903.

Diabetes Epidemiology Research International Study Group (1995). International analysis of insulin dependent diabetes mellitus mortality: a preventable mortality perspective. *American Journal of Epidemiology* **142**: 612–18.

Dorman JS, Laporte RE, Kuller LH, Cruikshanks KJ, Orchard TJ, Wagener DK, Becker DJ, Cavender DE, Drash AL (1984). The Pittsburgh insulin-dependent diabetes mellitus morbidity and mortality study. *Diabetes* **33**: 271–6.

EURODIAB IDDM Complications Study Group (1994). Microvascular and acute complications in IDDM patients: the EURODIAB IDDM complications study. *Diabetologia* **37**: 278–85.

Fisher M (2003). Diabetes: can we stop the time bomb? *Heart* **89** (Suppl 2): 28–30.

Fuller JH, Stevens LK, Wang SL (2001). Risk factors for cardiovascular mortality and morbidity: the WHO multinational study of vascular disease in diabetics. *Diabetologia* **44**: 554–64.

Gale E (2002). The rise of childhood type I diabetes in the 20th century. *Diabetes* **51**: 3353–61.

Garcia MJ, McNamara PM, Gordon T, Kannel W (1974). Morbidity and mortality in diabetics in the Framingham population. Sixteen year follow-up study. *Diabetes* **23**: 105–11.

Head J, Fuller JH (1990). International variations in mortality among diabetic patients: the WHO multinational study of vascular disease in diabetics. *Diabetologia* **33**: 477–81.

Kannel WB, McGee DL (1979). Diabetes and cardiovascular disease. The Framingham study. *Journal of the American Medical Association* **241**: 2035–8.

Kanters S, Banga JD, Stolk RP, Algra A (1999). Incidence and determinants of mortality and cardiovascular events in diabetes mellitus: a meta-analysis. *Vascular Medicine* **4**: 67–75.

Kessler I (1971). Mortality experience of diabetic patients. *American Journal of Medicine* **51**: 715–24.

Krolewski AS, Kosinski EJ, Warram JH, Leland OS, Busick EJ, Asmal AC, Rand LI, Christlieb AR, Bradley RF, Kahn CR (1987). Magnitude and determinants of coronary artery disease in juvenile-onset, insulin dependent diabetes mellitus. *American Journal of Cardiology* **59**: 750–5.

Laakso M (1998). Hypertension and macrovascular disease – the killing fields of NIDDM. *Diabetes Research and Clinical Practice* **39** (Suppl 98): S27–33.

Laakso M, Kuusisto J (1996). Epidemiological evidence for the association of hyperglycaemia and atherosclerotic vascular disease in non-insulin-dependent diabetes mellitus. *Annals of Medicine* **28**: 415–18.

Laakso M, Lehto S (1997). Epidemiology of macrovascular disease in diabetes. *Diabetic Reviews* **5**: 294–308.

Laakso M, Pyorala K (1985). Age of onset and type of diabetes. *Diabetes Care* **8**: 114–17.

Laing SP, Swerdlow AJ, Slater SD, Botha JL, Burden AC, Waugh NR, Smith AWM, Hill RD, Bingley PJ, Patterson CC, Qiao Z, Keen H (1999a). The BDA Cohort Study I: All-cause mortality in patients with insulin-treated diabetes mellitus. *Diabetic Medicine* **16**: 459–65.

Laing SP, Swerdlow AJ, Slater S, Botha JL, Burden AC, Waugh NR, Smith AWM, Hill RD, Bingley PJ, Patterson CC, Qiao Z, Keen H (1999b). The BDA Cohort Study II: Cause-specific mortality in patients with insulin-treated diabetes mellitus. *Diabetic Medicine* **16**: 466–71.

Laing SP, Swerdlow AJ, Carpenter LM, Slater SD, Burden AC, Botha JL, Morris AD, Waugh NR, Gatling W, Gale EAM, Patterson CC, Qiao Z, Keen H (2003a). Mortality from cerebrovascular disease in a cohort of 23 000 patients with insulin-treated diabetes. *Stroke* **34**: 418–21.

Laing SP, Swerdlow AJ, Slater SD, Burden AC, Morris AD, Waugh NR, Gatling W, Bingley PJ, Patterson CC (2003b). Mortality from heart disease disease in a cohort of 23 000 patients with insulin-treated diabetes. *Diabetologia* **46**: 760–5.

Lehto S, Ronnemaa T, Pyorala K, Laakso M (1996). Predictors of stroke in middle-aged patients with non-insulin-dependent diabetes. *Stroke* **27**: 63–8.

Lloyd CE, Becker D, Ellis D, Orchard TJ (1996a). Incidence of complications in insulin-dependent diabetes mellitus: a survival analysis. *Americal Journal of Epidemiology* **143**: 431–41.

Lloyd CE, Kuller LH, Ellis D, Becker DJ, Wing RR, Orchard TJ (1996b). Coronary artery disease in IDDM. Gender differences in risk factors but not in risk. *Arteriosclerosis, Thrombosis and Vascular Biology* **16**: 720–6.

Lounamaa P, Lounama R, Tuomilehto J, Reunanen A (1991). Mortality of Type I diabetes: the relative risk is higher in females but the absolute increased risk is higher in males. *Diabetologia* **34** (Suppl 2): A178.

Manson JE, Colditz GA, Stampfer MJ, Willett WC, Krolewski AS, Rosner B, Arky AR, Speizer FE, Hennekens CH (1991). A prospective study of maturity onset diabetes mellitus and risk of coronary heart disease and stroke in women. *Archives of Internal Medicine* **151**: 1141–47.

Morris AD, Boyle DI, MacAlpine R, Emslie-Smith A, Jung RT, Newton RW, MacDonald TM (1997). The diabetes audit and research in Tayside Scotland (DARTS) study: electronic record linkage to create a diabetes register. DARTS/MEMO collaboration. *British Medical Journal* **315**: 524–8.

Morris AD, McAlpine R, Steinke D, Boyle DI, Ebrahim AR, Vasudev N, Stewart CP, Jung RT, Leese GP, MacDonald TM, Newton RW (1998). Diabetes and lower-limb amputations in the community. A retrospective cohort study. DARTS/MEMO collaboration. *Diabetes Care* **21**: 738–43.

Morrish NJ, Wang SL, Stevens LK, Fuller JH, Keen H (2001). Mortality and causes of death in the WHO multinational study of vascular disease in diabetes. *Diabetologia* **44** (Suppl 2): S14–21.

Moss SE, Klein R, Klein BEK (1991). Cause-specific mortality in a population based study of diabetes. *American Journal of Public Health* **81**: 1158–62.

Muggeo M, Verlato G, Bonora E, Bressan F, Girotto S, Corbellini M, Gemma ML, Moghetti P, Zenere M, Cacciatori V, Zoppini G, De Marco R (1995). The Verona Diabetes Study: a population-based survey on known diabetes mellitus prevalence and 5 year all-cause mortality. *Diabetologia* **38**: 318–25.

Nathan DM, Meigs J, Singer DE (1997). The epidemiology of cardiovascular disease in type 2 diabetes mellitus; how sweet it is... or is it? *Lancet* **350** (Suppl 1): 4–9.

Neaton JD, Wentworth DN, Cutler J, Stamler J, Kuller L (1993). Risk factors for death from different types of stroke. *Annals of Epidemiology* **3**: 493–9.

Orchard TJ, Dorman JS, Maser RE, Becker DJ, Drash AL, Ellis D, La Porte RE, Kuller LH (1990). Prevalence of complications in IDDM by sex and duration. Pittsburgh epidemiology of diabetes complications study II. *Diabetes* **39**: 1116–24.

Stamler J, Vaccaro O, Neaton JD, Wentworth D (1993). Diabetes, other risk factors and 12 year cardiovascular mortality for men screened in the Multiple Risk Factor Intervention Trial. *Diabetes Care* **16**: 434–45.

Sultz HA, Schlesinger ER, Mosner WE, Fieldman JG (1972). *Longterm Childhood Illness*. Pittsburgh: University of Pittsburgh Press, pp. 223–248.

UK Prospective Diabetes Study (UKPDS) Group (1998). Intensive blood-glucose control with sulphonylureas or insulin compared with conventional treatment and risk of complications in patients with type 2 diabetes (UKPDS 33). *Lancet* **352**: 837–53.

Wong JS, Pearson DW, Murchison LE, Williams MJ, Narayan V (1991). Mortality in diabetes mellitus: experience of a geographically defined population. *Diabetic Medicine* **8**: 135–9.

2 Pathogenesis of Atherosclerosis and Vascular Disease in Type 2 Diabetes

Naveed Sattar and *Alistair Cormack*

2.1 Introduction

As described extensively elsewhere in this book, vascular disease is the major cause of morbidity and mortality in individuals with type 2 diabetes, with up to 75% of all such individuals succumbing to some form of cardiovascular disease (CVD). Most recent evidence from a large-scale study in Canada has shown that the transition to a high-risk CVD category occurs at a younger age for men and women with diabetes than for those without diabetes (mean difference 14.6 years) (Booth *et al.*, 2006). In other words, diabetes confers an equivalent vascular risk to aging 15 years.

It is now clear that type 2 diabetes mellitus cannot be regarded simply as a state of hyperglycaemia but as part of a spectrum of metabolic disorders, most of which are associated with cardiovascular risk. For the vast majority (~90%), type 2 diabetes is a state of insulin resistance and the frank diabetic state is often manifest after many years (i.e. 10–20 years) of insulin resistance (Warram *et al.*, 1990). Insulin resistance, in turn, is associated with many risk factor abnormalities that commonly precede the development of hyperglycaemia and these typically include central obesity, a dyslipidaemia characterised by high triglyceride and low HDL-cholesterol, higher blood pressure, low-grade inflammation, haemostatic changes, oxidative stress, endothelial dysfunction and alterations in circulating concentrations of adipokines, in particular adiponectin, an adipocyte-derived protein with insulin-sensitising and anti-inflammatory properties (Figure 2.1) (Sattar, 2005). Given that alterations in many of these risk factors are directly or indirectly linked to vascular disease, it is unsurprising that the atherosclerotic burden is enhanced many years before the frank hyperglycaemic

Diabetic Cardiology   Editors Miles Fisher and John J. McMurray
© 2007 John Wiley & Sons, Ltd.

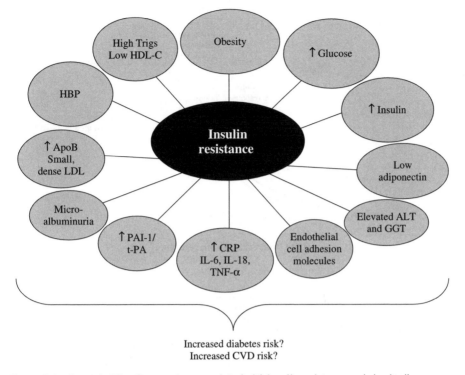

Figure 2.1 Expanded list of parameters associated with insulin resistance and obesity (by no mean comprehensive). Some of these parameters are more strongly associated with prediction of type 2 diabetes than CVD. (HBP = high blood pressure; HDL-C = HDL-cholesterol; Trigs = triglycerides.)

state of type 2 diabetes manifests. In other words, the ticking clock for vascular disease begins well before diagnosis of diabetes (Haffner *et al.*, 1990) (Figure 2.2).

This chapter will examine proposed mechanisms for such increased vascular risk in individuals with type 2 diabetes. The contribution of both traditional risk factors, such as lipids and hypertension, as well as novel risk factors will be discussed. In addition, the potential relevance of hyperinsulinaemia, and of course hyperglycaemia, to the heightened CVD risk in individuals with diabetes will be reviewed. Finally, the concept of metabolic syndrome, an umbrella term for risk factors linked to insulin resistance and predictive of vascular disease, will be discussed.

2.2 What is Insulin Resistance?

The fundamental role of insulin is to facilitate cellular uptake of glucose in skeletal muscle and to limit hepatic gluconeogenesis, the other key determinant of steady-state plasma glucose levels. In the steady (or fasted) state the quantity of insulin required to maintain a plasma glucose level depends on muscle mass and hepatic glucose output. However, there is more than a twofold variation in the plasma insulin levels required to maintain identical plasma glucose levels in normal subjects (Hollenbeck and Reaven, 1987). This variation in insulin requirement for glucose disposal has been termed

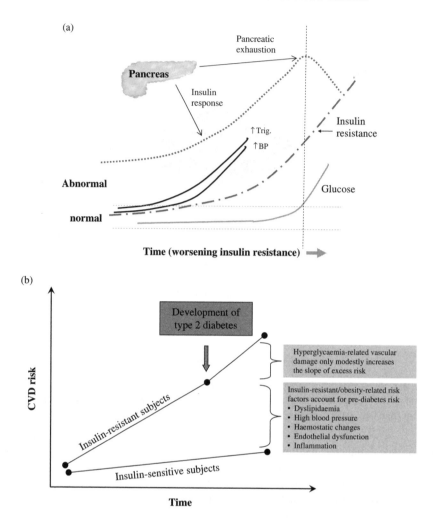

Figure 2.2 As insulin resistance worsens with age, the pancreas is often able to secrete increasing amounts of insulin over many years to maintain glucose homeostasis. In susceptible individuals, the pancreas eventually becomes 'exhausted' and subsequently glucose concentrations rise into the diabetic range. However, an array of other risk factor abnormalities such as elevations in triglyceride (Trig) or blood pressure (BP), and many novel parameters demonstrated in Figure 2.1 and detailed in the text, frequently accompany worsening insulin resistance. Since many of these are also CVD risk factors, this explains why CVD risk is already high at diagnosis of type 2 diabetes (b). It also explains why the hyperglycaemic element in type 2 diabetes is perhaps a late element in the excess risk of vascular disease in this condition. Of course, risk is further accelerated should individuals with diabetes subsequently develop renal disease. This simplified but conceptual model also illustrates why hyperglycaemia only modestly increases the already high established vascular risk in type 2 diabetes and why treating high glucose levels in isolation will only minimally attenuate vascular risk.

insulin resistance, whereby subjects needing higher amounts of insulin are 'insulin resistant' compared to those who need lesser amounts of insulin. Insulin response is a linear variable across populations; insulin resistance (or insulin sensitivity) is a relative concept in normal glucose-tolerant subjects, and there are no absolute cut-off values.

In pathogenic terms insulin resistance is a principal feature of type 2 diabetes and precedes the clinical development of the disease by 10–20 years (Warram *et al.*, 1990). Insulin resistance is caused by the decreased ability of peripheral target tissues (muscle and liver) to respond properly to normal insulin levels. Initially, increasing pancreatic insulin secretion is able to counteract insulin resistance and thus normal glucose homoeostasis can be maintained. However, pancreatic reserve eventually diminishes in the face of increasing peripheral demands and thus glucose concentrations rise, heralding a diagnosis of type 2 diabetes once plasma glucose concentrations go beyond universally agreed diagnostic cut-offs, whether fasting or post-glucose loading.

Multiple roles of insulin

One way to better understand the link between many risk parameters and elevated risk for type 2 diabetes is to appreciate that insulin imparts its effects on many tissues, not just skeletal muscle and liver but also adipose, endothelium and immune cells (Ritchie *et al.*, 2004; Bloomgarden, 2005; Reaven, 2005). Thus, insulin is relevant not simply to glucose uptake and metabolism, but it also:

- suppresses free fatty acid (FFA) release from adipose tissue;
- limits hepatic triglyceride synthesis;
- helps maintain endothelial homeostasis, with a net vasodilatory effect in insulin-sensitive subjects;
- is involved in regulating thrombotic cascades;
- may have a role in regulating inflammatory cascades (Figure 2.3).

It can thus be seen that a partial failure of insulin action, or a resistance to its normal actions at each of these tissues, could lead to a spectrum of metabolic abnormalities that individually and collectively accelerate the atherogenic process. Each of these pathways is now discussed in greater detail. It is important to appreciate that insulin may also have some apparent 'deleterious' actions but that the balance of effects is always protective in insulin-sensitive subjects. This is discussed later on.

2.3 Dyslipidaemia and Type 2 Diabetes

With increasing obesity, in particular visceral obesity, fat cells become enlarged and apparently less responsive to insulin, i.e. insulin resistant (Frayn, 2001). Some investigators argue that adipocyte sensitivity to insulin is maintained until well after other organs become insulin resistant but such work generally derives from studies on subcutaneous tissues rather than the generally accepted more relevant visceral

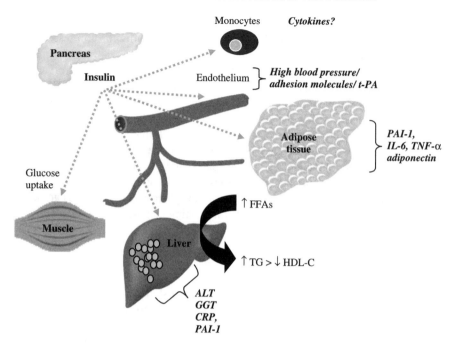

Figure 2.3 The relevance of insulin action extends beyond skeletal muscle, adipose tissue and liver, and includes effects on endothelium and immune cell function. In healthy insulin-sensitive subjects, it helps maintain low levels of free fatty acids (FFAs), and thus normal lipids, healthy endothelium and low cytokine levels. By contrast, in insulin-resistant subjects, such tissues respond less well to insulin, and thus derangements in the above pathways are favoured. (HDL-C = HDL-cholesterol; TG = triglycerides.)

adipose sites. Regardless of adipocyte insulin sensitivities, a simple increase in the mass of visceral fat tissue in obese individuals would in itself enhance FFA release. Such excess release of FFAs into the portal circulation drives excess hepatic triglyceride accumulation and synthesis, in the form of very-low-density lipoprotein (VLDL) particles, with a resultant increase in plasma triglyceride concentrations. It is clear that this process predates type 2 diabetes since, other than glucose, elevated plasma triglyceride concentration is arguably the strongest biochemical predictor of incident type 2 diabetes (Freeman *et al.*, 2002). Indeed, it is often not well appreciated but triglyceride levels are far stronger predictors of diabetes than of CVD (Wilson *et al.*, 2005).

The rise in triglyceride in the form of VLDL, in turn, promotes numerous atherogenic changes in other lipid particles. Critically, VLDL exchanges triglyceride for both LDL- and HDL-cholesteryl ester and this is one of the major mechanisms leading to a decline in HDL-cholesterol concentrations in the face of rising triglyceride concentrations. The cholesteryl esters transferred to triglyceride-rich lipoproteins (i.e. VLDL particles) render these 'remnant' particles more resistant to lipolytic breakdown and as a result more atherogenic, whereas hydrolysis of the accumulated triglyceride in LDL and HDL results in smaller, denser particles (Packard, 2006). Small, dense LDL particles are particularly atherogenic, whereas smaller HDL particles are less cardioprotective.

The above atherogenic lipoprotein perturbations are significantly exaggerated in the postprandial period, promoting enhanced plasma accumulation of cholesterol-enriched VLDL remnants, a further lowering in HDL-cholesterol and a further reduction in LDL particle size. Triglyceride intolerance (impaired clearance of postprandial lipaemia) is independently predictive of the presence of CVD (Eberly *et al.*, 2003). Overall, the pattern of elevated FFAs and triglyceride, low HDL-cholesterol and increased preponderance of small, dense LDL is strongly associated with type 2 diabetes and insulin resistance. There exist multiple mechanisms by which this lipid pattern can accelerate atherogenesis, as recently reviewed and described in detail in Table 2.1 (modified from Sattar *et al.*, 1998). In particular, small, dense LDL particles more

Table 2.1 Evidence linking atherogenic lipoprotein pertubations to endothelial dysfunction.

Particles	Potential mechanisms of endothelial damage
Triglyceride-rich lipoproteins and remnant particles	Increase oxidative burden
	Directly toxic to endothelium
	Can cross endothelial barrier
	Stimulate endothelial cell PAI-1 production
	Activate Factor VII
	Increase endothelial cell expression of adhesion molecules
Small, dense LDL	Increase susceptibility to oxidative damage
	Greater lysophosphatidylcholine content upon oxidisation
	Increase arterial residence time
	Increase penetration of arterial intima
	Increase affinity for endothelial proteoglycans
Free fatty acids	Increase oxidative stress
	Facilitate endothelial transfer of LDL and cholesterol-rich remnant particles
	Reduce albumin's protective properties, thereby allowing expression of VLDL toxicity
	Reduce endothelial cell production of prostacyclin and nitric oxide
	Impair ability of endothelial cells to inhibit platelet aggregation
High-density lipoproteins	Antioxidant roles bind free transition metals
	Intrinsic antioxidant enzymes
	Shuttle reactive hydroperoxides from endothelium to liver for excretion
	Limit endothelial toxicity of VLDL remnants

readily enter the arterial intima due to their smaller size. Once entered, they are more likely to be retained or anchored by proteoglycans, and thus more likely to be oxidised, whereupon they become antigenic and will release signals to recruit monocytes and favour their transformation into foam cells through a receptor-mediated intake (scavenger pathway). In other words, oxidised LDL is the key signal initiating the atherosclerotic plaque. Oxidised LDL particles also show cytotoxic potential, which is in part responsible for endothelial cell damage and macrophage degeneration in the atherosclerotic human plaque.

Of interest, recent prospective population studies have demonstrated better CVD prediction from a high apolipoprotein B (ApoB) to ApoAI ratio compared to the traditionally accepted cholesterol to HDL-cholesterol ratio (Walldius *et al.*, 2001; Sniderman, 2004). Apolipoprotein B is the key protein within LDL particles and rises with particle number, whereas ApoAI is the key protein within HDL particles responsible for its anti-atherogenic properties. It has recently been demonstrated that high ApoB correlates more strongly than LDL-cholesterol to insulin resistance, an observation that explains why ApoB levels are elevated in diabetes patients and why ApoB may better predict vascular events.

2.4 Hypertension

Hypertension is a much researched and documented risk factor for atherosclerosis and is discussed in relation to diabetes in far greater detail in Chapter 6. In the United Kingdom Prospective Diabetes Study (UKPDS), more than a third of patients at diabetes diagnosis were hypertensive (Matthews, 1999). Hypertension is pathogenic to the cardiovascular system in many ways, most obviously as a risk factor for atherogenesis by increasing shearing forces on plaques and hence plaque instability. Hypertension causes left ventricular hypertrophy, increasing myocardial blood flow requirements and impairing diastolic left ventricular filling, and hence is a risk factor also for cardiac failure. Perivascular fibrosis in hypertension impairs oxygen transport across the vessel wall and a combination of all of the above compromises subendocardial blood/oxygen supply.

Although it has been known for about 20 years that those with primary hypertension are more likely to be hyperinsulinaemic, have abnormal oral glucose tolerance tests and therefore be insulin resistant (Ferrari and Weidmann, 1990), the link between hypertension and insulin resistance is perhaps weaker than the association of the latter with dyslipidaemia or obesity (Reaven, 2006). Nevertheless, it has been estimated that insulin resistance is present in up to perhaps half of all patients with essential hypertension. In keeping with an association of blood pressure with diabetes, both high systolic and diastolic blood pressure predict incident diabetes in univariate analyses (Freeman *et al.*, 2002). Finally, recent meta-analyses have shown that throughout middle and old age, usual blood pressure is strongly and directly related to vascular (and overall) mortality, without any evidence of a threshold down to at least 115/75 mmHg (Lewington *et al.*, 2002). Hence, even small increases in blood pressure in the pre-diabetic phase are relevant to the heightened vascular risk in this population. The mechanism for higher blood pressure in diabetes or pre-diabetes is not precisely defined but will almost certainly be multifactorial. Relevant factors include endothelial dysfunction, adipocyte release of vasoactive substances such as angiotensin, hyperinsulinaemic activation of sympathetic nervous system and enhancement of renal sodium reabsorption (Mlinar *et al.*, 2007).

2.5 Endothelial Dysfunction and Type 2 Diabetes

The endothelium appears to play a critical role in the regulation of vascular tone and inhibiting leucocyte adhesion and platelet aggregation, through its release of mediators such as nitric oxide (NO) and prostacyclin. Nitric oxide is derived from L-arginine through the action of the constitutive form of the enzyme nitric oxide synthase (eNOS) (Schram and Stehouwer, 2005). It inhibits platelet aggregation and adhesion, modulates smooth-muscle-cell proliferation, attenuates the generation of endothelin and reduces leucocyte adhesion to the endothelium. Endothelial dysfunction is therefore characterised by altered permeability barrier function, enhanced adhesion molecule expression, increased leucocyte adhesion and impaired endothelium-dependent vasodilator responses (Schram and Stehouwer, 2005). Endothelial dysfunction is also associated with enhanced thrombosis and impaired fibrinolysis.

The concept of endothelial dysfunction has now been around for a number of years. Many researchers promote the notion that endothelial dysfunction is likely to be a critical early step in the process of atherogenesis, and as such they argue that endothelial dysfunction may represent an intermediate phenotype for vascular disease (McVeigh and Cohn, 2003). Its assessment has therefore assumed importance in clinical research, and relevant methods, including both blood measures and dynamic tests, are being tested as possible modalities to improve risk factor stratification.

Endothelial function measures as predictors of diabetes or in pre-diabetes

There is a wealth of data suggesting a potential role for endothelial dysfunction in insulin resistance (Fonseca and Jawa, 2005). Although the direction of causality remains somewhat debated, circulating elevations in several endothelial-derived factors, cell adhesion molecules and t-PA, have been shown to predict risk for type 2 diabetes independently of other predictors (Meigs *et al.*, 2006). Similar results have been seen with physiological tests of endothelial function. For example, Steinberg *et al.* (1996) showed that severely obese (mean body mass index $= 34\,\mathrm{kg/m^2}$) insulin-resistant individuals with normal glucose tolerance have the same degree of impairment in blood flow and vascular reactivity as those people with established type 2 diabetes. Similarly, when Caballero *et al.* examined endothelial function and vascular reactivity in two groups at risk for developing type 2 diabetes, subjects with impaired glucose tolerance and subjects with normal glucose tolerance but with a parental history of type 2 diabetes, they noted that both micro- and macrovascular reactivities were reduced in these two groups compared with healthy controls but were at a better level than in those with type 2 diabetes (Caballero *et al.*, 1999) (Figure 2.4). These findings suggest that vascular dysfunction may be an early feature of the insulin resistance syndrome.

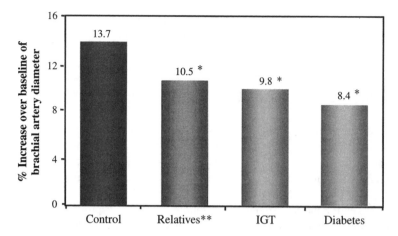

Figure 2.4 Impaired endothelium-dependent vasodilation in people at risk for type 2 diabetes. The brachial artery diameter change in response to reactive hyperaemia also known as flow-mediated dilation (endothelium-dependent vasodilation), is reduced in relatives of type 2 diabetic patients (Relatives), subjects with impaired glucose tolerance (IGT), and type 2 diabetic patients compared with healthy controls. Results are presented as mean percentage increase in diameter over baseline. *$P < 0.05$ vs. control; **one or both parents with diabetes. Reproduced with permission from Caballero AE (2003). Endothelial dysfunction in obesity and insulin resistance: a road to diabetes and heart disease. *Obesity Research* **11**: 1278–89.

Endothelial dysfunction in diabetes

There is now ample evidence from studies employing a variety of techniques in patients with type 2 diabetes for vascular endothelial dysfunction and impaired arterial stiffness at several sites including coronary vessels, brachial arteries and subcutaneous vessels (Tooke and Goh, 1999; Hink *et al.*, 2001). Many aspects of the insulin resistance syndrome may contribute to this dysfunction in patients with diabetes, including elevations in FFAs, characteristic lipid changes, obesity and hypertension, as well as the low-grade inflammation. Additionally, raised glucose concentrations can further damage vascular function. Finally, there is recent evidence that although insulin itself can stimulate both vasoconstrictor and vasodilator influences on the endothelium, the latter effects are likely diminished by factors common in diabetic individuals (Muis *et al.*, 2005) – discussed in greater detail below. It is clear that multiple risk factor pathways in diabetes adversely influence endothelial function, an observation once again emphasising multiple linkages between risk factor pathways.

Microalbuminuria as a clinical marker of endothelial dysfunction in diabetes?

There is considerable evidence to suggest that the presence of microalbuminuria signals a greater risk of CVD events in patients with and without diabetes. Microalbuminuria is defined as low levels of urinary albumin excretion of 30–300 mg/day.

Microalbuminuria is highly prevalent; in hypertensive and diabetic populations, its prevalence varies from 10 to 40%. It is interesting that microalbuminuria also is found frequently in seemingly healthy individuals (5–7%). Dysfunction of the vascular endothelium is regarded as an important factor in the pathogenesis of diabetic micro- and macroangiopathy (Basi and Lewis, 2006). The close linkage between microalbuminuria and endothelial dysfunction in diabetes has been used to explain the fact that microalbuminuria is a risk marker for atherothrombosis, and this topic has been widely reviewed by others (Schalkwijk and Stehouwer, 2005).

2.6 Inflammation

In recent years, inflammation has emerged as a new and important risk factor pathway in the pathogenesis of vascular disease. Acute phase markers such as white cell count, serum amyloid A and C-reactive protein (CRP) have been shown to be independent predictors of risk of vascular events in men and women. Much of the evidence for this association comes from studies measuring CRP and the term 'low-grade chronic inflammation' is now used since even modestly elevated CRP concentrations, within the traditionally accepted 'normal' range, predict myocardial infarction and ischaemic stroke in prospective studies (Sattar and Lowe, 2006). Other researchers use the term 'pro-inflammatory state' for this phenomenon, but essentially the terms are synonymous. The exact mechanisms for this association remain to be fully elaborated. One school of thought is that circulating markers of inflammation simply reflect the total plaque load in blood vessels since there is an abundance of inflammatory cells and molecules in plaques, particularly vulnerable plaques, with leakage into the circulation. However, CRP concentrations correlate poorly with extent of blood vessel occlusion as measured by angiography. Rather, factors such as age, smoking and, in particular, adiposity appear to be important determinants – the latter explains as much as 30% of the systemic inflammatory burden in population studies (Sattar and McInnes, 2005). Thus, the pro-inflammatory state, rather than presence of a specific marker, may be the contributory causative condition.

The balance of current evidence suggests that rather than CRP itself, upstream cytokines may be causally linked to vascular risk, since in addition to their role in regulating immune responses, cytokines mediate numerous metabolic effects. Cytokine-induced metabolic effects, which include transient alterations in lipids and peripheral insulin resistance, are favourable in the short term and function as part of the host response to infection and acute inflammation to target specific metabolic fuels to and from essential organs (Sattar *et al.*, 2003a). However, when these alterations are sustained, even if subtly elevated (as in obesity or in patients with diabetes), they appear to be deleterious and may promote accelerated atherogenesis via aggravation of several risk factor pathways, including lipoprotein metabolism, endothelial dysfunction and insulin resistance. Indeed, CRP concentration in population studies correlates with levels of many classical and novel coronary heart disease (CHD) risk factors in line with the pattern associated with the metabolic syndrome.

The latter observations linking chronically elevated cytokine concentrations to several features of the metabolic syndrome formed the basis for Pickup and Crook's original hypothesis (1998) suggesting that type 2 diabetes might be a disease of innate immunity. The extent to which elevations in serum concentrations of molecules usually associated with inflammation reflect the inflammatory response, i.e. a 'pro-inflammatory' state, remains unclear. Nevertheless, research in recent years, as detailed below, continues to add weight to the general hypothesis.

Elevated acute-phase markers in subjects at risk of type 2 diabetes

There are now robust data showing elevated inflammatory markers in obese men and women and in obese children. In addition, several other groups at risk of diabetes – including women with polycystic ovarian syndrome (PCOS), men and women of South Asian origin, Pima Indians, women with a family history of type 2 diabetes, and sedentary individuals – exhibit elevated inflammatory levels and do so independently of total body mass index (Ziegler, 2005; Sattar, 2006a). Markers of inflammation correlate with insulin resistance and predict type 2 diabetes, independently of other risk factors in several different populations (ARIC, WOSCOPS) (Schmidt et al., 1999; Freeman et al., 2002). Hence, it is clear that inflammatory perturbations predate diabetes by several years, and as such are potentially relevant to accelerated atherogenesis. The source for higher cytokine and acute-phase protein levels in pre-diabetes and diabetes remains unclear but will include adipocytes, endothelial cells and immune cells, with the function of the latter two cell types in particular being bi-directionally linked to perturbations in other risk factor pathways (Das, 2004). Whilst causal mechanisms linking systemic inflammatory markers and CVD remain to be fully elucidated, it is clear that inflammatory cells and molecules in abundance are critical constituents within unstable plaques, inhibiting collagen synthesis and deposition into cap and promoting cap erosion via release of metalloproteinases.

Finally, it should be recognised that whilst inflammatory parameters are clearly elevated in diabetes and almost certainly contribute to its accelerated atherogenesis, the current balance of evidence does not support the use of related markers, such as CRP, to enhance CVD risk prediction. This is partly due to the close relationship of CRP with existing risk factors and hence the magnitude of its independence in CVD prediction is too low to enhance risk factor stratification (Sattar and Lowe, 2006). That said, considerable efforts are being made to better understand the exact nature of the inflammatory insult in diabetes, in order to develop novel preventative measures. Moreover, many current modalities for treatment of diabetes and its vascular risk exhibit anti-inflammatory effects.

2.7 Adipokines – Adiponectin

There is considerable interest in the relationship between the adipocyte-derived protein adiponectin in both type 2 diabetes and CHD. Adiponectin is a 244-amino-acid protein that, despite being solely derived from adipose tissue, is paradoxically reduced in obesity (Greenberg and Obin, 2006). Circulating adiponectin levels, ranging from 0.5 to 30 μg/ml in humans, are reportedly around 1000-fold higher than circulating levels of other hormones such as insulin and leptin. Prospective epidemiological studies have consistently demonstrated that decreased adiponectin concentrations are associated with greater insulin resistance and increased risk of type 2 diabetes, apparently independent of obesity and other potential confounders (Lindsay *et al.*, 2002). Thus, the development of interventions that raise adiponectin levels has been proposed as a target to improve insulin sensitivity and glucose tolerance, and possibly to prevent CHD. Apart from a potentially protective role in diabetes, adiponectin could protect against cardiovascular disease by other proposed mechanisms. Adiponectin is strongly anti-inflammatory acting through the NFκB pathway, down-regulates adhesion molecule expression on endothelial cells and enhances lipid clearance in numerous animal models. In line with such observations, exogenous adiponectin administration protects against the development of atherosclerosis in ApoE-deficient mice (Greenberg and Obin, 2006). Such observations suggest that decreased synthesis and release of adiponectin in subjects destined to develop, or with, diabetes could be related to accelerated atherogenesis. In humans, however, the evidence so far has been somewhat conflicting. In the Health Professionals Study, a doubling of baseline adiponectin level was reported to be associated with a statistically significant 20% reduction in myocardial infarction (MI) risk in multivariate analyses, after adjustment for age, smoking, hypertension history, lipids, glycaemic control and CRP (Pischon *et al.*, 2004). The results from this study, based on 266 incident MI cases, have suggested that adiponectin is a major mechanistic link ('common soil') between diabetes and increased CHD risk. However, subsequent investigations in similarly sized studies have not reported significant associations between adiponectin levels and CHD risk. To help clarify the evidence, we recently reported new data from the prospective British Regional Heart Study, which involves almost 600 incident CHD deaths and events, more than twice as many as in the previous largest study (Sattar *et al.*, 2006). Our data suggested that adiponectin levels were not predictive of incident CHD events. Whilst these data suggest that adiponectin may not protect against vascular disease, it is premature to reach this conclusion for several reasons. For example, differing molecular forms of adiponectin may reflect differing biological effects (with the high molecular form being potentially associated with slightly greater insulin sensitivity). At present, there are no prospective studies relating high-molecular-weight adiponectin with vascular events but these are urgently required. In addition, several factors associated with greater CVD risk can increase adiponectin concentrations so that its relationship with incident CVD is potentially confounded. Such factors include impaired renal function, tissue wasting and brain natriuretic peptide, the latter released from ischaemic or damaged myocardium. Clearly, further data are needed to determine whether low adiponectin in diabetes is causal related to the accelerated atherogenesis in this condition.

2.8 Haemostatic Changes in Type 2 Diabetes

A full description of the haemostatic changes in diabetes is beyond the scope of this chapter and the reader is referred to some recent reviews on this topic (Juhan-Vague *et al.*, 2002; Grant, 2003). In simple terms, however, it is clear that type 2 diabetes is a pro-coagulant state, increasing the chance of vessel thrombosis and therefore acute coronary syndrome. This pro-coagulant and pro-thrombotic state is manifest through many arms of the coagulation process, including abnormal platelet function, increased levels of coagulation factors and decreased levels of endogenous anticoagulants. Some of these changes are intimately linked to endothelial dysfunction. For example, endothelial dysfunction results in decreased release of prostacyclin and NO – factors that normally inhibit platelet aggregation within normal vessels. Endothelial dysfunction also increases platelet activation by the release of von Willebrand factor. Fibrinogen and Factor VII levels are also increased in diabetes whilst endogenous anticoagulants, protein C and antithrombin III are reduced. Finally, circulating tissue factor levels appear to be increased in diabetes; tissue factor is one of the most potent pro-coagulants known and is found at the very top of the coagulation cascade and as such instigates coagulation. All changes collectively act to enhance blood stickiness and increase the chances of coronary thrombosis (Juhan-Vague *et al.*, 2002; Grant, 2003).

2.9 Hyperinsulinaemia

The role of insulin in the pathogenesis of vascular disease remains unclear. This is in part due to insulin diverse metabolic actions and in particular its complex interactions with the vasculature (Figure 2.5). In health, insulin has vasodilatory and anti-inflammatory properties via the endothelial NO pathway (Schalkwijk and Stehouwer, 2005). Insulin suppresses several pro-inflammatory transcription factors, such as NFκB, Egr-1 and activating protein-1 (AP-1). In the insulin-sensitive individual, insulin also suppresses expression on the leucocyte adhesion molecules and chemoattractant molecules (ICAM-1 and MCP-1) that are required for the migration and absorption of the monocyte into the vessel wall (Dandona *et al.*, 2003). With increasing resistance to insulin, its protective action is lost, thus contributing an inflammatory state and allowing unchecked expression of ICAM-1 and MCP-1.

In the insulin-resistant state, hyperinsulinaemia may also evoke a net vasoconstrictive rather than vasodilatory effect. Normally, hyperinsulinaemia activates

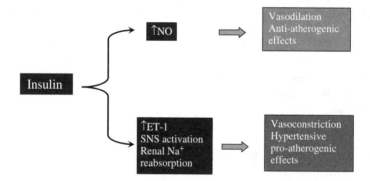

Figure 2.5 This simplified diagram demonstrates the diverse effects of insulin on vasculature. In insulin-sensitive subjects, insulin exerts a net vasodilatory and anti-atherogenic effect, predominantly via its stimulation of NO production in endothelial cells. Insulin may also be anti-inflammatory. However, in insulin-resistant subjects, insulin-mediated NO production becomes attenuated, due in part to local release of cytokines, and as a result the vasoconstrictor effects of insulin begin to dominate. (SNS = sympathetic nervous system.)

both the NO and the endothelin-1 pathways (Yudkin *et al.*, 2005). In insulin-resistant obese subjects, insulin-stimulated NO synthesis is impaired, resulting in unopposed vasoconstriction. Recently, based on some elegant animal work, Yudkin and colleagues have proposed that this vasoconstriction is the consequence of production of the adipocytokine TNF-α from the cuff of fat seen surrounding the origin of the arterioles. They suggested that this local release of TNF-α inhibits the PI3-K pathway of insulin signalling (and thus NO release), leaving unopposed vasoconstrictor effects of endothelin-1. They have termed this effect 'vasocrine' signalling (Yudkin *et al.*, 2005).

Insulin has additional vascular actions, such as the stimulation of vascular smooth-muscle cells and the production of plasminogen activator inhibitor-1 (PAI-1) through the mitogen-activated protein kinase (MAPK) pathway. Finally, as noted above, insulin can stimulate renal sodium retention and activation of the sympathetic nervous system, both effects that can contribute to elevations in blood pressure (Muis *et al.*, 2005).

2.10   Role of Hyperglycaemia

It is clear that intensive glycaemic control has a more modest effect on reducing macrovascular complications than microvascular complications (Stratton *et al.*, 2000). This is clearly because, as reviewed above, the development of CVD in diabetes is multifactorial, and hyperglycaemia is one of many risk factors. Moreover, the presence of elevated risk in the pre-diabetes phase, especially in those with insulin resistance-related features, suggests that development of hyperglycaemia has a lesser role in the macrovascular complications of diabetes. Nevertheless, there is an association – hyperglycaemia is clearly the major insult responsible for excess CVD risk in type 1 diabetes – and several mechanisms may link hyperglycaemia to accelerated vascular risk. Much of the relevant work relates to effects of hyperglycaemia on endothelial cells or function. *In vitro* experiments looking at normal aortic rings bathed in different concentrations of glucose solutions show that hyperglycaemia impairs nitric oxide-derived vasodilation (Tesfamariam *et al.*, 1991). Hyperglycaemia also reduces endothelium-dependent vasodilatation when healthy subjects are placed under hyperglycaemic conditions (Williams *et al.*, 1998). Hyperglycaemia increases levels of reactive oxygen species (ROS) such as the superoxide ion (Giardino *et al.*, 1996). It is thought that the production of ROS in hyperglycaemic states occurs, at least in part, at the mitochondrial level, via the NA(D)PH electron transport chain (Nishikawa *et al.*, 2000). One of the actions of the superoxide ion is to react with NO to inactivate it, forming peroxynitrite, hence attenuating the vasodilatatory, anti-inflammatory and antithrombotic effects of NO. Peroxynitrite oxidises tetrahydrobiopterin, the nitric oxide synthase (NOS) co-factor, and this in turn uncouples NOS. This uncoupling causes the enzyme to increase superoxide production instead of NO, thereby amplifying the oxidative stress at the expense of NO (Wever *et al.*, 1998).

High levels of glucose can also damage extracellularly and increase the production of advanced glycosylation end-products (AGEs) in the circulation and on matrix proteins. The AGEs directly affect cell function, arterial wall stiffness or gene expression of interacting cells. They are ligands for a number of scavenger receptors and the receptor for AGEs (RAGE). As reviewed by Goldberg and Dansky (2006), two lines of evidence strongly support the theory that AGEs mediate diabetic complications:

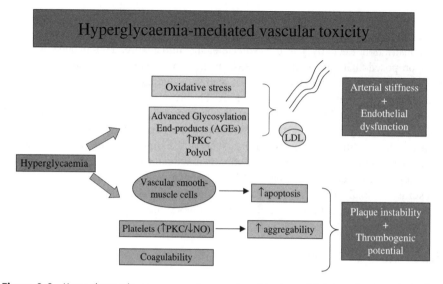

Figure 2.6 Hyperglycaemia can aggravate vascular risk via multiple mechanisms including: oxidative stress, leading to greater oxidation of LDL particles; endothelial dysfunction and arterial stiffness; effects on smooth-muscle cells; adverse effects on platelets; adverse effects on the coagulation cascade.

infusions of soluble RAGE, which is presumed to complex AGEs, reduce and stabilise atherosclerotic lesions, and inhibition of AGE formation reduces lesions; and diets enriched in AGEs promote lesions. Beyond AGEs, other mechanisms also link hyperglycaemia to oxidative stress and vascular dysfunction, as well as adverse effects on vascular smooth-muscle cells (Sundell, 2005) (Figure 2.6).

Finally, hyperglycaemia, at least at the experimental level, has also been shown to induce MMP expression in both endothelial cells and macrophages (Sundell, 2005). As discussed above, such changes are likely to render the plaque less stable and more susceptible to rupture and hence luminal thrombosis.

2.11 Metabolic Syndrome as a Link between Insulin Resistance and CVD?

Metabolic syndrome refers to a constellation of risk factors that is apparently associated with risk for both CVD and type 2 diabetes (Figure 2.7). Although a clustering of risk factors had been recognized as early as the 1920s, Gerald Reaven's Banting lecture in 1988 (Reaven, 1988) disseminated the concept to a wider audience and stimulated considerable further research. Reaven linked 'upstream' insulin resistance to a 'downstream' clustering of risk factors potentially responsible for the excess vascular risk in diabetes. He included glucose intolerance, hypertriglyceridaemia, low HDL-cholesterol and hypertension in his clustering, which he termed 'syndrome X', but interestingly obesity was not included (Reaven, 1988). The syndrome has since been variably termed the insulin resistance syndrome, Reaven's syndrome and the dysmetabolic syndrome. However, as it is not a discrete entity caused by a single

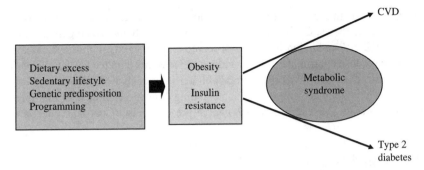

Figure 2.7 Scheme displaying the concept of metabolic syndrome as a link between obesity and insulin resistance (and related factors) with subsequent vascular disease and type 2 diabetes.

factor, but is likely caused by various factors in different individuals and racial groups, 'metabolic syndrome' has now become the preferred term. It should be stated at this point that some have questioned whether the collection of risk factors linked to obesity and insulin resistance truly constitutes a 'syndrome' (Kahn *et al.*, 2005). Regardless of such arguments, criteria for metabolic syndrome have been used to try to demonstrate increased CVD in subjects with a constellation of insulin resistance-related features. These studies have universally demonstrated that individuals with the metabolic syndrome do indeed have a higher risk of CVD, with greater risk with each additional criterion fulfilled (Sattar *et al.*, 2003b; Wilson *et al.*, 2005). However, it remains contentious whether metabolic syndrome criteria will be used in clinical practice (Sattar, 2006b). At present, the available prospective data do not suggest that metabolic syndrome criteria enhance risk prediction beyond traditional risk factor charts based on the Framingham risk score (Sattar, 2006b). Nevertheless, with specific reference to diabetes, it is of interest that subjects with type 2 diabetes who do not fulfil the criteria for metabolic syndrome do not appear at elevated CVD risk, whereas those who do fulfil the criteria are at increased risk (Alexander *et al.*, 2003). Such data concur with the observation that CVD risk is highest in the insulin-resistant patients with type 2 diabetes.

2.12 Effects of Anti-diabetic Drugs on Risk Factor Pathways

Of interest, there is now abundant evidence that insulin-sensitising therapies appear to offer benefits beyond just glucose lowering. Metformin, for example, has positive effects on FFAs, HDL-cholesterol, PAI-1 and vascular function, and may also lower markers of inflammation (Grant, 1995; Grant, 2003; Haffner *et al.*, 2005). Glitazones also benefit each of the above parameters, although their actions on HDL-cholesterol and inflammatory parameters are more pronounced and in addition they tend to raise adiponectin and lower the proportion of small, dense LDL particles (Haffner *et al.*, 2002). By contrast, sulphonylureas have far less and often negligible effects on such markers. Such observations emphasise once again the multiple linkages of insulin resistance on other risk factor pathways. They also concur with the greater benefits of metformin (and to a lesser extent glitazones) on CVD risk (Johnson *et al.*, 2005; Evans *et al.*,

2006). It is clear that by targeting glucose alone without attention to the many other risk factors in diabetes, CVD risk will be only modestly attenuated (Figure 2.7). Much stronger CVD risk reduction is clearly observed when patients with diabetes have, in addition to glucose control, their lipids and blood pressures targeted (Adler, 2003). That said, it is also clear that CVD risk remains higher in patients with diabetes even when current best therapies are employed. Such findings are in keeping with multiple risk factor abnormalities in diabetes, which can, at present, only be partially attenuated.

2.13 Conclusions

Patients with type 2 diabetes have multiple interrelated metabolic defects including derangement in lipids, blood pressure and haemostatic factors. Insulin resistance and obesity are linked closely to most (although not all) such defects, and as a result many pathway abnormalities are manifest in the pre-diabetes phase, often years before frank diabetes ensues. Such observations also help to explain why specific parameters (e.g. high triglyceride, high CRP, low adiponectin) beyond the obvious (e.g. obesity) predict incident diabetes. The development of frank hyperglycaemia once diabetes ensues adds another pathway towards vascular damage in those with type 2 diabetes but it is far more strongly associated with microvascular disease. Treatment of hyperglycaemia in isolation therefore will only minimally attenuate vascular risk in type 2 diabetes, whereas additional treatment of lipids, blood pressure and clotting abnormalities derives far greater benefit. However, despite best current therapies, CVD risk remains elevated in patients with diabetes compared to those without, emphasising the continued failure, despite best efforts, to reverse all of the multiple metabolic and vascular abnormalities in type 2 diabetes. Such observations also reiterate the need to develop better therapies to minimize CVD risk in this high-risk population.

References

Adler AI (2003). Managing diabetes: what to do about cardiovascular disease. *Diabetes Research and Clinical Practice* **61** (Suppl 1): S3–8.

Alexander CM, Landsman PB, Teutsch SM, Haffner SM (2003). NCEP-defined metabolic syndrome, diabetes, and prevalence of coronary heart disease among NHANES III participants age 50 years and older. *Diabetes* **52**: 1210–14.

Basi S, Lewis JB (2006). Microalbuminuria as a target to improve cardiovascular and renal outcomes. *American Journal of Kidney Disease* **47**: 927–46.

Bloomgarden ZT (2005). Inflammation, atherosclerosis, and aspects of insulin action. *Diabetes Care* **28**: 2312–19.

Booth GL, Kapral MK, Fung K, Tu JV (2006). Relation between age and cardiovascular disease in men and women with diabetes compared with non-diabetic people: a population-based retrospective cohort study. *Lancet* **368**: 29–36.

Caballero AE, Arora S, Saouaf R, Lim SC, Smakowski P, Park JY, King GL, Logerfo FW, Horton ES, Veves A (1999). Microvascular and macrovascular reactivity is reduced in subjects at risk for type 2 diabetes. *Diabetes* **48**: 1856–62.

Dandona P, Aljada A, Dhindsa S, Garg R (2003). Insulin as an anti-inflammatory and antiatherosclerotic hormone. *Clinical Cornerstone Supplement* **4**: S13–20.

Das UN (2004). Metabolic syndrome X: an inflammatory condition? *Current Hypertension Reports* **6**: 66–73.

Eberly LE, Stamler J, Neaton JD (2003). Relation of triglyceride levels, fasting and nonfasting, to fatal and nonfatal coronary heart disease. *Archives of Internal Medicine* **163**: 1077–83.

Evans JM, Ogston SA, Emslie-Smith A, Morris AD (2006). Risk of mortality and adverse cardiovascular outcomes in type 2 diabetes: a comparison of patients treated with sulfonylureas and metformin. *Diabetologia* **49**: 930–6.

Ferrari P, Weidmann P (1990). Insulin, insulin sensitivity and hypertension. *Journal of Hypertension* **8**: 491–500.

Fonseca V, Jawa A (2005). Endothelial and erectile dysfunction, diabetes mellitus, and the metabolic syndrome: common pathways and treatments? *American Journal of Cardiology* **96**: 13M–18M.

Frayn KN (2001). Adipose tissue and the insulin resistance syndrome. *Proceedings of the Nutrition Society* **60**: 375–80.

Freeman DJ, Norrie J, Caslake MJ, Gaw A, Ford I, Lowe GD, O'Reilly DS, Packard CJ, Sattar N (2002). C-reactive protein is an independent predictor of risk for the development of diabetes in the West of Scotland Coronary Prevention Study. *Diabetes* **51**: 1596–600.

Giardino I, Edelstein D, Brownlee M (1996). BCL-2 expression or antioxidants prevent hyperglycemia-induced formation of intracellular advanced glycation endproducts in bovine endothelial cells. *Journal of Clinical Investigation* **97**: 1422–8.

Goldberg IJ, Dansky HM (2006). Diabetic vascular disease: an experimental objective. *Arteriosclerosis, Thrombosis, and Vascular Biology* **26**: 1693–701.

Grant PJ (1995). The effects of metformin on cardiovascular risk factors. *Diabetes / Metabolism Reviews* **11** (Suppl 1): S43–50.

Grant PJ (2003). Beneficial effects of metformin on haemostasis and vascular function in man. *Diabetes and Metabolism* **29**: 6S44–52.

Greenberg AS, Obin MS (2006). Obesity and the role of adipose tissue in inflammation and metabolism. *American Journal of Clinical Nutrition* **83**: 461S–465S.

Haffner SM, Stern MP, Hazuda HP, Mitchell BD, Patterson JK (1990). Cardiovascular risk factors in confirmed prediabetic individuals. Does the clock for coronary heart disease start ticking before the onset of clinical diabetes? *Journal of the American Medical Association* **263**: 2893–8.

Haffner SM, Greenberg AS, Weston WM, Chen H, Williams K, Freed MI (2002). Effect of rosiglitazone treatment on nontraditional markers of cardiovascular disease in patients with type 2 Diabetes Mellitus. *Circulation* **106**: 679–84.

Haffner S, Temprosa M, Crandall J, Fowler S, Goldberg R, Horton E, Marcovina S, Mather K, Orchard T, Ratner R, Barrett-Connor, E (2005). Intensive lifestyle intervention or metformin on inflammation and coagulation in participants with impaired glucose tolerance. *Diabetes* **54**: 1566–72.

Hink U, Li H, Mollnau H, Oelze M, Matheis E, Hartmann M, Skatchkov M, Thais F, Stahl RA, Warnholtz A, Meinertz T, Griendling K, Harrison DG, Forstermann U, Munzel T (2001). Mechanisms underlying endothelial dysfunction in diabetes mellitus. *Circulation Research* **88**: E14–22.

Hollenbeck C, Reaven GM (1987). Variations in insulin-stimulated glucose uptake in healthy individuals with normal glucose tolerance. *Journal of Clinical Endocrinology and Metabolism* **64**: 1169–73.

Johnson JA, Simpson SH, Toth EL, Majumdar SR (2005). Reduced cardiovascular morbidity and mortality associated with metformin use in subjects with Type 2 diabetes. *Diabetic Medicine* **22**: 497–502.

Juhan-Vague I, Morange PE, Alessi MC (2002). The insulin resistance syndrome: implications for thrombosis and cardiovascular disease. *Pathophysiology of Haemostasis and Thrombosis* **32**: 269–73.

Kahn R, Buse J, Ferrannini E, Stern M (2005). The metabolic syndrome: time for a critical appraisal: joint statement from the American Diabetes Association and the European Association for the Study of Diabetes. *Diabetes Care* **28**: 2289–304.

Lewington S, Clarke R, Qizilbash N, Peto R, Collins R (2002). Age-specific relevance of usual blood pressure to vascular mortality: a meta-analysis of individual data for one million adults in 61 prospective studies. *Lancet* **360**: 1903–13.

Lindsay RS, Funahashi T, Hanson RL, Matsuzawa Y, Tanaka S, Tataranni PA, Knowler WC, Krakoff J (2002). Adiponectin and development of type 2 diabetes in the Pima Indian population. *Lancet* **360**: 57–8.

Matthews DR (1999). The natural history of diabetes-related complications: the UKPDS experience. United Kingdom Prospective Diabetes Study. *Diabetes, Obesity and Metabolism* **1** (Suppl 2): S7–13.

McVeigh GE, Cohn JN (2003). Endothelial dysfunction and the metabolic syndrome. *Current Diabetes Reports* **3**: 87–92.

Meigs JB, O'Donnell CJ, Tofler GH, Benjamin EJ, Fox CS, Lipinska I, Nathan DM, Sullivan LM, D'agostino RB, Wilson PW (2006). Hemostatic markers of endothelial dysfunction and risk of incident type 2 diabetes: the Framingham Offspring Study. *Diabetes* **55**: 530–7.

Mlinar B, Marc J, Janez A, Pfeifer M (2007). Molecular mechanisms of insulin resistance and associated diseases. *Clinica Chimica Acta* **375**: 20–35.

Muis MJ, Bots ML, Grobbee DE, Stolk RP (2005). Insulin treatment and cardiovascular disease; friend or foe? A point of view. *Diabetic Medicine* **22**: 118–26.

Nishikawa T, Edelstein D, Du XL, Yamagishi S, Matsumura T, Kaneda Y, Yorek MA, Beebe D, Oates PJ, Hammes HP, Giardino I, Brownlee M (2000). Normalizing mitochondrial superoxide production blocks three pathways of hyperglycaemic damage. *Nature* **404**: 787–90.

Packard CJ (2006). Small dense low-density lipoprotein and its role as an independent predictor of cardiovascular disease. *Current Opinion in Lipidology* **17**: 412–17.

Pickup JC, Crook MA (1998). Is type II diabetes mellitus a disease of the innate immune system? *Diabetologia* **41**: 1241–8.

Pischon T, Girman CJ, Hotamisligil GS, Rifai N, Hu FB, Rimm EB (2004). Plasma adiponectin levels and risk of myocardial infarction in men. *Journal of the American Medical Association* **291**: 1730–7.

Reaven GM (1988). Banting lecture 1988. Role of insulin resistance in human disease. *Diabetes* **37**: 1595–607.

Reaven GM (2005). Insulin resistance, the insulin resistance syndrome, and cardiovascular disease. *Panminerva Medica* **47**: 201–10.

Reaven GM (2006). The metabolic syndrome: is this diagnosis necessary? *American Journal of Clinical Nutrition* **83**: 1237–47.

Ritchie SA, Ewart MA, Perry CG, Connell JM, Salt IP (2004). The role of insulin and the adipocytokines in regulation of vascular endothelial function. *Clinical Science* **107**: 519–32.

Sattar N (2005). Insulin resistance and the metabolic syndrome as predictors of cardiovascular risk: where are we now? *Minerva Endocrinologica* **30**: 121–38.

Sattar N (2006a). High sensitivity C-reactive protein in cardiovasular disease and diabetes: evidence for a clinical role? *British Journal of Diabetes and Vascular Disease* **6**: 5–8.

Sattar N (2006b). The metabolic syndrome: should current criteria influence clinical practice? *Current Opinion in Lipidology* **17**: 404–11.

Sattar N, Lowe GD (2006). High sensitivity C-reactive protein and cardiovascular disease: an association built on unstable foundations? *Annals of Clinical Biochemistry* **43**: 252–6.

Sattar N, McInnes IB (2005). Vascular comorbidity in rheumatoid arthritis: potential mechanisms and solutions. *Current Opinion in Rheumatology* **17**: 286–92.

Sattar N, Petrie JR, Jaap AJ (1998). The atherogenic lipoprotein phenotype and vascular endothelial dysfunction. *Atherosclerosis* **138**: 229–35.

Sattar N, Gaw A, Scherbakova O, Ford I, O'Reilly DS, Haffner SM, Isles C, Macfarlane PW, Packard CJ, Cobbe SM, Shepherd, J (2003a). Metabolic syndrome with and without C-reactive protein as a predictor of coronary heart disease and diabetes in the West of Scotland Coronary Prevention Study. *Circulation* **108**: 414–19.

Sattar N, McCarey DW, Capell H, McInnes IB (2003b). Explaining how 'high-grade' systemic inflammation accelerates vascular risk in rheumatoid arthritis. *Circulation* **108**: 2957–63.

Sattar N, Wannamethee G, Sarwar N, Tchernova J, Cherry L, Wallace AM, Danesh J, Whincup PH (2006). Adiponectin and coronary heart disease: a prospective study and meta-analysis. *Circulation* **114**: 623–9.

Schalkwijk CG, Stehouwer CD (2005). Vascular complications in diabetes mellitus: the role of endothelial dysfunction. *Clinical Science* **109**: 143–59.

Schmidt MI, Duncan BB, Sharrett AR, Lindberg G, Savage PJ, Offenbacher S, Azambuja MI, Tracy RP, Heiss G (1999). Markers of inflammation and prediction of diabetes mellitus in adults (Atherosclerosis Risk in Communities study): a cohort study. *Lancet* **353**: 1649–52.

Schram MT, Stehouwer CD (2005). Endothelial dysfunction, cellular adhesion molecules and the metabolic syndrome. *Hormone and Metabolic Research* **37** (Suppl 1): 49–55.

Sniderman AD (2004). Applying apoB to the diagnosis and therapy of the atherogenic dyslipoproteinemias: a clinical diagnostic algorithm. *Current Opinion in Lipidology* **15**: 433–8.

Steinberg HO, Chaker H, Leaming R, Johnson A, Brechtel G, Baron AD (1996). Obesity/insulin resistance is associated with endothelial dysfunction. Implications for the syndrome of insulin resistance. *Journal of Clinical Investigation* **97**: 2601–10.

Stratton IM, Adler AI, Neil HA, Matthews DR, Manley SE, Cull CA, Hadden D, Turner RC, Holman RR (2000). Association of glycaemia with macrovascular and microvascular complications of type 2 diabetes (UKPDS 35): prospective observational study. *British Medical Journal* **321**: 405–12.

Sundell J (2005). Obesity and diabetes as risk factors for coronary artery disease: from the epidemiological aspect to the initial vascular mechanisms. *Diabetes, Obesity and Metabolism* **7**: 9–20.

Tesfamariam B, Brown ML, Cohen RA (1991). Elevated glucose impairs endothelium-dependent relaxation by activating protein kinase C. *Journal of Clinical Investigation* **87**: 1643–8.

Tooke JE, Goh KL (1999). Vascular function in Type 2 diabetes mellitus and pre-diabetes: the case for intrinsic endotheiopathy. *Diabetic Medicine* **16**: 710–15.

Walldius G, Jungner I, Holme I, Aastveit AH, Kolar W, Steiner E (2001). High apolipoprotein B, low apolipoprotein A-I, and improvement in the prediction of fatal myocardial infarction (AMORIS study): a prospective study. *Lancet* **358**: 2026–33.

Warram JH, Martin BC, Krolewski AS, Soeldner JS, Kahn CR (1990). Slow glucose removal rate and hyperinsulinemia precede the development of type II diabetes in the offspring of diabetic parents. *Annals of Internal Medicine* **113**: 909–15.

Wever RM, Luscher TF, Cosentino F, Rabelink TJ (1998). Atherosclerosis and the two faces of endothelial nitric oxide synthase. *Circulation* **97**: 108–12.

Williams SB, Goldfine AB, Timimi FK, Ting HH, Roddy MA, Simonson D C, Creager MA (1998). Acute hyperglycemia attenuates endothelium-dependent vasodilation in humans in vivo. *Circulation* **97**: 1695–701.

Wilson PW, D'Agostino RB, Parise H, Sullivan L, Meigs JB (2005). Metabolic syndrome as a precursor of cardiovascular disease and type 2 diabetes mellitus. *Circulation* **112**: 3066–72.

Yudkin JS, Eringa E, Stehouwer C (2005). 'Vasocrine' signalling from perivascular fat: a mechanism linking insulin resistance to vascular disease. *Lancet* **365**: 1817–20.

Ziegler D (2005). Type 2 diabetes as an inflammatory cardiovascular disorder. *Current Molecular Medicine* **5**: 309–22.

3 Coronary Heart Disease and Diabetes

Colin Berry, Miles Fisher and *John J. McMurray*

3.1 Nature of Coronary Heart Disease in Diabetes

Case–control studies have demonstrated that diabetic patients with angiographically normal coronary arteries have smaller calibre coronary arteries than non-diabetic control subjects (Mosseri *et al.*, 1998). Diabetes is an aetiological factor for the pathogenesis of coronary heart disease (CHD) and an adverse prognostic marker (Kip *et al.*, 1996). Diabetic patients with coronary disease have a higher prevalence of other risk factors for CHD, and related vascular co-morbidity (Kip *et al.*, 1996).When CHD is present diabetic patients typically have more severe disease as evidenced by more extensive coronary artery calcification compared with non-diabetic patients (Wong *et al.*, 1994; Arad *et al.*, 2001), with more arteries involved (Dortimer *et al.*, 1978; Moise *et al.*, 1984; Abaci *et al.*, 1999; Melidonis *et al.*, 1999; Waldecker *et al.*, 1999; Cariou *et al.*, 2000; Natali *et al.*, 2000) and a higher prevalence of left main stem disease. These features have also been found at postmortem investigations (Waller *et al.*, 1980). Surprisingly, it is not known whether diabetic patients have more complex coronary lesions, such as those occurring at bifurcations (Morgan *et al.*, 2004).

Coronary artery collateral development is an adaptive response in CHD. In one retrospective cohort study of patients who underwent coronary angiography, the coronary collateral score was significantly less in diabetic patients (Abaci *et al.*, 1999). In another study inducible collateral coronary blood flow was assessed in 18 diabetic and 38 non-diabetic patients undergoing elective percutaneous coronary intervention (PCI) for a single vessel proximal stenosis of 50–90%, and the mean coronary wedge pressure increased by a similar degree in diabetic and non-diabetic patients (Kyriakides *et al.*, 2002).

Typically, type 1 diabetes is linked with microvascular disease, and type 2 diabetes is associated with macrovascular disease. Nevertheless, type 1 diabetes is also associated with premature CHD (see also Chapter 1). One angiographic study of 31 young,

Diabetic Cardiology Editors Miles Fisher and John J. McMurray
© 2007 John Wiley & Sons, Ltd.

symptomatic patients with type 1 diabetes found that the severity of CHD, in terms of the number of coronary arteries affected, the number of segments involved, the degree to which these arteries were narrowed angiographically and the distribution of these narrowings, was more pronounced in diabetic patients compared with control subjects (Valsania et al., 1991). Furthermore, the diabetic pattern of small-calibre coronary arteries, with diffuse disease and a high proportion of arteries with distal stenoses, rendered more diabetic patients unsuitable for surgical revascularisation.

The severity of CHD in diabetes is related to glycaemic control (Aronson et al., 1996). Although insulin resistance is associated with CHD severity in non-diabetic patients, it is less certain whether this relationship exists in diabetic patients (Takezako et al., 1999). Conventional risk factors for atherosclerosis are also related to the severity of angiographic disease in diabetics. Observational studies have found that plasma concentrations of intermediate-density lipoprotein are a positive predictor of disease severity, whereas high-density lipoprotein concentrations are a negative predictor in patients with type 2 diabetes (Syvanne et al., 2001).

Although the presence of increasingly severe obstructive coronary artery lesions is associated with an adverse outcome in the longer term (Moise et al., 1984), recent work has demonstrated that most myocardial infarctions occur as a result of the rupture of non-obstructive plaque (Mann and Davies, 1996; Maseri and Fuster, 2003). Thus, the extent of plaque disease, or 'plaque burden', rather than the number of obstructive lesions, may be a determinant of prognosis. Given that atherosclerotic coronary disease tends to be more widespread in diabetic patients, their greater risk for plaque rupture may be greater, and there is some postmortem evidence that plaque is more inflamed and necrotic in patients with diabetes, and so more likely to rupture (Burke et al., 2004).

3.2 Presentation of CHD in Diabetes

Diabetic patients may experience symptoms caused by CHD in the same way as non-diabetic patients. Other symptoms attributable to obstructive CHD include breathlessness, manifesting as 'angina-equivalent', and ischaemia-related left ventricular dysfunction. Palpitations, presyncope and syncope may arise because of ischaemia-related arrhythmia, such as atrial fibrillation/flutter, and ventricular arrhythmia, including ectopy and tachycardia. A characteristic feature of diabetes is the absence or muted intensity of angina. This 'silent ischaemia' is partly related to diabetic autonomic neuropathy (Findlay, 2003). The prognosis of patients with 'silent ischaemia', as evidenced by ischaemic changes on an electrocardiogram (ECG) on exercise testing without symptoms and good prognostic features, is similar to those with symptomatic angina (Lotan et al., 1994; Marwick, 1995).

Other presentations

Coronary heart disease may be first suspected in a diabetic patient who presents with a complication of this disease. For example, a diabetic patient may present with symptomatic heart failure, the aetiology of which is obstructive CHD. Alternatively, the cause of a peripheral embolic event may be thrombus arising within a dilated, ischaemic left ventricle. Coronary heart disease may be detected in diabetic patients who present with a stroke (Chapter 7) or with obstructive peripheral vascular disease (Chapter 8). It may also be detected in diabetic patients who present for management of a non-cardiovascular problem, e.g. an abnormal ECG obtained as part of a routine work-up for an elective surgical procedure.

3.3   Non-invasive Investigation

Stress testing

According to Bayes' theorem, the greater the likelihood that the CHD is present (pretest probability), the greater the validity of a positive test and the likelihood that it is a true positive. Furthermore, a negative result is more likely to represent a true negative (Gibbons *et al.*, 1997). The positive predictive value of stress testing is greater in individuals who have a higher absolute risk of CHD, such as in diabetes. Stress testing is a fundamental method for assessing both diabetic and non-diabetic patients. Although stress testing will detect a large number of abnormalities in truly asymptomatic people with diabetes, the long-term effect of intervention for asymptomatic CHD in diabetic patients is not certain, so stress testing is not currently recommended as a screening test, and should be used where there is a clinical suspicion of CHD.

Nuclear stress testing

These tests may be more informative in diabetic patients than with stress testing without information about myocardial perfusion, particularly in patients with silent ischaemia. In one multicentre series of 4755 patients (20% diabetic subjects), fixed and reversible defects, as revealed by stress single-photon emission computed tomography (SPECT) myocardial perfusion imaging, were independently predictive of cardiac death, and the predictive value of SPECT in this population was greatest for diabetic women (Giri *et al.*, 2002).

Stress tests in diabetic patients may be falsely negative because asymptomatic ischaemia is more likely in diabetic patients, compared with non-diabetic patients. Furthermore, in those with positive stress tests, the specificity is less than in non-diabetic patients.

Stress echo

Stress echocardiography is a useful method to test for the presence of inducible myocardial ischaemia. This form of stress testing assesses left ventricular systolic function at rest, and during pharmacologically induced stress. This method can also assess for hibernation, which is viable but hypocontractile myocardium perfused by inadequate coronary blood flow. Pharmacological stress echocardiography may be particularly useful in diabetic patients, with enhanced specificity and sensitivity compared with standard exercise ECG testing (Albers *et al.*, 2006).

3.4 Pharmacological Treatment of CHD in People with Diabetes

In the management of stable angina pectoris the first aim of treatment is to relieve symptoms (morbidity) by reducing myocardial oxygen demand, with a further aim of reducing mortality if possible. Nitrates, calcium channel blockers and the potassium channel opening agent nicorandil are all of symptomatic benefit. In the IONA study nicorandil reduced hospital admissions with angina (IONA Study Group, 2002). Eight per cent of the study subjects had diabetes, and there was similar benefit in the diabetes subgroup (IONA Study Group, 2004). As in non-diabetic subjects there are relatively few data that show prognostic benefit of pharmacological treatments for patients with stable angina, in contrast to patients following acute myocardial infarction (see Chapter 4). The most compelling evidence for prognostic benefit in diabetic subjects comes from subgroup analysis of multicentre studies for beta-blockers and ACE inhibitors, and from subgroup and meta-analysis of antiplatelet therapy.

Beta-blockers

The prognostic benefits of beta-blockers following myocardial infarction in patients with myocardial infarction are described in Chapter 4. A retrospective analysis of the prognostic effects of beta-blockers in 2723 patients with diabetes and stable CHD was performed as part of the Bezafibrate Infarction Prevention (BIP) study (Jonas *et al.*, 1996). About one-third of the diabetic patients were categorised as receiving chronic beta-blocker therapy, mostly cardioselective. There was a significant 44% reduction in mortality in the beta-blocker group, with a 42% reduction in cardiac mortality. The low use of beta-blockers in diabetic subjects with CHD has been demonstrated in several registries, and probably reflects erroneous fears about hypoglycaemia in this group of patients. Hypoglycaemia is uncommon in diabetic patients with CHD as many of these patients have severe insulin resistance. If hypoglycaemia occurs cardioselective beta-blockers may slightly reduce the symptoms of hypoglycaemia, but have no appreciable effect on the recovery from hypoglycaemia (see also Chapter 5, p. 119). In non-diabetic subjects the metabolic effects of beta-blockers include worsening of glucose tolerance and the possible development of overt diabetes in people with impaired glucose tolerance. In people with established diabetes, however, the metabolic effects are negligible and the introduction of beta-blocker therapy does not usually require any adjustment of diabetic therapy.

ACE inhibitors

The prognostic benefits of ACE inhibitors following myocardial infarction in patients with diabetes are also described in Chapter 4. The ACE inhibitors ramipril and perindopril have been used to treat diabetic patients with CHD in the absence of left ventricular dysfunction in the HOPE and EUROPA studies, both of which included diabetic patients either following previous myocardial infarction or with stable CHD, and both of which showed a significant reduction in cardiac events and total mortality

(Heart Outcomes Prevention Evaluation (HOPE) Study Investigators, 2000; Daly *et al.*, 2005). These studies remain controversial because of the differences in blood pressure between the ACE inhibitor and placebo groups, and debate whether the prognostic benefit was related to reductions in blood pressure in a very-high-risk group of patients, or whether it was to an effect of ACE inhibition, which is supported in various clinical and animal models? The PEACE study with quinapril did not show similar benefit in lower risk patients with CHD, but the diabetic patients in this study were withdrawn when it was felt unethical not to treat these diabetic patients with an open-label ACE inhibitor (PEACE Trial Investigators, 2004). To date, similar cardiovascular risk reduction has not yet been proven with angiotensin receptor blockers (ARBs).

A few studies have shown that the use of ACE inhibitors may reduce insulin resistance and slightly improve glycaemic control in diabetic patients, and a couple of studies have shown an increase in the frequency of admission for hypoglycaemia in diabetic patients treated with ACE inhibitors compared to those not treated. In a population-based study from Scotland ACE inhibitor use was associated with an increased frequency of hospital admission for hypoglycaemia, with an odds ratio of 3.2 (Morris *et al.*, 1997). In non-diabetic subjects the use of ACE inhibitors (and ARBs) has been associated with a lesser progression to diabetes as a secondary outcome in several cardiovascular studies, mostly when used to treat hypertension, and this is discussed further in Chapter 6, p. 158.

Antiplatelet therapy

Antiplatelet therapy is widely used as a preventative agent in cardiovascular disease (CVD). Aspirin is the most commonly used antiplatelet agent, and a substantial evidence base exists for its role in the prevention of cardiovascular events. It would seem intuitive that if diabetic individuals are at an increased risk of cardiovascular events, it would be reasonable to try to diminish the risk by giving antiplatelet therapy to all diabetic patients. The evidence base for the possible benefit of antiplatelet therapy to reduce events in diabetic patients with stable CHD, as distinct from following acute coronary syndromes, is remarkably small. The Antiplatelet Trialists' Collaboration (ATC) has performed two meta-analyses of antiplatelet therapy. In 1994 they demonstrated a significant reduction in vascular events (non-fatal myocardial infarction, non-fatal stroke or vascular death) in diabetic patients with vascular disease treated with antiplatelet therapy (Antiplatelet Trialists' Collaboration, 1994). The reduction was similar to that seen in other high-risk cohorts (e.g. previous myocardial infarction, transient ischaemic attack or stroke). A second analysis of 1365 diabetic patients whose sole vascular risk factor was diabetes (i.e. primary prevention) showed no benefit from antiplatelet therapy.

The larger 2002 ATC meta-analysis again showed no benefit where diabetes alone was the risk factor (Antithrombotic Trialists' Collaboration, 2002). It included data from the diabetic subgroup of the Hypertension Optimal Treatment (HOT) study, and the Early Treatment Diabetic Retinopathy Study (ETDRS). In the HOT study 75 mg of aspirin reduced symptomatic myocardial infarction (MI) in diabetic patients with hypertension, but total and cardiovascular mortality were not reduced (Hansson *et al.*,

1998). In the ETDRS 650 mg of aspirin produced a reduction in symptomatic MI (ETDRS Investigators, 1992). Both HOT and ETDRS therefore showed benefits only in terms of decreased symptomatic MI, but show no impact on reducing cardiovascular death in patients with diabetes. Similar lack of benefit has been observed in other studies when using aspirin for the primary prevention of CVD in people with diabetes.

Clopidogrel

The thienopyridine clopidogrel blocks platelet aggregation by irreversibly inhibiting platelet ADP receptors. A *post hoc* analysis of the diabetic patients randomised in the Clopidogrel versus Aspirin in Patients at Risk of Ischaemic Events (CAPRIE) study found that clopidogrel therapy reduced the relative risk of death, MI, stroke or rehospitalisation compared with aspirin therapy (Bhatt *et al.*, 2002). However, specific randomised trials will be needed to determine whether clopidogrel alone or clopidogrel plus aspirin are superior to aspirin alone in the prevention of cardiovascular events in diabetic patients with established CVD. In the CHARISMA trial, the effect of clopidogrel versus placebo when added to background aspirin was assessed in high-risk individuals and four-fifths of the subjects had diabetes (Bhatt *et al.*, 2006). The primary endpoint was a composite of MI, stroke or cardiovascular death and this was not significantly different in the clopidogrel and placebo groups, and there was no benefit in the diabetes patients when analysed as a separate subgroup.

3.5 Coronary Revascularisation in Diabetes

Patients with diabetes account for approximately one-quarter of all patients undergoing coronary revascularisation procedures each year, and they experience worse outcomes compared with non-diabetic subjects. Although surgical revascularisation remains the recommended strategy for diabetic multivessel CHD, recent advances in percutaneous coronary intervention (PCI) may be challenging this approach.

Coronary artery bypass grafting (CABG)

No clinical trials to date of surgical revascularisation versus medical therapy have been performed exclusively in diabetic patients. Three landmark trials of surgical revascularisation versus medical therapy in multivessel CHD were the European Coronary Surgery Study (ECSS) (European Coronary Surgery Study Group, 1982), the Veterans Administration Cooperative Study of Surgery for Coronary Artery Disease (VACSS) (Veterans Administration Coronary Artery Bypass Surgery Cooperative Study Group, 1984) and the Coronary Artery Surgery Study (CASS) (Alderman *et al.*, 1990). Collectively, these trials demonstrated that surgery improved survival in patients with multivessel CHD and reduced left ventricular function. Compared with medical therapy, surgical revascularisation conferred a mortality benefit in patients with left main stem or at least two-vessel CHD, particularly where the proximal left anterior descending coronary artery was involved. The magnitude of this benefit was greater in those with impaired left ventricular systolic function, and was evident in patients who were asymptomatic or who had mild angina.

A meta-analysis of the long-term outcomes of patients who participated in seven randomised trials of CABG versus medical therapy demonstrated that mortality was lower in the CABG group compared with the medical therapy group at 5 years, 7 years and 10 years (Yusuf *et al.*, 1994). The risk reduction was greatest in patients with left main artery disease. Patients with proximal left anterior descending disease also derived prognostic benefit from surgery, regardless of the number of vessels involved. Importantly, the risk reduction conferred by surgery was similar for patients with normal or reduced left ventricular function. Of the 2649 patients included in this analysis, 10% had diabetes and no interaction of diabetic status with outcome was found (Yusuf *et al.*, 1994).

One explanation for the survival benefit of CABG may be a reduced mortality after ischaemic events occurring subsequent to the revascularisation. Peduzzi *et al.* (1991) demonstrated that although the 10-year *incidence* of MI was greater in patients who underwent surgery, the *survival* of surgical patients was substantially greater than medically treated patients. The reduction in postinfarction mortality with surgery was 99% in the first month and 49% subsequently. No information was provided about diabetes in this report, but subsequently similar findings were reported for BARI diabetic subjects by Detre *et al.* (2000).

This improved cardiac prognosis of CABG-treated patients after MI probably occurs for a number of reasons:

- When a native vessel or graft occlusion occurs, collateral blood flow provided by the non-occluded bypass-grafts can maintain myocardial perfusion.

- The distal location of a graft can ensure myocardial perfusion despite the presence of more widespread proximal disease.

- The improved myocardial perfusion, and protection in the face of further occlusive native vessel or graft disease, can explain the reduction in angina, MI and repeat revascularisation with CABG.

- Surgical revascularisation may also reduce the risk of sudden death, especially for patients with triple-vessel CHD (Holmes *et al.*, 1986).

These prognostic benefits probably reflect the impact of revascularisation with improved distal myocardial perfusion, but the importance of the extent of revascularisation remains unclear.

Although revascularisation for prognostically important coronary disease, such as left main stem or double-vessel disease including the proximal left anterior descending artery, should represent standard practice, recent evidence-based advances in secondary prevention therapies and advances in surgical techniques, such as off-pump revascularisation, raise the question of the applicability of these data some 10 years on.

Complications after surgical revascularisation

Diabetic patients fare less well after CABG compared with non-diabetic patients, and early and long-term morbidity and mortality are higher in diabetic patients (Higgins *et al.*, 1992). Compared with non-diabetic patients, diabetic patients have:

- Increased perioperative mortality

- Increased 30-day mortality

- Increased in-hospital mortality

- Increased long-term mortality.

And increased postoperative complications including:

- Increased repeat revascularisations

- Increased wound infections and sternal wound infection (Slaughter *et al.*, 1993)

- Increased postoperative arrhythmias

- Increased respiratory failure

- Increased renal failure (Mangano *et al.*, 1998).

This leads to greater resource utilisation in diabetic patients undergoing CABG (Mangano *et al.*, 1998). There is recent evidence that tight glycaemic control in diabetic CABG patients may improve perioperative outcomes, decrease wound complications and may even improve survival (Lazar *et al.*, 2004).

Percutaneous transluminal coronary angioplasty (PTCA)

Since percutaneous transluminal coronary angioplasty (PTCA) was first described by Andreas Grüntzig in 1981, percutaneous coronary intervention (PCI) has become a fundamental anti-ischaemic therapy for CHD, with the principal gain being improvements in symptoms and quality of life. Several trials, including the Randomised Intervention Treatment of Angina (RITA) (Hampton *et al.*, 1993, Henderson *et al.*, 1998), the German Angioplasty Bypass Investigation (GABI) (Hamm *et al.*, 1994), the Emery Angioplasty versus Surgery Trial (EAST) (King *et al.*, 1994, 2000) and the Bypass Angioplasty Revascularisation Investigation (BARI) (Rogers *et al.*, 1995; Alderman *et al.*, 1996) essentially confirmed that CABG was superior to PTCA for the treatment of symptomatic multivessel CHD, especially in diabetic patients. The BARI trial continues to have a particularly important influence on the approach to revascularisation in diabetic CHD patients, and for this reason this trial is discussed in detail below.

Bypass Angioplasty Revascularisation Investigation (BARI)

The Bypass Angioplasty Revascularisation Investigation (BARI) study enrolled. patients with severe angina or evidence of ischaemia requiring revascularisation, and angiographic evidence of two- or three-vessel CHD (Rogers *et al.*, 1995; Alderman *et al.*, 1996). The hypothesis was that an initial strategy of PTCA would result in comparable outcomes to CABG, and the primary endpoint was all-cause mortality at

5 years. Importantly, diabetes was not one of the prespecified subgroups for analysis at the outset of this trial.

Overall 4107 patients were eligible and 1829 patients were randomly assigned to an initial treatment strategy of CABG ($n = 914$) or PTCA ($n = 915$). In the PTCA group, stents could be used as 'bailout' management of complications. Another 2010 patients underwent revascularisation on the basis of a recommendation by their physician, and were entered into a registry (see below). A total of 268 patients declined all follow-up. Of the 1829 randomised patients, 353(19%) had diabetes as defined by a history of diabetes with use of oral anti-diabetic agents or insulin at study entry.

Patients in the PTCA group had a shorter mean postprocedure hospital stay of 5 days compared with 9 days for the CABG group. The respective in-hospital event rates for CABG and PTCA were 1.3% and 1.1% for mortality, 4.6% and 2.1% for Q-wave MI ($P < 0.01$) and 0.8% and 0.2% for stroke. The 5-year survival rate was similar at 89% for those assigned to CABG and 86% for those assigned to PTCA. By 5 years 8% of the patients assigned to CABG had undergone additional revascularisation procedures, compared with 54% of those assigned to PTCA, and the use of anti-ischaemic medication was higher in patients assigned to PTCA (Alderman *et al.*, 1997a).

Among the 1476 patients without treated diabetes, survival was virtually identical by assigned treatment and the cardiac mortality rate was also similar, demonstrating that compared with CABG an initial strategy of PTCA did not compromise 5-year survival in non-diabetic patients with multivessel disease, although subsequent revascularisation was required more often with this strategy.

Diabetes subgroup analysis

Diabetic patients in BARI differed from non-diabetic patients in many ways; heart failure, hypertension, chronic kidney disease, peripheral vascular disease, mean triglyceride concentration and mean body mass index were all higher in diabetic patients compared with non-diabetic patients. Within 1 year, the Data and Safety Monitoring Board detected a difference in event rates between diabetic patients treated with CABG or PTCA that met the prespecified significance for subgroup analysis. Among diabetic patients who were being treated with insulin or oral anti-diabetic agents at baseline, the 5-year survival was 81% for the CABG group as compared with 66% for the PTCA group ($P = 0.003$) (Figure 3.1). The excess in mortality in diabetic patients who underwent PTCA was largely attributable to an excess of cardiac death (21% in the PTCA group vs. 6% in the CABG group). This mortality difference was mainly due to the low mortality rate of CABG-treated diabetic patients who received an internal mammary artery (IMA) graft. Based on these observations, the US National Institutes of Health (the sponsors of BARI) issued an alert in September 1995 that was intended to guide clinicians toward surgical revascularisation in diabetic patients.

The intention-to-treat analysis was extended to 7 years, at which time the survival rates in diabetic patients were 76% after CABG and 56% after PTCA ($P = 0.0011$) (Alderman *et al.*, 2000). The survival advantage in the CABG group was largely confined to patients who had received an IMA graft compared to those who had received only saphenous vein grafting (SVG), and the survival rate in patients who

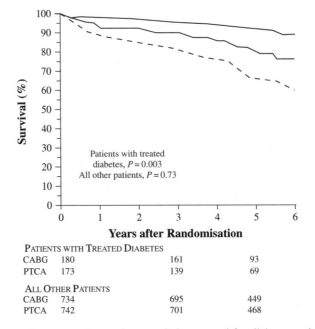

Figure 3.1 Survival among patients who were being treated for diabetes at baseline (heavy lines) and all other patients (light lines). Patients assigned to CABG are indicated by solid lines, and those assigned to PTCA by dashed lines. The numbers of patients at risk are shown below the graph at baseline, 3 years and 5 years. Reproduced from Alderman EL, Andrews K, Bost J, Bourassa M, Chaitman BR, Detre K, et al. (1996). Comparison of coronary bypass surgery with angioplasty in patients with multivessel disease. *New England Journal of Medicine* **335**: 217–25.

underwent PTCA was similar to that in patients who underwent SVG. Furthermore, the difference between the two groups was explained by 353 patients with diabetes for whom the 7-year survival was 76% and 56% in those treated by CABG and PTCA, respectively ($P = 0.0011$). Repeat revascularisation in CABG-treated patients was similar in diabetic and non-diabetic patients, but in PTCA-treated patients repeat revascularisations were much more common in diabetic patients than in non-diabetic patients. Predictors of mortality in BARI included insulin-treated diabetes, heart and renal failure, Black race and older age (Brooks *et al.*, 2000). The only significant interaction term for survival was insulin-treated diabetes.

In summary, this trial showed that where an IMA graft could be used, CABG conferred a survival benefit in diabetic patients with angina or inducible ischaemia and at least two-vessel CHD.

The BARI registry

By contrast with the BARI randomised patients, in the BARI registry survival with PTCA and CABG was similar (Alderman *et al.*, 1997b; Detre *et al.*, 1999). Registry patients had a better risk profile, including less heart failure and cigarette smoking. Compared with CABG-treated registry patients, PTCA-treated registry patients had a lower prevalence of three-vessel CHD and proximal and ostial left anterior descending disease. Thus the PTCA registry patients were at lower risk than the CABG registry patients.

At 5 years, mortality rates were higher in randomised diabetic patients compared to registry diabetic patients (Alderman *et al.*, 1997b). However, the diabetic registry patients treated by PTCA or CABG had similar cardiac mortality and total mortality rates (Detre *et al.*, 1999). The differences in the randomised group for diabetic patients undergoing PTCA were due to an early increase in death in insulin-treated diabetics, with tablet-treated patients experiencing a greater death rate during mid-late follow-up. Survival was dependent on insulin use at baseline in PTCA (but not CABG)-treated patients. In other words, the benefit of CABG was greater early on for insulin-treated diabetes (who probably had more severe disease).

Subsequent analysis of the BARI population, dichotomised according to diabetic status, was performed to compare PTCA vs. CABG in the group of patients in whom surgical revascularisation has been proven to be superior to medical therapy, i.e. patients with three-vessel coronary disease or two-vessel coronary disease including the left anterior descending artery (Berger *et al.*, 2001).

In the BARI registry, 5-year mortality was similar for diabetic patients who underwent PTCA or CABG (Alderman *et al.*, 1997b). With longer term follow-up of the randomised patients, 7-year survival amongst those with three-vessel disease undergoing PTCA and CABG was 79% versus 84% ($P = 0.06$), respectively, and 85% versus 87% ($P = 0.36$) when only non-diabetic subjects were analysed (Alderman *et al.*, 2000). The 7-year survival of diabetic patients undergoing CABG was 76% and in those undergoing PTCA it was 58%. The survival advantage of surgically treated diabetic patients was almost exclusively confined to those who received an IMA graft (7-year survival 83%) compared to those who received SVG only (7-year survival 54%). This observation supports earlier findings that IMA grafts confer a survival advantage compared with saphenous vein conduits (Loop *et al.*, 1986). This latter outcome was similar to diabetic patients who underwent multivessel PTCA (7-year survival 55%). The survival rates among non-diabetic patients were very similar (86% IMA vs. 85% SVG vs. 87% PTCA). Furthermore, in high-risk anatomic subsets (e.g. three-vessel disease) in which survival is prolonged by CABG versus medical therapy, revascularisation by PTCA and CABG yielded equivalent survival over 7 years.

This suggests that maintained myocardial blood flow, which is preserved to a greater extent by arterial rather than venous conduits, was associated with a reduction in recurrent ischaemia cardiac events and a reduced risk of death.

Other registries

A total of 3220 patients (24% diabetes) at the Duke Medical Center who had undergone cardiac catheterisation had symptomatic two- or three-vessel CHD suitable for either CABG or PTCA, and had undergone revascularisation within 30 days of the initial angiogram. The unadjusted 5-year survival rates were 74% in diabetic and 86% in non-diabetic patients and, after adjustment for imbalances in baseline characteristics, diabetes remained a significant predictor of poorer survival in patients undergoing revascularisation. Diabetic patients receiving PTCA had an adjusted 5-year survival rate of 86%, whereas in PTCA patients without diabetes the survival rate was greater at 92%. Similarly, after CABG, diabetic patients had a lower 5-year survival rate compared with non-diabetic patients (89% versus 93%) (Barsness *et al.*, 1997).

The Emory registry included 834 and 1805 diabetic patients with multivessel disease treated by PTCA and CABG, respectively (Weintraub *et al.*, 1998). After CABG there were more in-hospital deaths and a trend toward more Q-wave myocardial infarctions than after PTCA. Five-and 10-year survival rates were 78% and 45% after PTCA and 76% and 48% after CABG, respectively ($P = 0.47$). At 5 and 10 years, insulin-treated patients had lower survival rates of 72% and 31% after PTCA and 70% and 48% after CABG, respectively ($P = 0.54$). Multivariate predictors of long-term mortality were older age, low left ventricular ejection fraction, heart failure and hypertension. Overall, insulin treatment was a predictor of long-term mortality. After adjustment for differences in baseline characteristics, the 5- and 10-year survival rates were 68% and 36% after PTCA and 75% and 47% after CABG, respectively, in the insulin-treated subgroup. Non-fatal events were more common after PTCA, especially additional revascularisation. These results again underline the superiority of CABG for insulin-treated diabetic patients.

It is likely that differences existed between the clinical characteristics of patients in the BARI, Duke and Emory registries. In BARI, of the patients who were eligible for either form of revascularisation, but elected to choose one over another, 60% versus 40% chose CABG versus PTCA in BARI, whereas 81% versus 19% chose CABG versus PTCA in Duke, with a similar proportion in Emory (Kelsey, 1999). In the DUKE registry 32% of the CABG-treated patients had three-vessel CHD (including proximal left anterior descending disease), whereas only 4% of the PTCA-treated patients had this form of disease. These differences highlight the fact that a registry is comprised of a non-randomised population, and this should be considered when interpreting the findings of registries such as these.

Mechanisms to explain the survival benefits of CABG versus PTCA in diabetic patients in BARI

Diabetic patients undergoing CABG had more extensive revascularisation with, on average, 3.0 grafts placed, compared with 2.7 grafts in non-diabetic patients ($P = 0.04$) (Alderman *et al.*, 1997b). In contrast to the PTCA group, diabetic and non-diabetic CABG patients who underwent repeat coronary angiography by 30 months for any reason had a similar prevalence of obstructive stenosis (and jeopardised myocardium, defined as the proportion of the myocardium jeopardised by stenosis of 50% or more) in terminal epicardial coronary arteries (20% diabetic patients vs. 19% non-diabetic patients).

Detre *et al.* (1999) undertook further studies of the BARI population to determine the reasons why diabetic patients experienced a survival benefit with CABG, compared with PTCA. Diabetic patients have a greater mortality risk with acute MI compared with non-diabetic patients, and they hypothesised that previous CABG might impact upon this risk. In this analysis, randomised and registry patients who underwent either CABG or PTCA were studied together. Diabetic patients, regardless of whether they underwent PTCA or CABG, were more likely to be female and Black and were more likely to have a history of congestive heart failure, hypertension, renal dysfunction and peripheral vascular disease than the patients without diabetes. In other words, patients who underwent PTCA had different socio-demographic characteristics, and less severe CHD, compared to those who underwent CABG. These baseline differences reflect the influences of patient and physician choice in those patients who were not randomised. Consequently, the randomised diabetic patients represent a selected population. Thus, firm conclusions that CABG is the superior treatment for all diabetic patients with symptomatic multivessel coronary disease cannot be reached.

In this combined population, 1512 ($n = 290$ diabetes) of the 3603 patients underwent CABG as their initial revascularisation procedure (42%), and an additional 442 of the remaining 2091 patients (i.e., those who underwent PTCA first) underwent CABG some time during the first year of follow-up (Detre $et\,al.$, 1999). Thereafter, the rate of crossover to CABG decreased to an average annual incidence of 2.8%. A larger proportion of the patients with diabetes than of the patients without diabetes initially underwent revascularisation by CABG (45% vs. 41%, $P = 0.08$). Among the patients who initially underwent revascularisation by PTCA, 34% of those with diabetes compared with 29% of those without diabetes underwent CABG within 5 years (relative risk of crossover to CABG among patients with diabetes, 1.25; $P = 0.04$). At 5 years, 64% of the patients with diabetes and 58% of those without diabetes had undergone CABG. Diabetic patients were 1.9 times more likely compared to those without diabetes to experience a Q-wave MI during follow-up.

Overall, this protective effect of CABG for a patient with an MI explained only about 50% of the overall reduction in mortality attributable to the procedure. The remaining benefit of CABG among the patients with diabetes was demonstrated by a further reduction in mortality during follow-up, perhaps a result of the reduction in the degree of chronic ischaemia. This can probably be explained by the more extensive revascularisation provided by CABG, and the protection provided by these conduits with recurrent coronary events. The absence of this effect in non-diabetic patients may be explained in part by the greater potential of non-diabetic subjects for coronary collateral artery formation (Abaci $et\,al.$, 1999).

Other reasons why CABG might confer a survival benefit compared with PTCA in diabetic patients in BARI

The BARI investigators undertook a follow-up analysis of all patients undergoing either protocol-driven coronary angiography at years 1 and 5, or angiography performed because of recurrent ischaemia (within 30 months) (Kip $et\,al.$, 2002). The amount of ischemic myocardial territory was quantified by identifying terminal arteries with evidence of a stenoses $\geq 50\%$ of the reference diameter. Myocardial scores after surgery were calculated assuming complete revascularisation. Among PTCA patients, the mean percentage increase in total jeopardised myocardium was greater in diabetic patients than in non-diabetic patients. In contrast, among CABG patients, diabetes was not associated with percentage increase in jeopardised myocardium. On multivariate analyses, diabetes conferred a twofold risk of an increased percentage of jeopardised myocardium during follow-up for either the first protocol- or ischaemia-driven angiogram during the first 30 months. This result reflects the increased risk of restenosis and disease progression in PTCA-treated diabetic patients. This $post\ hoc$ analysis is subject to selection bias, as patients who died, and who probably had more severe CHD, were not included in this analysis and only a small proportion of CABG patients underwent repeat angiography. However, this phenomenon was evident in diabetic patients regardless of whether repeat angiography was performed for protocol- or ischaemia-driven reasons.

Summary of findings comparing CABG with PTCA in diabetic patients

Recurrent ischaemia leading to angina, repeat revascularisation and cardiac mortality is more common after PTCA than with CABG, because PTCA more commonly results in incomplete revascularisation and an appreciable risk of ischaemia. Incomplete revascularisation is an independent predictor of adverse outcome (Cowley *et al.*, 1993). Whilst several trials have found CABG to be superior to PTCA in diabetes (O'Keefe *et al.*, 1998; Weintraub *et al.*, 1998, 1999), whereas one other trial (Halon *et al.*, 2000) and the Duke University registry (Barsness *et al.*, 1997) did not. Overall, surgical revascularisation for multivessel CHD in diabetic patients, particularly in insulin-treated patients, is associated with a survival advantage compared with PTCA.

However, studies with long-term follow-up beyond 10 years have indicated that the survival benefits of surgery may be attenuated. van Domburg *et al.* (2002) reported on 1041 surgically treated patients (8% diabetes) and 704 (11%) medically treated patients who underwent first PTCA or CABG at the Thorax Centre in Rotterdam. During the first 10 years after revascularisation, survival and revascularisation rates in diabetic and non-diabetic patients who had multivessel disease were better in surgically treated patients, compared to those who underwent PTCA. On follow-up at 10–20 years, revascularisation rates in surgically treated patients were higher whereas survival was similar in both groups (Figure 3.2).

Thus, whilst restenosis rates and survival are poorer in diabetic patients undergoing PTCA compared to those undergoing surgery, this is not the case for non-diabetic patients with multivessel disease, and these differences appear to dissipate with follow- up in the longer term, most likely due to late graft failure.

3.6 Stents for Coronary Artery Disease in Diabetes

Adjunctive devices, such as stents, and novel antithrombotic therapies were generally not used in the clinical trials described above. Early cohort studies derived from a non-randomised setting demonstrated that restenosis rates at 6 months after single- vessel balloon angioplasty, as measured by quantitative coronary angiography, were twice as high in diabetic patients (63%) compared with non-diabetic patients due to higher rates of late lumen loss and late vessel occlusion, but no differences were observed in stented diabetic patients (25%), compared with stented non-diabetic patients (27%) (Van Belle *et al.*, 1997).

Stent usage is associated with reductions in the risk of acute complications, such as coronary artery dissection, and reduced restenosis in the longer term. Studies in the stenting era have clearly shown that diabetic patients have worse outcomes in the short and longer term compared with non-diabetic patients (Abizaid *et al.*, 1998; Elezi *et al.*, 1998; Cutlip *et al.*, 2002). In a reasonably large cohort of patients with

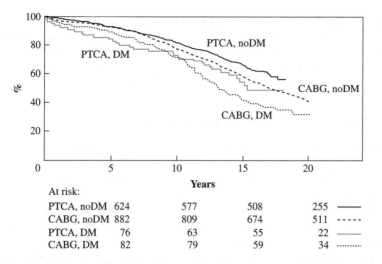

At risk:

PTCA, noDM	624	577	508	255 ——
CABG, noDM	882	809	674	511 - - - - -
PTCA, DM	76	63	55	22 ——
CABG, DM	82	79	59	34 ·········

Figure 3.2 Cumulative survival following coronary bypass surgery (CABG) and coronary angioplasty (PTCA) after initial CABG and PTCA, according to patients with diabetes (DM) and without diabetes (noDM). Reproduced from van Domburg RT, Foley DP, Breeman A, van Herwerden LA, Serruys PW (2002). Coronary artery bypass graft surgery and percutaneous transluminal coronary angioplasty. Twenty-year clinical outcome. *European Heart Journal* **23**: 543–9. Figure 4, p. 547. By permission of the European Society of Cardiology.

native coronary artery lesions treated with Palmatz-Schatz stent implantation using conventional methods, the in-hospital mortality was 2% in insulin-treated patients, which was higher than in non-insulin-treated patients (0%) and non-diabetic subjects (0.3%) (Abizaid *et al.*, 1998). Stent thrombosis did not differ among groups. During follow-up, target lesion revascularisation (TLR) was 28% in insulin-treated patients, which is significantly higher than in non-insulin-treated patients (18%) and non-diabetic subjects (16%). Late cardiac event-free survival (including death, MI and any coronary revascularisation procedure) was significantly lower in insulin-treated patients (60%) compared with non-insulin-treated patients (70%) and non-diabetic patients (76%). Insulin-treated diabetes was an independent predictor for cardiac events in general and TLR during long-term follow-up. Whilst clinical event rates were higher in insulin-treated patients, acute and long-term procedural outcome were found to be similar for non-insulin-treated patients compared with non-diabetic patients.

Clinical trials of stents versus CABG involving diabetic patients

Coronary Angioplasty versus Bypass Revascularisation Investigation (CABRI)

The Coronary Angioplasty versus Bypass Revascularisation Investigation (CABRI) was one of the largest trials of PTCA versus CABG and had follow-up over a 4-year period (Kurbaan *et al.*, 2001). Complete revascularisation was mandatory, and in the percutaneous group new devices such as atherectomy or stents were allowable at the operator's discretion. A total of 1054 subjects, of whom 125 (12%) had diabetes, were randomised to CABG or PTCA; 37% of the CABG group received an

IMA graft. Diabetic patients had a higher mortality rate than non-diabetic patients. Diabetic patients randomised to PTCA had a higher mortality rate than diabetic patients randomised to CABG (CABG vs. PTCA: 8/63(12%) vs. 14/62(23%)). Post-revascularisation angiographic evidence of residual CHD was consistently significantly greater in PTCA than in respective CABG subgroups.

Arterial Revascularisation Therapy Study (ARTS)

The Arterial Revascularisation Therapy Study (ARTS) trial randomised 1205 patients with multivessel coronary artery disease to stent implantation ($n = 600$; diabetic = 112(19%)) or CABG ($n = 605$; diabetic = 96(16%)) (Abizaid et al., 2001). At 1 year the event-free survival overall was 74% in the stented group and 88% in the surgical group, largely due to a higher rate of revascularisation in the stented group (17% vs. 4%). Interestingly, 40% of the major adverse events in the first 30 days after intervention were due to stent thrombosis. In the future, the incidence of this problem might be expected to fall with a greater use of new adjunctive therapies, such as clopidogrel and glycoprotein IIb/IIIa inhibitors, neither of which were used in this trial.

At 1 year, diabetic patients treated with stenting had the lowest event-free survival rate (63%) because of a higher incidence of repeat revascularisation (typically CABG) as compared with both diabetic patients treated with CABG (84%) and non-diabetic patients treated with stents (76%). This difference was largely due to a higher rate of incomplete revascularisation in patients who underwent PCI (70%), compared to those who had a CABG (84%). Conversely, diabetic and non-diabetic patients experienced similar 1-year event-free survival rates when treated with CABG (84% and 88%). Multivessel diabetic patients treated with stenting had a worse 1-year outcome than patients assigned to CABG or non-diabetics treated with stenting. Alternatively, diabetic patients had an increased risk of stroke with CABG versus PCI (4% vs. 0%).

Other studies

At least three additional trials have compared PCI with bare metal stents versus bypass surgery in patients with multivessel CHD (Rodriguez et al., 2001; Sedlis et al., 2002; Sigwart et al., 2002; Rodriguez et al., 2003). The SOS (Stent or Surgery) trial showed less repeat revascularisation with CABG than with PCI overall at 2 years, but the diabetic group was not analysed separately (Sigwart et al., 2002). The other trials showed mixed results.

Registry information for PCI with stenting in diabetic patients

Other data also suggest that outcomes after PCI can be similar to those after CABG in diabetic patients with multivessel CHD. In one registry of 9586 patients ($n = 1714$ (18%) diabetes), 970 patients had multivessel disease; CABG was performed in 318 (33%), PCI in 351 (36%) and 301 (31%) were treated medically (Kapur et al., 2003). In-hospital mortality was 3% in the CABG group and 2% in the PCI group, and 1-year mortality was 7% in the CABG group, 9% in the PCI group and 10% in the medical therapy group ($P = NS$). The rates of repeat revascularisation at 1 year were 2% in the CABG group and 23% in the PCI group ($P < 0.0001$). These non-randomised data suggest that survival after PCI in the stent-era is better than previously, but the rate of recurrent ischaemic and repeat revascularisation remains high, compared with CABG.

Predictors of restenosis after stenting in diabetic patients

Intravascular ultrasound studies have shown that restenosis in both stented and non-stented lesions is due to intimal hyperplasia (Kornowski *et al.*, 1997; Levine *et al.*, 1997; Van Belle *et al.*, 1997), which is a smooth-muscle-cell proliferative response. In one series of 241 patients ($n = 63$ with diabetes) who had 251 native lesions stented, follow-up angiography with intravascular ultrasound demonstrated the late lumen loss was more pronounced in both stented and non-stented lesions of diabetic patients (Kornowski *et al.*, 1997).

Results from registries and clinical trials indicate that diabetic patients have an increased risk of restenosis, repeat revascularisation and death after PCI (Rozenman *et al.*, 2000; Van Belle *et al.*, 2001). A useful retrospective study of clinical trial participants was performed at the Cardialysis Core Laboratory in Rotterdam (West *et al.*, 2004). Restenosis occurred in 550 of 2672 (21%) non-diabetic and 130 of 418 (31%) diabetic patients ($P < 0.001$). Reduced body mass index (BMI), larger reference diameter before stenting and longer stented length of vessel were multivariate predictors of restenosis.

In the ARTS trial, the incidence of death/stroke/MI at 3 years was similar in stented patients who, according to the BMI, were normal (BMI 18.5–24.9 kg/m²), overweight (BMI 25–30 kg/m²) or obese (BMI > 30 kg/m²; $n = 124$) at 30%, 37% and 32%, respectively (Gruberg *et al.*, 2005). The rates for these respective groups managed by surgical revascularisation were 24%, 16% and 11%. The rates of repeat revascularisation, although much higher in PCI-treated patients than CABG-treated patients, were unrelated to BMI. Thus, in this trial BMI was unrelated to outcome in both PCI- and CABG-treated patients.

3.7 Drug-eluting Stents

Drug-eluting stents (DES) are a recent development in interventional cardiology, and are currently the subject of intense investigation. These are standard stents such as the Bx Velocity (Cordis Corporation) or Express Stent, which have been treated with a polymer-containing antiproliferative compound (by inhibition of the cell cycle / replication), thereby attenuating restenosis. The polymer-mediated slow release of antiproliferative agents that elute from stents at the site of arterial injury attenuates neointima formation and reduces the risk of restenosis and revascularisation. Recently, attention has focused on the potential for DES thrombosis.

SIRIUS was a double-blind randomised trial of 1058 patients undergoing clinically indicated percutaneous coronary intervention who were randomly assigned to sirolimus-eluting stent ($n = 533$) or control bare stent ($n = 525$) (Moses *et al.*, 2003). Repeat angiography was planned for 6 months, with baseline and follow-up angiograms analysed by a core laboratory in Boston. Both stent groups were well matched in terms of clinical and angiographic profiles and 26.4% were diabetic. Procedural success and in-hospital outcomes did not differ between the two groups. At 9 months, clinical restenosis, defined as target lesion revascularisation, was 4% in the sirolimus limb versus 17% in the control limb. At 12 months, the absolute difference in target lesion revascularisation continued to increase and was 5% versus 20%. There were no differences in death or MI rates. In high-risk patient subsets, defined by vessel size, lesion length and presence of diabetes mellitus, there was a 70–80% reduction in clinical restenosis (i.e. TLR) at 1 year. Diabetes (odds ratio 1.677; $P = 0.0152$) was second only to previous CABG (1.972; $P = 0.0219$) as a predictor of restenosis. Diabetic patients with a reference vessel diameter of < 2.5 mm and a lesion length of > 15 mm had the highest risk of clinical restenosis by 1 year, although in these patients DES therapy reduced this risk by 71%. Compared with the control intervention, treatment with this DES resulted in 180 events being prevented for 1000 patients treated, compared with 138 events being prevented in non-diabetics.

These data are consistent with results from other clinical trials with a sirolimus-eluting stent (Abizaid et al., 2004; Fajadet et al., 2005) and diabetes is therefore a risk factor for restenosis with DES (Scheen and Warzee, 2004). Compared with the other trials patients in SIRIUS were older and a higher proportion had diabetes, or had undergone previous intervention. These patients also more often had multivessel coronary disease. Thus, the patients randomised in SIRIUS were somewhat more representative of the type of patient usually encountered in clinical practice.

The clinical development of DES has been associated with a number of problems, including initial limited availability of stents with diameter > 3 mm. Late stent thrombosis (> 12 months' postimplantation) is a complication increasingly associated with use of DES. Diabetes is a predictor of stent thrombosis and this presents a dilemma for interventional cardiologists who must evaluate both the risk of restenosis against the risk of stent thrombosis on an individual basis. In general terms, DES remains the best treatment for diabetic patients undergoing PCI.

Angiographic follow-up of patients who received a sirolimus DES for a target lesion stenosis $< 50\%$ was associated with survival free of major cardiovascular events of 95%, with no target lesion revascularisation (Hoye et al., 2004). These data raise the question of whether the grounds for stenting could be expanded. Thus, patients who have angiographic evidence of CHD may undergo stenting with a DES not just for flow-limiting disease, but also where this is evidence of a 'vulnerable plaque'. This strategy is presently undergoing assessment in the ongoing PROSPECT trial.

Clinical data with a DES, which elutes paclitaxel, are also encouraging. The TAXUS IV study investigated whether the paclitaxel-eluting Express stent (Boston Scientific Corp.) would be associated with lower rates of restenosis, target vessel revascularisation and major adverse cardiac events (MACE) than treatment with the bare-metal (control) Express stent (Stone et al., 2004). A total of 1314 patients were enrolled in 73 US centres. Randomisation of patients in TAXUS IV was stratified by the presence of treated diabetes and vessel size < 3.0 mm or ≥ 3.0 mm. Procedural therapy also included standardisation of techniques, including a mandatory predilatation and an appropriately sized single stent deployed at 12 atmospheres or more. Stent postdilatation was at the operator's discretion, and additional stents were allowable for edge dissections (Type B) or otherwise suboptimal results. Clinical follow-up was at 1, 4, 9 and 12 months, and yearly thereafter till 5 years. Follow-up angiography was prespecified in a subset of 732 patients. A total of 662 patients were randomised to a TAXUS stent and 663 to a bare-metal control Express stent and follow-up was available in 639 and 633 patients, respectively. Treated diabetic patients represented 23% (8% insulin-treated) in the DES group and 25% (8% insulin-treated) in the control group. Cardiac death occurred in 1.4% of paclitaxel-treated patients and 1.3% of bare-metal-stented patients ($P = 0.83$). The MACE was 11% in paclitaxel-treated patients and 20% in the control group ($P < 0.001$); this was driven by a reduction in target vessel revascularisation (10% vs. 19%).

A few more recent trials have compared the effects of sirolimus- and paclitaxel-eluting stents. In the SIRTAX trial the major adverse cardiac event rate was less with sirolimus-eluting stents compared with paclitaxel-eluting stents, and this difference was more pronounced in diabetic patients (Windecker et al., 2005). In the ISAR diabetes trial PCI with sirolimus-eluting stents resulted in less in-segment restenosis in insulin-treated and non-insulin-treated diabetic patients (Dibra et al., 2005).

Contemporary trials of percutaneous versus surgical revascularisation

CARDIA (Kapur et al., 2005) is a prospective, multicentre, randomised controlled trial of PCI versus surgery in diabetic patients with prognostically significant CHD, in whom, in the opinion of the operator, either strategy could be performed from a technical point of view.

BARI 2D (Sobel et al., 2003) is a 2×2 factorial industry-sponsored trial, which will result in 50% of patients randomised to medical therapy or revascularisation, and within each of these two groups an additional randomisation will take place to insulin-administered or insulin-sensitising agents, in an anticipated sample size of 2800 patients and a 5-year follow-up period. Enrolment criteria will include diabetes, documented ischaemia on stress testing and at least one obstructive ($> 50\%$) narrowing of a major epicardial coronary artery on angiography. Its first hypothesis is that revascularisation (according to conventional practices based on data from the BARI registry) performed 'early' in diabetic patients with asymptomatic ischaemia (as determined by non-invasive stress testing) or mild angina may be associated with superior outcomes compared with medical therapy. One other comparison will be of intensive pharmacological therapy alone or in combination with revascularisation, the type being directed by the physician. BARI 2D will also compare outcomes of patients treated with insulin versus those treated with insulin-sensitising agents. In this case, the target HbA1c is $\leq 7.0\%$.

FREEDOM is a superiority trial that will compare a multivessel stenting strategy using sirolimus-eluting stents with CABG. Diabetic patients should have multivessel coronary artery disease (CAD) (two or more stenotic lesions in at least two major epicardial coronary arteries), amenable to either PCI with DES (at the discretion of the operator) or surgical revascularisation. The projected sample size is 2400. The follow-up period is 5 years and the primary endpoint is all-cause mortality, non-fatal MI and stroke. This trial should provide important information for the future management of diabetic patients with obstructive CAD.

3.8   Drug Therapy and PCI in Diabetic Patients

Aspirin

Aspirin reduces the risk of acute closure in PCI by approximately 50% and the magnitude of this benefit appears similar in diabetic and non-diabetic patients.

Clopidogrel

PCI-CURE

The efficacy of clopidogrel for the prevention of cardiovascular death, MI or stroke, in the setting of acute coronary syndromes, was tested in the Clopidogrel in Unstable Angina to Prevent Recurrent Events (CURE) study, and is described in Chapter 4, p. 70 (Yusuf *et al.*, 2001). PCI-CURE was a prespecified substudy of the CURE study, and included 1315 patients (diabetes $n = 249$ (19%)) in the clopidogrel group and 1345 patients (diabetes $n = 255$ (19%)) in the placebo group, who underwent PCI (Mehta *et al.*, 2001). Following PCI, patients were treated with open-label thienopyridine (clopidogrel or ticlopidine) for 1 month, and then resorted to their original study drug (placebo or clopidogrel) for an average of 8 months. The primary endpoint (death/non-fatal MI/target vessel revascularisation within 30 days of PCI) occurred in 59 (4%) patients in the clopidogrel-treated group and 86 (6%) of the placebo-treated group ($P = 0.03$). Of the 504 diabetic patients, 32 (13%) of clopidogrel-treated patients and 42(16%) of placebo-treated patients experienced cardiovascular death or MI during follow-up (hazard ratio 0.77, 95% CI 0.48–1.22), whereas in non-diabetic patients a benefit in favour of clopidogrel was apparent (hazard ratio 0.66, 95% CI 0.50–0.87). The lack of apparent effect in the diabetic subgroup may be due to small numbers, although there is increasing evidence that people with diabetes might be resistant to the antiplatelet effects of aspirin and clopidogrel in currently used doses.

CREDO

The Clopidogrel for Reduction of Events During Observation (CREDO) trial compared short-term (1 month) versus longer term (1 year) maintenance therapy after coronary stenting (Steinhubl *et al.*, 2002). In this trial, 2116 patients were randomised to receive 300 mg of clopidogrel ($n = 1053$; diabetes $n = 290$ (27.5%)) or placebo ($n = 1063$; diabetes $n = 270$ (25.4%)) prior to PCI. After the PCI, all patients received 75 mg per day of clopidogrel to day 28. After that, patients in the loading dose group continued to receive 75 mg of clopidogrel daily till 1 year, whereas the other group received placebo. All patients received aspirin. Clopidogrel therapy was associated with an absolute risk reduction of 3% and a significant relative risk reduction of 27% in the combined risk of death, MI or stroke. Pretreatment with clopidogrel at least 6 h (but not 3 h) before the PCI resulted in a 39% relative risk reduction for death/MI/TLR. Major bleeding with clopidogrel tended to be more common (9% vs. 7%), but minor bleeding was similar in both groups.

CURE, PCI-CURE and CREDO raise a number of important issues, all of which are relevant to diabetic acute coronary patients. The population of patients in this study programme was highly selected. For example, patients with a predisposition to bleeding were excluded, leading to bias and a minimisation of the pro-bleeding effects of clopidogrel. Also, these results relate only to high-risk acute coronary patients presenting with ECG changes or significant changes in plasma biomarker concentrations. Thus, the effects of clopidogrel in acute coronary patients without these features are uncertain. Furthermore, the benefits of clopidogrel in the longer term (beyond 9 months after starting treatment) are uncertain.

Glycoprotein IIb/IIIa inhibitor therapy and PCI in diabetic patients

Abciximab, tirofiban and eptifibitide are platelet glycoprotein (Gp) IIb/IIIa integrin receptor blockers that prevent fibrinogen molecules binding to platelets, thus inhibiting thrombus formation. Abciximab is a Fab fragment of a monoclonal antibody, whereas tirofiban and eptifibitide are 'small molecule', synthetic, high-affinity inhibitors of this receptor that have a shorter half-life (< 2 h) and are suitable for intravenous administration. Abciximab reduces restenosis through non-platelet effects, which are anti-inflammatory and antiproliferative.

The Evaluation of Platelet IIb/IIIa Inhibition in Stenting (EPISTENT) trial was designed to assess the role of platelet GpIIb/IIIa blockade for use in elective stenting (Marso *et al.*, 1999). A total of 2399 patients with ischaemic heart disease and suitable coronary artery lesions were randomly assigned to stenting plus placebo ($n = 809$; 173 diabetes (21%)), stenting plus abciximab ($n = 794$; 162 diabetes (20%)), or balloon angioplasty plus abciximab ($n = 796$; 156 diabetes (20%)). The primary endpoint was a combination of death, MI or need for urgent revascularisation in the first 30 days, and this occurred in 87 (11%) of patients in the stent plus placebo group, 42 (5%) in the stent plus abciximab group and 55 (7%) in the balloon plus abciximab group. In diabetic patients, the primary endpoint occurred in 12% of patients who received stent plus placebo compared with 6% in diabetics who received stent + GpIIb/IIIa inhibitor therapy ($P = 0.04$). These results indicated that platelet GpIIb/IIIa blockade with abciximab can improve early outcomes after coronary stenting in people with diabetes (Marso *et al.*, 1999).

The Enhanced Suppression of the Platelet IIb/IIIa Receptor with Integrilin Therapy (ESPRIT) trial was designed to test the efficacy and safety of a high-dose regimen of eptifibitide as an adjunct to elective coronary stenting (Tcheng *et al.*, 2000). This more recent trial was undertaken at a time of contemporary stenting techniques. The primary endpoint was the composite of death, non-fatal MI, urgent target vessel revascularisation and bailout with GpIIb/IIIa inhibitor therapy at 48 h. A total of 2064 patients were randomised to eptifibitide ($n = 1064$; 208(20%) diabetes) or placebo ($n = 1024$; 211(21%) diabetes). This trial was stopped early on the recommendation of the data and safety monitoring board because an interim analysis showed a 43% relative risk reduction associated with eptifibitide therapy compared with placebo-treated patients. This event rate was driven by a reduction in MI associated with GpIIb/IIIa therapy. The primary endpoint in diabetic patients was 4% in the eptifibitide group, compared with 7% in the placebo group ($P = 0.2$), which translated into a relative risk of 0.58 (95% CI 0.25–1.35). A subsequent meta-analysis including data from EPISTENT and ESPRIT demonstrated a survival advantage conferred by abciximab in people with diabetes (Bhatt *et al.*, 2000).

The Do Tirofiban and ReoPro Give Similar Efficacy Trial (TARGET) compared the effectiveness of tirofiban and abciximab in 5308 patients undergoing PCI with the intention to perform coronary stenting (Topol *et al.*, 2001). Patients were stratified according to diabetic status at enrolment. Compared with non-diabetic patients, patients with diabetes ($n = 1117$) showed similar 30-day ischaemic outcomes, an increased incidence of any target vessel revascularisation at 6 months (10% versus 8%; $P = 0.008$) and a trend toward higher 1-year mortality (2.5% versus 1.6%; $P = 0.056$). The primary endpoint was a composite of death, non-fatal MI and urgent target vessel revascularisation at 30 days, which occurred less frequently in the abciximab group (6%) compared with the tirofiban group (8%; $P = 0.038$). At 6 months and 1 year, however, there were no differences between the two diabetic groups in terms of ischaemic outcomes or death (Roffi *et al.*, 2002)

Most of the GpIIb/IIIa inhibitor trials excluded thienopyridine use. These limitations have resulted in questions about the effectiveness of GpIIb/IIIa receptor inhibition in clopidogrel-treated patients. The Intracoronary Stenting and Antithrombotic Regimen – Rapid Early Action for Coronary Treatment (ISAR-REACT) addressed this question (Kastrati *et al.*, 2004). A total of 2159 patients who were planned to undergo elective PCI were pretreated with 600 mg of clopidogrel at least 2 h before the procedure, followed by 75 mg of clopidogrel for at least 1 month and subsequently randomised to treatment with either abciximab or placebo. Insulin-requiring diabetic patients and those with unstable symptoms or a bleeding diathesis were not included in this study; 221/1079 (21%) subjects randomised to abciximab and 214/1080(20%) subjects randomised to placebo had diabetes. There was no difference in survival or recurrent ischaemia in either treatment group, either for the population as a whole or in the diabetic subgroup.

More recently, the Is Abciximab a Superior Way to Eliminate Elevated Thrombotic Risk in Diabetics (ISAR-SWEET) enrolled 701 diabetic patients (351 abciximab and 350 patients to placebo) who underwent elective PCI and were administered 600 mg of clopidogrel at least 2 h before the procedure (Mehilli *et al.*, 2004). Of these patients, approximately 29% were insulin-treated, 51% were on oral hypoglycaemic drugs only and 20% were on no diabetic therapy at all (with equal proportions in each group). The primary endpoint of this trial (death or MI at 1 year) occurred with similar frequency in both groups, whereas the angiographic restenosis occurred in 101(29%) patients in the abciximab group and in 137(38%) patients in the placebo group ($P = 0.01$). The incidence of target lesion revascularisation was 23% in the abciximab group and 30% in the placebo group. In lesions treated with drug-eluting stents the incidence of angiographic restenosis was 7% in the abciximab group and 5% in the placebo group. Thus, although the addition of abciximab does not affect the risk of death or MI, there is a beneficial effect on the risk of restenosis and recurrent angina. The attenuation by clopidogrel pretreatment of some of the effect of abciximab on clinical events is likely to be due to the antiplatelet and anti-inflammatory effects of clopidogrel. Contemporary PCI guidelines recommend GpIIb/IIIa inhibitors in patients with unstable CHD and in elective PCI patients with risk factors such as diabetes.

Impact of anti-diabetic therapies on coronary intervention

Thiazolidinediones improve insulin sensitivity, particularly in skeletal muscle, the liver and adipocytes (see Chapter 11). In a randomised study of troglitazone in consecutive diabetic patients undergoing elective PCI, 55 patients with 60 lesions were randomised to troglitazone ($n = 30$ stents) or control (conventional therapy, $n = 26$) (Takagi *et al.*, 2002). Treatment with troglitazone reduced angiographic in-stent restenosis and target lesion revascularisation rates after coronary stent implementation, and serial intravascular ultrasound assessment demonstrated a reduction in neointimal tissue proliferation in the troglitazone group.

A case–control study involving 83 patients with type 2 diabetes randomised patients to either rosiglitazone (8 mg daily pre-PCI and 4 mg daily thereafter) or placebo. Angiographic follow-up was performed at 6 months. The restenosis rates were 18% in the rosiglitazone group and 38% in the control group ($P = 0.002$). The minimum lumen stent diameter was 2.49 (0.88) mm compared with 1.91(0.05) mm in the control group ($P = 0.0009$), and target lesion revascularisation rates were lower in the rosiglitazone group (10%) compared with the control group (20%; $P = 0.244$) (Choi *et al.*, 2004).

A smaller study of 54 patients who were randomised to pioglitazone or placebo has shown similar results, with less late luminal loss and in-stent restenosis in the pioglitazone group (Nishio *et al.*, 2006). Leptin concentrations independently correlated with the late luminal loss on multiple regression analysis.

Longer term studies on the effects of glitazones on other cardiovascular outcomes following PCI in patients with diabetes areclearly required.

3.9 Conclusions

Early clinical trials demonstrated surgical revascularisation to be superior to medical therapy in patients with angina and prognostically significant CHD. Subsequent trials demonstrated PTCA to have similar effects on survival compared with medical therapy, but CABG conferred a survival advantage for patients with multivessel CHD, particularly in those with diabetes. Revascularisation rates were consistently greater after PTCA than after CABG. Stenting reduced the need for revascularisation, compared with PTCA, but had no effect on survival or recurrent MI. Recent developments in percutaneous revascularisation, particularly with regard to adjunctive antithrombotic therapies and drug-eluting stents, raise the possibility that the effects of multivessel stenting on survival, and possibly revascularisation in the long term, may be non-inferior to surgical revascularisation.

References

Abaci A, Oguzhan A, Kahraman S, Eryol NK, Unal S, Arinc H, Ergin A (1999). Effect of diabetes mellitus on formation of coronary collateral vessels. *Circulation* **99**: 2239–42.

Abizaid A, Kornowski R, Mintz GS, Hong MK, Abizaid AS, Mehran R *et al.* (1998). The influence of diabetes mellitus on acute and late clinical outcomes following coronary stent implantation. *Journal of the American College of Cardiology* **32**: 584–9.

Abizaid A, Costa MA, Centemero M, Abizaid AS, Legrand VMG, Limet RV *et al.* (2001). Clinical and economic impact of diabetes mellitus on percutaneous and surgical treatment of multivessel coronary disease patients: insights from the Arterial Revascularization Therapy Study (ARTS) trial. *Circulation* **104**: 533–8.

Abizaid A, Costa MA, Blanchard D, Albertal M, Eltchaninoff H, Guagliumi G *et al.* (2004). Sirolimus-eluting stents inhibit neointimal hyperplasia in diabetic patients. Insights from the RAVEL Trial. *European Heart Journal* **25**: 107–12.

Albers AR, Krichavsky MZ, Balady GJ (2006). Stress testing in patients with diabetes mellitus diagnostic and prognostic value. Circulation 113: 583–92.

Alderman EL, Bourassa MG, Cohen LS, Davis KB, Kaiser GG, Killip T *et al.* (1990). Ten-year follow-up of survival and myocardial-infarction in the randomized Coronary-Artery Surgery Study. *Circulation* **82**: 1629–46.

Alderman EL, Andrews K, Bost J, Bourassa M, Chaitman BR, Detre K *et al.* (1996). Comparison of coronary bypass surgery with angioplasty in patients with multivessel disease. *New England Journal of Medicine* **335**: 217–25.

Alderman EL, Andrews K, Brooks MM, Detre K, Kelsey SF, Rosen AD *et al.* (1997a). Five-year clinical and functional outcome comparing bypass surgery and angioplasty in patients with multivessel coronary disease. A multicenter randomized trial. *Journal of the American Medical Association* **277**: 715–21.

Alderman E, Bourassa M, Brooks MM, Califf R, Chaitman B, Detre K *et al.* (1997b). Influence of diabetes on 5-year mortality and morbidity in a randomized trial comparing CABG and PTCA in patients with multivessel disease: the Bypass Angioplasty Revascularization Investigation (BARI). *Circulation* **96**: 1761–9.

Alderman EL, Brooks MM, Bourassa M, Califf RM, Chaitman BR, Detre K *et al.* (2000). Seven-year outcome in the Bypass Angioplasty Revascularization Investigation (BARI) by treatment and diabetic status. *Journal of the American College of Cardiology* **35**: 1122–9.

Antiplatelet Trialists' Collaboration (1994). Collaborative overview of randomised trials of antiplatelet therapy – I: Prevention of death, myocardial infarction, and stroke by prolonged antiplatelet therapy in various categories of patients. *British Medical Journal* **308**: 81–106

Antithrombotic Trialists' Collaboration (2002). Collaborative meta-analysis of randomised trials of antiplatelet therapy for prevention of death, myocardial infarction and stroke in high risk patients. *British Medical Journal* **324**: 71–86.

Arad Y, Newstein D, Cadet F, Roth M, Guerci AD (2001). Association of multiple risk factors and insulin resistance with increased prevalence of asymptomatic coronary artery disease by an electron-beam computed tomographic study. *Arteriosclerosis Thrombosis and Vascular Biology* **21**: 2051–8.

Aronson D, Bloomgarden Z, Rayfield EJ (1996). Potential mechanisms promoting restenosis in diabetic patients. *Journal of the American College of Cardiology* **27**: 528–35.

Barsness GW, Peterson ED, Ohman EM, Nelson CL, DeLong ER, Reves JG *et al.* (1997). Relationship between diabetes mellitus and long-term survival after coronary bypass and angioplasty. *Circulation* **96**: 2551–6.

Berger PB, Velianou JL, Aslanidou Vlachos H, Feit F, Jacobs AK, Faxon DP *et al.* (2001). Survival following coronary angioplasty versus coronary artery bypass surgery in anatomic subsets in which coronary artery bypass surgery improves survival compared with medical therapy. Results from the Bypass Angioplasty Revascularization Investigation (BARI). *Journal of the American College of Cardiology* **38**: 1440–9.

Bhatt DL, Marso SP, Lincoff AM, Wolski KE, Ellis SG, Topol EJ (2000). Abciximab reduces mortality in diabetics following percutaneous coronary intervention. *Journal of the American College of Cardiology* **35**: 922–8.

Bhatt DL, Marso SP Hirsch AT Ringleb PA Hacke W Topol EJ (2002). Amplified benefit of clopidogrel versus aspirin in patients with diabetes mellitus. *American Journal of Cardiology* **90**: 625–8.

Bhatt DL, Fox KA, Hacke W, Berger PB, Black HR, Boden WE *et al.* (2006). Clopidogrel and aspirin versus aspirin alone for the prevention of atherothrombotic events. *New England Journal of Medicine* **354**: 1706–17.

Brooks MM, Jones RH, Bach RG, Chaitman BR, Kern MJ, Orszulak TA *et al.* (2000). Predictors of mortality and mortality from cardiac causes in the bypass angioplasty revascularization investigation (BARI) randomized trial and registry. *Circulation* **101**: 2682–9.

Burke AP, Kolodgie FD, Zieske A, Fowler DR, Weber DK, Varghese PJ *et al.* (2004). Morpholgical findings of coronary atherosclerotic plaques in diabetics: a postmortem study. *Arteriosclerosis Thrombosis and Vascular Biology* **24**: 1266–71.

Cariou B, Bonnevie L, Mayaudon H, Dupuy O, Ceccaldi B, Bauduceau B (2000). Angiographic characteristics of coronary artery disease in diabetic patients compared with matched non-diabetic subjects. *Diabetes Nutrition and Metabolism* **13**: 134–41.

Choi D, Kim S-K, Choi s-H, Ko y-G, Ahn C-W, Jang Y *et al.* (2004). Preventative effects of rosiglitazone on restenosis after coronary stent implantation in patients with type 2 diabetes. *Diabetes Care* **27**: 2654–60.

Cowley MJ, Vandermael M, Topol EJ, Whitlow PL, Dean LS, Bulle TM, Ellis SG (1993). Is traditionally defined complete revascularization needed for patients with multivessel disease treated by elective coronary angioplasty. Multiplevessel Angioplasty Prognosis Study (MAPS). *Journal of the American College of Cardiology* **22**: 1289–97.

Cutlip DE, Chauhan MS, Baim DS, Ho KKL, Popma JJ, Carrozza JP *et al.* (2002). Clinical restenosis after coronary stenting: perspectives from multicenter clinical trials. *Journal of the American College of Cardiology* **40**: 2082–9.

Daly CA, Fox KM, Remme WJ, Bertrand ME, Ferrari R, Simmoons ML; EUROPA Investigators (2005). The effect of perindopril on cardiovascular morbidity and mortality in patients with diabetes in the EUROPA study: results from the PERSUADE substudy. *European Heart Journal* **26**: 1369–78.

Detre KM, Guo P, Holubkov R, Califf RM, Sopko G, Bach R *et al.* (1999). Coronary revascularization in diabetic patients: a comparison of the randomized and observational components of the Bypass Angioplasty Revascularization Investigation (BARI). Circulation **99**: 633–40.

Detre KM, Lombardero MS, Brooks MM, Hardison RM, Holubkov R, Sopko G *et al.* (2000). The effect of previous coronary-artery bypass surgery on the prognosis of patients with diabetes who have acute myocardial infarction. *New England Journal of Medicine* **342**: 989–97.

Dibra A, Kastrati A, Mehilli J, Pache J, Schulen H, von Beckerath N *et al.* (2005). Paclitaxel-eluting or sirolimus-eluting stents to prevent restenosis in diabetic patients. *New England Journal of Medicine* **353**: 663–70.

Dortimer AC, Shenoy PN, Shiroff RA, Leaman DM, Babb JD, Liedtke AJ, Zelis R (1978). Diffuse coronary artery disease in diabetic patients: fact or fiction? *Circulation* **57**: 133–6.

Elezi S, Kastrati A, Pache J, Wehinger A, Hadamitzky M, Dirschinger J *et al.* (1998). Diabetes mellitus and the clinical and angiographic outcome after coronary stent placement. *Journal of the American College of Cardiology* **32**: 1866–73.

ETDRS Investigators (1992). Aspirin effects on mortality and morbidity in patients with diabetes mellitus. Early Treatment Diabetic Retinopathy Study report 14. *Journal of the American Medical Association* **268**: 1292–300.

European Coronary Surgery Study Group (1982). Long-term results of prospective randomised study of coronary artery bypass surgery in stable angina pectoris. *Lancet* **ii**: 1173–80.

Fajadet J, Morice MC, Bode C, Barragan P, Serruys PW, Wijns W *et al.* (2005). Maintenance of long-term clinical benefit with sirolimus-eluting coronary stents: three-year results of the RAVEL trial. *Circulation* **111**: 1040–4.

Findlay I (2003). Silent myocardial ischaemia in people with diabetes. In: Fisher M (ed.) *Heart Disease and Diabetes*. London: Martin Dunitz, pp. 65–92.

Gibbons RJ, Balady GJ, Beasley JW, Bricker JT, Duvernoy WFC, Froelicher VF *et al.* (1997). ACC/AHA guidelines for exercise testing. A report of the American College of Cardiology American Heart Association task force on practice guidelines (Committee on Exercise Testing). *Journal of the American College of Cardiology* **30**: 260–311.

Giri S, Shaw LJ, Murthy DR, Travin MI, Miller DD, Hachamovitch R *et al.* (2002). Impact of diabetes on the risk stratification using stress single-photon emission computed tomography myocardial perfusion imaging in patients with symptoms suggestive of coronary artery disease. *Circulation* **105**: 32–40.

Gruberg L, Mercado N, Milo S, Boersma E, Disco C, van Es GA *et al.* (2005). Impact of body mass index on the outcome of patients with multivessel disease randomized to either coronary artery bypass grafting or stenting in the ARTS trial: the obesity paradox II? *American Journal of Cardiology* **95**: 439–44.

Halon DA, Flugelman MY, Merdler A, Rennert HS, Weisz G, Shahla J, Lewis BS (2000). Similar late revascularization rates 10 to 12 years after angioplasty or bypass surgery for multivessel coronary artery disease: a report from the Lady Davis Carmel Medical Center (LDCMC) Registry. *American Journal of Cardiology* **86**: 1131–4.

Hamm CW, Reimers B, Ischinger T, Rupprecht HJ, Berger J, Bleifeld W (1994). A randomized study of coronary angioplasty compared with bypass surgery in patients with symptomatic multivessel coronary disease. German Angioplasty Bypass Investigation (GABI). *New England Journal of Medicine* **331**: 1037–43.

Hampton JR, Henderson RA, Julian DG, Parker J, Pocock SJ, Sowton E, *et al.* (1993). Coronary angioplasty versus coronary artery bypass surgery: the Randomized Intervention Treatment of Angina (RITA) trial. *Lancet* **341**: 573–80.

Hansson L, Zanchetti A, Carruthers SG, Dahlof B, Elmfeldt D, Julius S *et al.* (1998). Effects of intensive blood-pressure lowering and low-dose aspirin in patients with hypertension: principal results of the Hypertension Optimal Treatment (HOT) randomised trial. HOT Study Group. *Lancet* **351**: 1755–62.

Heart Outcomes Prevention Evaluation (HOPE) Study Investigators (2000). Effect of ramipril on cardiovascular and microvascular outcomes in people with diabetes mellitus: results of the HOPE study and MICRO-HOPE substudy. *Lancet* **355**: 253–9.

Henderson RA, Pocock SJ, Sharp SJ, Nanchahal K, Sculpher MJ, Buxton MJ, Hampton JR (1998). Long-term results of RITA-1 trial: clinical and cost comparisons of coronary angioplasty and coronary-artery bypass grafting. *Lancet* **352**: 1419–25.

Higgins TL, Estafanous FG, Loop FD, Beck J Blum JM, Paranandi L (1992). Stratification of morbidity and mortality outcome by preoperative risk-factors in coronary-artery bypass patients. A clinical severity score. *Journal of the American Medical Association* **267**: 2344–8.

Holmes DR, Davis KB, Mock MB, Fisher LD, Gersh BJ, Killip T, Pettinger M (1986). The effect of medical and surgical treatment on subsequent sudden cardiac death in patients with coronary-artery disease: a report from the Coronary-Artery Surgery Study. *Circulation* **73**: 1254–63.

Hoye A, Lemos PA, Arampatzis CA, Saia F, Tanabe K, Degertekin M, *et al.* (2004). Effectiveness of sirolimus-eluting stent implantation for coronary narrowings < 50% in diameter. *American Journal of Cardiology* **94**: 112–4.

IONA Study Group (2002). Effect of nicorandil on coronary events in patients with stable angina: the Impact Of Nicorandil in Angina (IONA) randomised trial. *Lancet* **359**: 1269–75.

IONA Study Group (2004). Impact of nicorandil in angina: subgroup analyses. *Heart* **90**: 1427–30.

Jonas M, Reicher-Reiss H, Boyko V, Shotan A, Mandelzweig L, Goldbourt U, Behar S (1996). Usefulness of beta-blocker therapy in patients with non-insulin-dependent diabetes mellitus and coronary artery disease. Bezafibrate Infarction Prevention (BIP) Study Group. *American Journal of Cardiology* **77**: 1273–7.

Kapur A, Bartolini D, Mostafavi E, Rickard MC, Hall RJ, Beatt KJ (2003). Percutaneous coronary intervention versus coronary bypass surgery in diabetes – 1 year follow-up results from a prospective registry 1998–2001. *European Heart Journal* **24**: 474.

Kapur A, Malik IS, Bagger JP, Anderson JR, Kooner JS, Thonas M *et al.* (2005). The Coronary Arterry Revascularisation in Diabetes (CARDia) trial: background, aims, and design. *American Heart Journal* **149**: 13–9.

Kastrati A, Mehilli J, Schuhlen H, Dirschinger J, Dotzer F, ten Berg JM *et al.* (2004). A clinical trial of abciximab in elective percutaneous coronary intervention after pretreatment with clopidogrel. *New England Journal of Medicine* **350**: 232–8.

Kelsey SF (1999). Patients with diabetes did better with coronary bypass graft surgery than with percutaneous transluminal coronary angioplasty: Was this BARI finding real? *American Heart Journal* **138**: S387–93.

King SB, Lembo NJ, Weintraub WS, Kosinski AS, Barnhart HX, Kutner NH *et al.* (1994). A randomized trial comparing coronary angioplasty with coronary bypass surgery. *New England Journal of Medicine* **331**: 1044–50.

King SB, Kosinski AS, Guyton RA, Lembo NJ, Weintraub WS (2000). Eight-year mortality in the Emory Angioplasty versus Surgery Trial (EAST). *Journal of the American College of Cardiology* **35**: 1116–21.

Kip KE, Faxon DP, Detre KM, Yeh WL, Kelsey SF, Currier JW (1996). Coronary angioplasty in diabetic patients. The National Heart, Lung, and Blood Institute Percutaneous Transluminal Corollary Angioplasty Registry. *Circulation* **94**: 1818–25.

Kip KE, Alderman EL, Bourassa MG, Brooks MM, Schwartz L, Holmes DR *et al.* (2002). Differential influence of diabetes mellitus on increased jeopardized myocardium after initial angioplasty or bypass surgery: Bypass angioplasty revascularization investigation. *Circulation* **105**: 1914–20.

Kornowski R, Mintz GS, Kent KM, Pichard AD, Satler LF, Bucher TA, *et al.* (1997). Increased restenosis in diabetes mellitus after coronary interventions is due to exaggerated intimal hyperplasia. A serial intravascular ultrasound study. *Circulation* **95**: 1366–9.

Kurbaan AS, Bowker TJ, Ilsley CD, Sigwart U, Rickards AF (2001). Difference in the mortality of the CABRI diabetic and nondiabetic populations and its relation to coronary artery disease and the revascularization mode. *American Journal of Cardiology* **87**: 947–50.

Kyriakides ZS, Psychari S, Chrysomallis N, Georgiadis M, Sbarouni E, Kremastinos DT (2002). Type II diabetes does not prevent the recruitment of collateral vessels and the normal reduction of myocardial ischaemia on repeated balloon inflations during angioplasty. *Heart* **87**: 61–6.

Lazar HL, Chipkin SR, Fitzgerald CA, Bao Y, Cabral H, Apstein CS (2004). Tight Glycaemic control in diabetic coronary artery bypass graft patients improves perioperative outcomes and decreases recurrent ischaemic events. *Circulation* **109**: 1497–502.

Levine GN, Jacobs AK, Keeler GP, Whitlow PL, Berdan LG, Leya F, *et al.* (1997). Impact of diabetes mellitus on percutaneous revascularization (CAVEAT-I). *American Journal of Cardiology* **79**: 748–55.

Loop FD, Lytle BW, Cosgrove DM, Stewart RW, Goormastic M, Williams GW *et al.* (1986). Influence of the internal-mammary-artery graft on 10-year survival and other cardiac events. *New England Journal of Medicine* **314**: 1–6.

Lotan C, Lokovitsky L, Gilon D, Manor O, Gotsman MS (1994). Silent myocardial ischemia during exercise testing: does it indicate a different angiographic and prognostic syndrome? *Cardiology* **85**: 407–14.

Mangano CM, Diamondstone LS, Ramsay JG, Aggarwal A, Herskowitz A, Mangano DT (1998). Renal dysfunction after myocardial revascularization: risk factors, adverse outcomes, and hospital resource utilization. *Annals of Internal Medicine* **128**: 194–203.

Mann JM, Davies MJ (1996). Vulnerable plaque. Relation of characteristics to degree of stenosis in human coronary arteries. *Circulation* **94**: 928–31.

Marso SP, Lincoff AM, Ellis SG, Bhatt DL, Tanguay JF, Kleiman NS *et al.* (1999). Optimizing the percutaneous interventional outcomes for patients with diabetes mellitus – Results of the EPISTENT (Evaluation of Platelet IIb/IIIa Inhibitor for Stenting Trial) diabetic substudy. *Circulation* **100**: 2477–84.

Marwick TH (1995). Is silent ischemia painless because it is mild? *Journal of the American College of Cardiology* **25**: 1513–5.

Maseri A, Fuster V (2003). Is there a vulnerable plaque? *Circulation* **107**: 2068–71.

Mehilli J, Kastrati A, Schühlen H, Dibra A, Dotzer F, von Beckerath H *et al.* (2004). Randomized clinical trial of abciximab in diabetic patients undergoing elective percutaneous coronary interventions after treatment with a high loading dose of clopidogrel. *Circulation* **110**: 3727–35.

Mehta SR, Yusuf S, Peters RJG, Bertrand ME, Lewis BS, Natarajan MK *et al.* (2001). Effects of pretreatment with clopidogrel and aspirin followed by long-term therapy in patients undergoing percutaneous coronary intervention: the PCI-CURE study. *Lancet* **358**: 527–33.

Melidonis A, Dimopoulos V, Lempidakis E, Hatzissavas J, Kouvaras G, Stefanidis A, Foussas S (1999). Angiographic study of coronary artery disease in diabetic patients in comparison with nondiabetic patients. *Angiology* **50**: 997–1006.

Moise A, Theroux P, Taeymans Y, Waters DD, Lesperance J, Fines P *et al.* (1984). Clinical and angiographic factors associated with progression of coronary artery disease. *Journal of the American College of Cardiology* **3**: 659–67.

Morgan KP, Kapur A, Beatt KJ (2004). Anatomy of coronary disease in diabetic patients: an explanation for poorer outcomes after percutaneous coronary intervention and potential target for intervention. *Heart* **90**: 732–8.

Morris AD, Boyle DI, McMahon AD, pearce H, Evans JM, Newton RW *et al.* (1997). ACE inhibitor use is associated with hospitalization for severe hypoglycemia in patients with diabetes. DARTS/MEMO Collaboration. Diabetes Audit and Research in Tayside, Scotland. Medicines Monitoring Unit. *Diabetes Care* **20**: 1363–7.

Moses JW, Leon MB, Popma JJ, Fitgerald PJ, Holmes DR, O'Shaunessy C *et al.* (2003). Sirolimus-eluting stents versus standard stents in patients with stenosis in a native coronary artery. *New England Journal of Medicine* **349**: 1315–23.

Mosseri M, Nahir M, Rozenman Y, Lotan C, Admon D, Raz I, Gotsman MS (1998). Diffuse narrowing of coronary arteries in diabetic patients: the earliest phase of coronary artery disease. *Cardiology* **89**: 103–10.

Natali A, Vichi S, Landi P, Severi S, L'Abbate A, Ferrannini E (2000). Coronary atherosclerosis in Type II diabetes: angiographic findings and clinical outcome. *Diabetologia* **43**: 632–41.

Nishio K, Sakurai M, kusuyama T, Shigemitsu M, Fukui T, Kawamura K *et al.* (2006). A randomized comparison of pioglitazone to inhibit restenosis after coronary stenting with type 2 diabetes. *Diabetes Care* **29**: 101–6.

O'Keefe JH, Blackstone EH, Sergeant P, McCallister BD (1998). The optimal mode of coronary revascularization for diabetics. A risk-adjusted long-term study comparing coronary angioplasty and coronary bypass surgery. *European Heart Journal* **19**: 1696–703.

PEACE Trial Investigators (2004). Angiotensin-converting enzyme inhibition in stable coronary artery disease. *New England Journal of Medicine* **351**: 2058–68.

Peduzzi P, Detre K, Murphy ML, Thomsen J, Hultgren H, Takaro T (1991). 10-year incidence of myocardial-infarction and prognosis after infarction. Department of Veterans Affairs Cooperative Study of Coronary Artery Bypass Surgery. *Circulation* **83**: 747–55.

Rodriguez A, Bernardi V, Navia J, Baldi J, Grinfeld L, Martinez J *et al.* (2001). Argentine Randomized Study: Coronary Angioplasty with Stenting versus Coronary Bypass Surgery in patients with Multiple-Vessel Disease (ERACI II): 30-day and one-year follow-up results. *Journal of the American College of Cardiology* **37**: 51–8.

Rodriguez A, Rodriguez Alemparte M, Baldi J, Navia J, Delacasa A, Vogel D *et al.* (2003). Coronary stenting versus coronary bypass surgery in patients with multiple vessel disease and significant proximal LAD stenosis: results from the ERACI II study. *Heart* **89**: 184–8.

Roffi M, Moliterno DJ, Meier B, Powers ER, Grines CL, DiBattiste PM *et al.* (2002). Impact of different platelet glycoprotein IIb/IIIa receptor inhibitors among diabetic patients undergoing percutaneous coronary intervention: do Tirofiban and ReoPro Give Similar Efficacy Outcomes Trial (TARGET) 1-year follow-up. *Circulation* **105**: 2730–6.

Rogers WJ, Alderman EL, Chaitman BR, DiSciascio G, Horan M, Lytle B *et al.* (1995). Bypass Angioplasty Revascularization Investigation (BARI): baseline clinical and angiographic data. *American Journal of Cardiology* **75**: C9–17.

Rozenman Y, Sapoznikov D, Gotsman MS (2000). Restenosis and progression of coronary disease after balloon angioplasty in patients with diabetes mellitus. *Clinical Cardiology* **23**: 890–4.

Scheen AJ, Warzee F (2004). Diabetes is still a risk factor for restenosis after drug-eluting stent in coronary arteries. *Diabetes Care* **27**: 1840–1.

Sedlis SP, Morrison DA, Lorin JD, Esposito R, Sethi G, Sacks J *et al.* (2002). Percutaneous coronary intervention versus coronary bypass graft surgery for diabetic patients with unstable angina and risk factors for adverse outcomes with bypass: outcome of diabetic patients in the AWESOME randomized trial and registry. *Journal of the American College of Cardiology* **40**: 1555–66.

Sigwart U, Stables RH, Booth J, Erbel R, Wahrborg P, Lubsen J *et al.* (2002). Coronary artery bypass surgery versus percutaneous coronary intervention with stent implantation in patients with multivessel coronary artery disease (the Stent or Surgery trial): a randomised controlled trial. *Lancet* **360**: 965–70.

Slaughter MS, Olson MM, Lee JT, Ward HB (1993). A 15-year wound surveillance study after coronary artery bypass. *Annals of Thoracic Surgery* **56**: 1063–8.

Sobel BE, Frye R, Detre KM (2003). Burgeoning dilemmas in the management of diabetes and cardiovascular disease: rationale for the Bypass Angioplasty Revascularization Investigation 2 Diabetes (BARI 2D) trial. *Circulation* **107**: 636–42.

Steinhubl SR, Berger PB, Mann JT, Fry ETA, DeLago A, Wilmer C, Topol EJ (2002). Early and sustained dual oral antiplatelet therapy following percutaneous coronary intervention: a randomized controlled trial. *Journal of the American Medical Association* **288**: 2411–20.

Stone GW, Ellis SG, Cox DA, Hermiller J, O'Shaughnessy C, Mann JT, *et al.* (2004). One-year clinical results with the slow-release, polymer-based, paclitaxel-eluting TAXUS Stent. The TAXUS-IV trial. *Circulation* **109**: 1942–7.

Syvanne M, Pajunen P, Kahri J, Lahdenpera S, Ehnholm C, Nieminen MS, Taskinen MR (2001). Determinants of the severity and extent of coronary artery disease in patients with type-2 diabetes and in nondiabetic subjects. *Coronary Artery Disease* **12**: 99–106.

Takagi T, Yamamuro A, Tamita K, Yamabe K, Katayama M, Morioka S *et al.* (2002). Impact of troglitazone on coronary stent implantation using small stents in patients with type 2 diabetes mellitus. *American Journal of Cardiology* **89**: 318–22

Takezako T, Saku K, Zhang B, Shirai K, Arakawa K (1999). Insulin resistance and angiographical characteristics of coronary atherosclerosis. *Japanese Circulation Journal* **63**: 666–73.

Tcheng JE, O'Shea JC, Cohen EA, Pacchiana CM, Kitt MM, Lorenz TJ *et al.* (2000). Novel dosing regimen of eptifibatide in planned coronary stent implantation (ESPRIT): a randomised, placebo-controlled trial. *Lancet* **356**: 2037–44.

Topol EJ, Moliterno DJ, Herrmann HC, Powers ER, Grines CL, Cohen DJ *et al.* (2001). Comparison of two platelet glycoprotein IIb/IIIa inhibitors, tirofiban and abciximab, for the prevention of ischemic events with percutaneous coronary revascularization. *New England Journal of Medicine* **344**: 1888–94.

Valsania P, Zarich SW, Kowalchuk GJ, Kosinski E, Warram JH, Krolewski AS (1991). Severity of coronary artery disease in young patients with insulin-dependent diabetes mellitus. *American Heart Journal* **122**: 695–700.

Van Belle E, Bauters C, Hubert E, Bodart JC, Abolmaali K, Meurice T *et al.* (1997). Restenosis rates in diabetic patients: a comparison of coronary stenting and balloon angioplasty in native coronary vessels. *Circulation* **96**: 1454–60.

Van Belle E, Ketelers R, Bauters C, Perie M, Abolmaali K, Richard F *et al.* (2001). Patency of percutaneous transluminal coronary angioplasty sites at 6-month angiographic follow-up: A key determinant of survival in diabetics after coronary balloon angioplasty. *Circulation* **103**: 1218–24.

van Domburg RT, Foley DP, Breeman A, van Herwerden LA, Serruys PW (2002). Coronary artery bypass graft surgery and percutaneous transluminal coronary angioplasty. Twenty-year clinical outcome. *European Heart Journal* **23**: 543–9.

Veterans Administration Coronary Artery Bypass Surgery Cooperative Study Group (1984). Eleven year survival in the Veterans Administration randomized trial of coronary artery bypass surgery for stable angina. *New England Journal of Medicine* **311**: 1333–9.

Waldecker B, Waas W, Haberbosch W, Voss R, Steen-Muller MK, Hiddessen A *et al.* (1999). Type 2 diabetes and acute myocardial infarction. Angiographic findings and results of an invasive therapeutic approach in type 2 diabetic versus nondiabetic patients. *Diabetes Care* **22**: 1832–8.

Waller BF, Palumbo PJ, Lie JT, Roberts WC (1980). Status of the coronary arteries at necropsy in diabetes mellitus with onset after age 30 years. Analysis of 229 diabetic patients with and without clinical evidence of coronary heart disease and comparison to 183 control subjects. *American Journal of Medicine* **69**: 498–506.

Weintraub WS, Stein B, Kosinski A, Douglas JS, Ghazzal ZMB, Jones EL *et al.* (1998). Outcome of coronary bypass surgery versus coronary angioplasty in diabetic patients with multivessel coronary artery disease. *Journal of the American College of Cardiology* **31**: 10–9.

Weintraub WS, Kosinski A, Culler S (1999). Comparison of outcome after coronary angioplasty and coronary surgery for multivessel coronary artery disease in persons with diabetes. *American Heart Journal* **138**: S394–9.

West NEJ, Ruygrok PN, Disco CMC, Webster MW, Lindeboom WK, O'Neill WW *et al.* (2004). Clinical and angiographic predictors of restenosis after stent deployment in diabetic patients. *Circulation* **109**: 867–73.

Windecker S, Remondino A, Eberli FR, Juni P, Raber L, Wenaweser P *et al.* (2005). Sirolimus-eluting and paclitaxel-eluting stents for coronary revascularization. *New England Journal of Medicine* **353**: 653–62.

Wong ND, Kouwabunpat D, Vo AN, Detrano RC, Eisenberg H, Goel M, Tobis JM (1994). Coronary calcium and atherosclerosis by ultrafast computed tomography in asymptomatic men and women: relation to age and risk-factors. *American Heart Journal* **127**: 422–30.

Yusuf S, Zucker D, Peduzzi P, Fisher LD, Takaro T, Kennedy JW *et al.* (1994). Effect of coronary artery bypass graft surgery on survival: overview of 10-year results from randomized trials by the Coronary-Artery Bypass Graft-Surgery Trialists Collaboration. *Lancet* **344**: 563–70.

Yusuf S, Zhou F, Mehta SR, Chrolavicius S, Togoni G, Fox KK; Clopidogrel In Unstable Angina to Prevent Recurrent Events Trial Invetsigators (2001). Effects of clopidogrel in addition to aspirin in patients with acute coronary syndromes without ST-segment elevation. *New England Journal of Medicine* **345**: 494–502.

4 Diabetes and Acute Coronary Syndromes

Colin Berry, Miles Fisher and *John J. McMurray*

4.1 Introduction

Diabetic patients have a worse prognosis after an acute coronary syndrome (ACS), due to an increased risk of both cardiovascular and non-cardiovascular death. Early cardiovascular death is most often due to heart failure, whereas death in the medium term (up to 15 years) is more often due to reinfarction (Aronson *et al.*, 1997; Vaccaro *et al.*, 2004). In the longer term, beyond 20 years, this increased risk of cardiovascular death normalises, but the risk of non-cardiovascular death remains elevated (Vaccaro *et al.*, 2004). Platelet activation is a feature of ACS (Merlini *et al.*, 1994) and platelet activation and thrombin-generation are more pronounced in diabetes, compared with non-diabetic subjects, and are related to glycaemic control (Aoki *et al.*, 1996).

4.2 Antiplatelet Agents

Aspirin

Aspirin irreversibly inhibits platelet thromboxane A2, which in turn inhibits platelet aggregation. The Second International Study of Infarct Survival (ISIS-2) was a placebo-controlled, factorial study involving streptokinase alone, or in combination with aspirin (160 mg daily), in 17 187 subjects with suspected acute myocardial infarction (MI) (ISIS-2 Collaborative Group, 1988). Of the diabetic patients randomised to aspirin, 94/645 (15%) died from a vascular cause, compared with 94/642 (15%) deaths in the placebo-treated diabetic patients. This result was at odds with the rest of the findings in this study, where aspirin significantly reduced mortality, and the authors argued for a lack of heterogeneity between subgroups. Consequently, as for non-diabetic subjects, aspirin is a first-line therapy in ACS in diabetic subjects.

Diabetic Cardiology   Editors Miles Fisher and John J. McMurray
© 2007 John Wiley & Sons, Ltd.

Clopidogrel

CURE

The efficacy of clopidogrel in addition to aspirin for the prevention of cardiovascular death, MI or stroke, in the setting of ACS (non-ST-segment elevation), was tested in the Clopidogrel in Unstable Angina to Prevent Recurrent Events (CURE) study (Yusuf *et al.*, 2001). Patients were eligible for enrollment in this multicentre trial if they presented within 24 h after the onset of ischaemic chest pain, and had either electrocordiograph (ECG) evidence of ischaemia or elevation of cardiac biomarkers (greater than twice the upper limit of normal). CURE took place in 482 hospitals that were characterised as not having a policy for early intervention in patients with unstable coronary disease. This intended bias reduced any confounding effect of revascularisation on the study's primary aim.

Of the 6259 patients randomised to clopidogrel ($n = 1405$ (22%) with diabetes) and 6303 patients randomised to placebo ($n = 1435$ (23%) with diabetes), 9% and 11%, respectively, experienced the composite primary endpoint ($P < 0.001$). Of the three components, clopidogrel had a statistically significant effect on MI, but not on cardiovascular death or stroke. Alternatively, clopidogrel increased the risk of major bleeding and minor bleeding. Diabetic and non-diabetic patients benefited from clopidogrel therapy to a similar extent. Of note, glycoprotein (Gp)IIb/IIIa inhibitor therapy use within the preceding 3 days was an exclusion criterion for participation in this study. Overall, only 10% of patients in CURE received quadruple therapy with aspirin, clopidogrel, heparin and GpIIb/IIIa therapy, thus evidence to support this treatment regime is lacking. Furthermore, because of the low intervention rate (23%) during the index admission, the findings of CURE are most relevant to unstable angina with non-ST-elevation MI (UA-NSTEMI) patients who do not undergo invasive management.

PCI-CURE

In PCI-CURE, a prespecified substudy of CURE patients who underwent interventional management, 1315 patients ($n = 249$ (19%) with diabetes) in the clopidogrel group and 1345 patients ($n = 255$ (19% with diabetes) in the placebo group underwent percutaneous coronary intervention (PCI) (Mehta *et al.*, 2001). These patients were pretreated with the study drug for a median time of 10 days before PCI. Following PCI, patients were treated with open-label thienopyridine (clopidogrel or ticlopidine) for 1 month, and then resorted to their original study drug (placebo or clopidogrel) for an average of 8 months. The primary endpoint (death/non-fatalMI/target vessel revascularisation within 30 days of PCI) occurred in 59 (4.5%) patients in the clopidogrel-treated group and 86 (6.4%) of the placebo-treated group ($P = 0.03$). When events that occurred before PCI were included there was a 31% relative risk reduction for cardiovascular death or MI with assignment to clopidogrel ($P = 0.002$). Of the 504 diabetic patients, 32 (13%) of clopidogrel-treated patients and 42 (16%) of placebo-treated patients experienced cardiovascular death or MI during follow-up (hazard ratio 0.77, 95% CI 0.48–1.22), whereas in non-diabetic patients a significant benefit in favour of clopidogrel was apparent (hazard ratio 0.66, 95% CI 0.50–0.87).

The lack of apparent effect in the diabetic subgroup may be due to small numbers.

Both CURE and PCI-CURE raised a number of important issues, all of which are relevant to diabetic patients with ACS. The population of patients in this study programme was highly selected. For example, patients with a predisposition to bleeding were excluded, leading to bias and a minimisation of the pro-bleeding effects of clopidogrel. Also, these results relate only to high-risk ACS patients presenting with ECG changes or significant changes in plasma biomarker concentrations. Thus, the effects of clopidogrel in ACS patients without these features are uncertain. Furthermore, the benefits of clopidogrel in the longer term (beyond 9 months after starting treatment) are uncertain.

Other studies

Two other large trials have now demonstrated similar benefits in combining clopidogrel with aspirin in patients with ST-elevation MI (STEMI). CLARITY-TIMI 28 randomised 3491 patients within 12 h of a STEMI to clopidogrel or placebo in addition to thrombolytic therapy and aspirin (Sabatine et al., 2005). There was a statistically significant 36% reduction in the composite endpoint of death, recurrent MI or an occluded infarct-related artery on angiography; 16% of the subjects had diabetes, but subgroup analysis was not included. COMMIT enrolled 45 852 randomised patients with acute STEMI to clopidogrel or placebo in addition to aspirin for the duration of their hospital stay, and this produced a 9% relative risk reduction in the primary endpoint of death, reinfarction or stroke during the scheduled treatment period (COMMIT Collaborative Group, 2005). Surprisingly, no information about the numbers of patients with diabetes, or the responses in the diabetic subgroup, was provided.

4.3 Thrombolysis

Thrombolysis, or clot degradation, is mediated by plasmin, a serine protease that degrades fibrin and fibrinogen. Thrombolytic agents such as streptokinase may promote the conversion of plasminogen to plasmin, or may be fibrin-specific, such as tissue plasminogen activator (tPA). This latter agent, produced commercially using recombinant DNA technology, is converted by plasmin in vivo, to a molecule with potent fibrinolytic activity. It is also non-antigenic, but has a short half-life necessitating continous infusion. Reteplase is a modified form of tPA that has a longer half-life and can be given by bolus administration.

In ISIS-2, streptokinase therapy combined either with placebo or 160 mg of aspirin as described above reduced early and late vascular deaths (ISIS-2 Collaborative Group, 1988). Of the diabetic patients who were randomised to 1.5 MU of intravenous streptokinase, 73/619 (12%) died compared with 115/666 (17%) who received placebo. In ISIS-3, streptokinase and the fibrin-specific agents anisoylated purified streptokinase activator complex (anistreplase or APSAC) and tissue plasminogen activator (tPA) were compared (ISIS-3 Collaborative Group, 1992). Reinfarction occurred less frequently in tPA-treated patients (397/13569, 2.9%) compared with streptokinase-treated patients (472/13607, 3.5%; $P < 0.02$). In GISSI-2, streptokinase and tPA were also compared in a 2×2 factorial design (Gruppo Italiano per lo Studio della Sprovvivenza nell'Infarto Micardico, 1990).When the results of these trials were combined, there were no differences in survival at 6 months between the two treatment groups, although postinfarct angina and recurrent MI were lower. No information was provided on outcomes in diabetic patients in either of these trials. Other trials of fibrin-selective thrombolytic agents in acute MI have found similar efficacy in diabetic and non-diabetic patients (Bode *et al.*, 1996; Van de Werf *et al.*, 1999, 2001; Braunwald *et al.*, 2000).

GUSTO I

The Global Utilisation of Streptokinase and Tissue Plasminogen Activator for Occluded Coronary Arteries I (GUSTO I) trial was a randomised, open label, multicentre trial involving 41 021 patients with acute STEMI presenting within 6 h after the onset of symptoms and ST elevation of ≥ 0.1 mV in ≥ 2 limb leads, or ≥ 0.2 mV in ≥ 2 praecordial leads, and was designed to determine the effects of four thrombolytic strategies on outcome after acute MI (GUSTO Investigators, 1993). The findings of this large-scale trial indicated that accelerated tPA given with intravenous heparin provided a survival benefit over previous standard thrombolytic regimens. Subgroup analysis was perfomed of diabetic patients, and the 30-day mortality was 12.5% and 9.7% for insulin and non-insulin-treated patients, respectively, compared with 6.2% for non-diabetic patients (Mak *et al.*, 1997). Diabetes was also a predictor of non-haemorrhagic stroke, which was one of the secondary endpoints.

An angiographic substudy was performed, in which patients were randomised to angiography at 90 min, 180 min, 24 h or 5–7 days (GUSTO Angiographic Investigators, 1993). The patients who underwent coronary angiography at 90 min had repeat angiography performed after 5–7 days. All follow-up beyond this was clinical. This study demonstrated that mortality was related to 90-min patency: 8.9% in patients with no/minimal distal myocardial perfusion in the infarct-related artery (IRA) territory (thrombolysis in MI (TIMI) O–I) compared with 4.4% in patients with TIMI grade III flow ($P = 0.009$). Infarct artery patency occurred earlier and was more complete in non-Q MI. Left ventricular function was also greater in patients who achieved early IRA patency. In the diabetic patients restoration of flow (TIMI III) at 90 min post-thrombolysis was similar in diabetic (40.3%) and non-diabetic (37.6%) patients. Furthermore, the reocclusion rate of an initially patent (TIMI II or III at 90 min) IRA, although not statistically significant, tended to be more common in diabetic patients (9.2% vs. 5.3%; $P = 0.17$). The 30-day mortality rate of diabetic patients with TIMI III flow at 90 min was much higher compared with non-diabetic patients (8.6% vs. 3.4%; relative risk 2.7, 95% CI 0.9–7.8).

It was uncertain whether the higher mortality in diabetic patients was due to a lower rate of successful thrombolysis, increased reocclusion after successful thrombolysis, greater ventricular injury or a more adverse angiographic or clinical profile in diabetic patients. The GUSTO investigators therefore investigated the relationships of diabetes mellitus with early IRA patency and reocclusion rates, global and regional ventricular function indexes and mortality (Woodfield *et al.*, 1996; Mak *et al.*, 1997). The diabetic cohort had a higher proportion of female and elderly patients, and they were more often hypertensive, came to the hospital later and had more congestive heart failure and a higher number of previous MIs and bypass surgery procedures. Ninety-minute patency (TIMI III) rates in patients with and without diabetes were 40% and 38%, respectively ($P = 0.7$). Reocclusion rates were 9.2% vs. 5.3% ($P = 0.17$). The ejection fraction at 90 min after thrombolysis was similar in diabetic and non-diabetic patients (mean $\pm$ SEM $= 61.0 \pm 1.6\%$ vs. $60.1 \pm 0.7\%, P = 0.7$), as was regional ventricular function (number of abnormal chords: 19.1 ± 2.0 vs. $17.5 \pm 0.8, P = 0.3$; SD/chord: -2.3 ± 0.2 vs. $-2.4 \pm 0.1, P = 0.6$). Diabetic patients had less compensatory hyperkinesia in the non-infarct zone (SD/ chord: 1.3 ± 0.2 vs. $1.7 \pm 0.1, P \leq 0.01$). No significant difference in ventricular function was noted at 5- to 7-day follow-up. The 30-day mortality rate was 11.3% in diabetic versus 5.9% in non-diabetic patients ($P \leq 0.0001$). After adjustment for clinical and angiographic variables, diabetes remained an independent determinant of 30-day mortality ($P = 0.02$). The investigators concluded that early (90-min) IRA patency, as well as regional and global ventricular function, do not differ between patients with and without diabetes after thrombolytic therapy, except for reduced compensatory hyperkinesia in the non-infarct zone among patients with diabetes. Diabetes remained an independent determinant of 30-day mortality after correction for clinical and angiographic variables.

4.4 Beta-blockers

In the First International Study of Infarct Survival (ISIS-1 Collaborative Group, 1986) 16 027 patients with suspected acute MI who presented within 12 h after symptom onset and who were not already taking a beta-blocker or verapamil were randomised to placebo or 5 mg of intravenous atenolol followed by a further dose of 5 mg after 10 min if the heart rate was 60 beats per minute or more. The target maintenance dose of atenolol was 100 mg per day. Six per cent of randomised patients had known diabetes. Of these patients, 30/463 (6.5%) treated with atenolol died by 7 days compared with 40/495 (8.1%). This result is consistent with the overall mortality reduction of 15% (95% CI 1–27%) conferred by atenolol therapy in the study population. The mechanisms for this atenolol effect were in the main due to reductions in vascular mortality (cardiac rupture, ventricular arrhythmia). Interestingly, reinfarctions also tended to be less, although inotrope use and heart block occurred more commonly in beta-blocked patients. At one year, 866/8037 atenolol treated patients died, compared with 951/7990 placebo-treated patients, and total mortality was also reduced. Although no detailed information was provided about the effects of atenolol in diabetic and non-diabetic patients, no heterogeneity of effect was reported. Several other studies of beta-blockers following acute coronary syndromes have shown similar benefits in diabetic and non-diabetic subjects.

The underprescription of beta-blockers in diabetic patients post-MI may be due to several reasons. First, it could be that clinicians may avoid prescribing beta-blockers because of an erroneous belief that beta-blockers may provoke hypoglycaemia (discussed in Chapter 5, p. 119). Second, diabetic patients may experience left heart failure more often in ordinary clinical practice (which can at least delay the introduction of beta-blocker therapy). Third, the presence of co-morbidities, such as chronic obstructive pulmonary disease and peripheral vascular disease, may be more common in diabetic MI patients. Finally, the underprescription of beta-blockers could simply suggest non-adherence to evidence-based guidelines.

4.5 ACE Inhibitors

ISIS-4 was a randomised factorial trial of early oral captopril, oral mononitrate and intravenous magnesium sulphate in 58 050 patients with suspected acute MI (ISIS-4 Collaborative Group, 1995). Captopril treatment conferred a small but significant reduction in 5-week mortality, and this survival advantage was maintained in the longer term. No subgroup treatment heterogeneity was observed, although the results in diabetic subjects were not described in detail.

In the Survival and Ventricular Enlargement (SAVE) trial patients who were within 3–16 days after an acute MI and a left ventricular ejection fraction < 40%, but without overt heart failure or recurrent myocardial ischaemia, were randomised to captopril or placebo (Pfeffer et al., 1992). A test-dose of 6.25 mg of captopril was administered to 2250 patients, which resulted in 19 patients being excluded because of symptomatic hypotension or ischaemia. Thus, 2231 patients were randomised to either placebo or captopril, 12.5 mg initially, followed by titration to a maximum dose of 50 mg three times daily. The primary endpoint was all-cause mortality. The mean age of the patients was 59 years. Of the 1115 patients randomised to captopril therapy and the 1116 patients randomised to placebo therapy, 21% and 23% had diabetes. After 42 (range 24–60) months, follow-up, 275(25%) patients died in the placebo group and 228(20%) died in the captopril group (relative risk reduction 19%, 95% CI 3–32%; $P = 0.019$). Fewer captopril-treated patients died ($n = 234$) from cardiovascular causes than placebo-treated ($n = 188$) patients (relative risk reduction 21% (5–35%); $P = 0.014$). The incidence of recurrent fatal or non-fatal MI was lower in the captopril-treated group ($n = 133$) compared with the placebo group ($n = 170$) (relative risk 25% (5–40%); $P = 0.015$). The risk reduction of progressive heart failure was 36% (4–58%; $P = 0.032$). Alternatively, no between-group differences were observed in the incidence of sudden unexpected death. These effects were consistent across different subgroups, including diabetes.

In the GISSI-3 trial the effects of lisinopril alone, or in combination with nitrate therapy, were studied in 19 394 patients with suspected acute MI (Devita et al., 1994). Of those patients randomised to lisinopril ($n = 9435$) or placebo ($n = 9460$), 15% and 16%, respectively, had diabetes. A subsequent analysis of the diabetic subgroup showed similar improvements in survival with lisinopril in people with diabetes and non-diabetic subjects (Zuanetti et al., 1997).

4.6 Angiotensin Receptor Blockers

In the Valsartan in Acute Myocardial Infarction Trial (VALIANT), patients 0.5–10 days post-acute MI complicated by clinical or radiological evidence of heart failure, or a reduced left ventricular ejection fraction (<40% on radionuclide ventriculography or ≤ 35% on echocardiography or contrast angiography), or both, were randomised to monotherapy with captopril or valsartan, or combination therapy with both of these drugs (Pfeffer *et al.*, 2003). At randomisation, patients were required to have a systolic blood pressure of > 100 mmHg and a serum creatinine concentration of < 2.5 mg/dl (220 μmol/l). Of the 4909, 4885 and 4909 patients randomised to the valsartan, valsartan + captopril and captopril groups, 23.1%, 23.5% and 22.8% had diabetes, respectively. All-cause mortality rates were similar for all three groups, and a prespecified analysis in diabetes demonstrated valsartan to be non-inferior to captopril. There was no interaction between diabetes status and treatment group. Patients with a new or known diagnosis of diabetes had a worse prognosis than non-diabetic patients (Aguilar *et al.*, 2004) (Figure 4.1).

In the Optimal Therapy in Myocardial Infarction with the Angiotensin II Antagonist Losartan (OPTIMAAL) trial, the angiotensin receptor blocker losartan (50 mg once daily) was compared with captopril (50 mg three times daily) in 5477 patients (mean age 67.4 years, SD 9.8) with a new Q-wave MI and heart failure detected (Dickstein and Kjekhus, 2002). In this trial, mortality tended to be higher in losartan-treated patients than in captopril-treated patients, and no interaction with diabetes was detected.

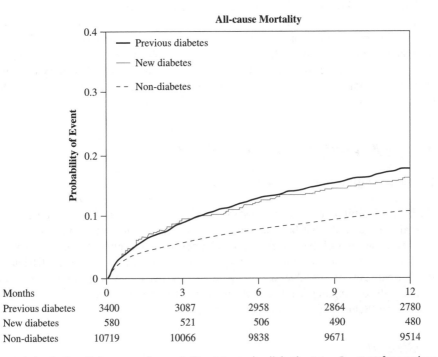

Months	0	3	6	9	12
Previous diabetes	3400	3087	2958	2864	2780
New diabetes	580	521	506	490	480
Non-diabetes	10719	10066	9838	9671	9514

Figure 4.1 Kaplan–Meier curves for mortality at 1 year by diabetic status $P = 0.43$ for previous versus new diabetes; $P < 0.001$ for previous versus no diabetes diagnosis; $P < 0.001$ for new versus no diabetes diagnosis. Reproduced from Aguilar *et al.* (2004). Newly diagnosed and previously known diabetes mellitus and 1-year outcomes of acute myocardial infarction – The VALsartan In Acute myocardial iNfarcTion (VALIANT) trial. *Circulation* 110: 1572–8. Figure 2, p. 1575.

4.7 Heparin

Unfractionated heparins are high-molecular-weight polysaccharides that, when given intravenously, potentiate antithrombin activity and prolong the activated thrombin time. The anticoagulant effect of low-molecular-weight heparins (LMWH) occurs mainly through inhibition of Factor Xa. LMWH have a more predictable, longer lasting anticoagulant effect than unfractionated heparin. A meta-analysis of 12 randomised trials of LMWH and unfractionated heparin in 17 157 aspirin-treated patients with an acute coronary syndrome found that short-term therapy (up to 7 days) with either form of heparin reduced the risk of death or MI by nearly half (hazard ratio 0.53, 95% CI 0.38–0.73; $P = 0.0001$) (Eikelboom $et\,al.$, 2000). Although these drugs have comparable efficacy (hazard ratio 0.88, 95% CI 0.69–1.12; $P = 0.34$) LMWH have a more predictable anticoagulant effect and are more straightforward to administer. Meta-analysis has demonstarted that LMWH have similar effects in diabetic and non-diabetic patients (Eikelboom $et\,al.$, 2000). LMWH are recommended as 'first line' therapies, in conjunction with aspirin and/or clopidogrel, for patients with UA-NSTEMI. LMWH can also be used safely and effectively when combined with GpIIb/IIIa, and efficacy data indicate enoxaparin to be superior to unfractionated heparin in this setting (Cohen $et\,al.$, 2000).

Recently, the Fifth Organization to Assess Strategies in Acute Ischaemic Syndromes (OASIS-5) evaluated whether the synthetic pentasaccharide fondaparinux could be safer and more effective than enoxaparin in the treatment of 20 078 ($n = 5078$ (25%) with diabetes) high-risk patients with UA-NSTEMI (Yusuf $et\,al.$, 2006). Fondaparinux was $non\text{-}inferior\ to$ enoxaparin for the outcome of death, MI and refractory ischaemia at 9 days. Notably, fondaparinux reduced the risk of major bleeding by nearly half (hazard ratio 0.52; $P < 0.01$).

4.8 Glycoprotein IIb/IIIa Inhibitors

Unstable angina and non-ST-elevation MI

GpIIb/IIIa inhibitor therapies in unstable coronary disease have now been tested in several clinical trials that have included a considerable numbers of diabetic patients. The administration of these agents should be considered as either a primary treatment for UA-NSTEMI, or as an adjunctive therapy for revascularisation (see also Chapter 3). Early treatment of unstable angina with GpIIb/IIIa inhibitor therapy can reduce the severity of ongoing cardiac ischaemia, as detected by continuous ECG Holter monitoring (Schulman $et\,al.$, 1996).

PRISM-PLUS

The Platelet Receptor Inhibition in Ischaemic Syndrome Management in Patients Limited by Unstable Signs and Symptoms (PRISM-PLUS) was a multinational trial involving 14 countries that took place between November 1994 and September 1996 (Bazzino $et\,al.$, 1998). In this trial, 1570 subjects with unstable angina or non-ST-elevation MI (NSTEMI), including 228 men and 134 women with diabetes, were treated with aspirin and unfractionated heparin and randomised to tirofiban therapy ($n = 773$) or placebo ($n = 797$). The study drugs were administered for a minimum of 48 h, and continued thereafter if intervention was performed. Investigators were encouraged to refrain from any invasive management for the first 48 h (unless refractory ischaemia or a new MI occurred), but then to perform coronary angiography 48–72 h after randomisation. The heparin dose was adjusted according to body weight rather than the level of anticoagulation. The primary endpoint was death, non-fatal MI or refractory ischaemia within 7 days of randomisation. Coronary angiography was performed during the index hospitalisation in 90% of patients; 30% underwent a PCI and 23% underwent coronary artery bypass grafting (CABG). At 48 h, death, MI or refractory ischaemia occurred with comparable frequency in the tirofiban- and placebo-treated groups (19(5.7%) vs. 24(6.9%); $P = NS$). At 7 days, the tirofiban-treated group had a lower incidence of death or MI than the placebo group (13% vs. 18%; relative risk ratio 0.68, 95% CI 0.53–0.88; $P = 0.004$). This difference was due to a reduction in MI and refractory ischaemia, chiefly driven by a difference in patients who underwent PCI.

As in ESPRIT (Tcheng et al., 2000), PRISM-PLUS was also stopped early because of an apparent early treatment effect. At 6 months, the primary event rates for the tirofiban- and placebo-treated patients were 28% and 32%, respectively ($P = 0.002$). The mortality rates in both groups at 7 days (1.9%) and 6 months (7%) were identical. In a subgroup analysis of the diabetic patients at 6 months, treatment with tirofiban reduced the number of deaths or MI (19/169 (11%) vs. 37/193 (19%); absolute risk benefit 8%, 95% CI 0.7–15.3%; $P = 0.03$) (Theroux et al., 2000). There was no excess bleeding in the tirofiban-treated patients. The diabetic subgroup data indicate that Gp IIb/IIIa inhibitor therapy may be beneficial in diabetic patients who present with unstable angina or acute MI.

PURSUIT

The Platelet Glycoprotein IIb/IIIa in Unstable Angina: Receptor Suppression Using Integrilin Therapy (PURSUIT) trial (PURSUIT Trial Investigators, 1998) was designed to test whether treatment with eptifibitide could have incremental benefit beyond that with aspirin and heparin in reducing the incidence of death or recurrent non-fatal MI within 30 days in patients with an acute NSTEMI. A total of 4722 patients (22% of whom were diabetic) were randomised to treatment with eptifibitide and 4739 patients (23% of whom were diabetic) were randomised to placebo therapy. The patients were enrolled a median time of 11 h after the onset of symptoms, and the median duration of therapy was 72 h. The index event was MI in 45% of eptifibitide-treated patients and in 46% of the placebo group. Compared with placebo, treatment with eptifibitide was associated with a 1.5% reduction in the absolute event of death/MI (14.2% vs. 15.7%; $P = 0.04$). This difference was apparent at 96 hs and maintained at 30 days. The greater part of this treatment effect occurred in patients undergoing PCI (30-day event rate: 11.6% vs. 16.7%; $P = 0.01$) whereas the event rate was 14.5% vs. 15.6% ($P = 0.23$) in those patients who did not undergo PCI. The incidence of death or non-fatal MI was comparable in diabetic patients and non-diabetic patients treated with eptifibitide, compared with placebo. Adverse bleeding events (mostly minor) were more common in eptifibitide-treated patients, compared with the placebo group.

ESPRIT

Although ESPRIT was an efficacy trial of eptifibitide as an adjunct to stenting, a small proportion of the patients enrolled had experienced an ACS (Tcheng *et al.*, 2000). Thus, 139 (13%) patients in the eptifibitide group and 140 (14%) patients in the placebo group had either unstable angina or NTSTEMI (Tcheng *et al.*, 2000). In patients with an ACS ≤ 2 days, the primary endpoint occurred in 8% of patients in the eptifibitide group and 15% of patients in the placebo group (relative risk 0.53, 95% CI 0.26–1.05; $P = 0.063$). These data are of interest since ESPRIT patients were treated with clopidogrel, in contrast to patients enrolled in earlier trials of eptifibitide in UA-NSTEMI, such as PURSUIT, who did not receive clopidogrel.

GUSTO IV-ACS

The Global Utilisation of Strategies to Open Occluded Coronary Arteries Trial IV in Acute Coronary Syndromes (GUSTO IV-ACS) enrolled 7800 patients with more than 5 min of chest pain, who also had either ST-segment depression and/or elevated troponin T or I concentrations, and in whom revascularisation was not planned (Simoons *et al.*, 2001). Patients were randomised to abciximab or placebo in addition to conventional therapy with aspirin and heparin (unfractionated or low molecular weight) and the respective primary endpoint (death/MI at 30 days) was 8.0% in the placebo-treated patients and 8.2% and 9.2% in the abciximab-treated patients.

In the meta-analysis of six randomised, placebo-controlled trials that involved 31 402 patients with UA-NSTEMI who were not routinely scheduled to undergo invasive management, GpIIb/IIIa inhibitor therapy was associated with a reduction in the risk of death or MI (11.8% vs. 10.8%; odds ratio 0.91, 95% CI 0.84–0.98; $P = 0.015$) (Boersma *et al.*, 2002). The benefits of active treatment were confined to those patients who underwent PCI (odds ratio (95% CI): 0.89(0.80–0.98)), whereas patients who did not undergo PCI derived no benefit (odds ratio(95%CI): 0.95(0.86–1.05)). Current guidelines indicate that GpIIb/IIIa inhibitor therapy is indicated for patients at high risk of thrombotic events, in particular those who are troponin positive. Short-term treatment (for 12 h) with abciximab or longer term treatment (24–108 h) with tirofiban or eptifibitide can be initiated as part of a PCI-based strategy.

GpIIb/IIIa therapy in STEMI

GpIIb/IIIa inhibitor therapy may be used as an adjunctive reperfusion therapy in the management of STEMI. These drugs may be particularly useful during PCI, particularly where intracoronary thrombus is evident, or when a 'no-reflow' phenomenon occurs because of microvascular embolisation. In the ESPRIT trial, STEMI was the index event in a small proportion of patients: 44(4%) eptifibitide group and 49(5%) in the placebo group (Tcheng *et al.*, 2000). Of these patients, 11.4% experienced the primary endpoint in the eptifibitide group compared with 20.4% in the placebo group (relative risk 0.56, 95% CI 0.21–1.50; $P = 0.24$). These data relate to subgroup analyses. The types and distribution of reperfusion therapy according to study drugs are not reported, thus these data should be interpreted with caution.

There may be a role for GpIIb/IIIa inhibitor therapy as an adjunctive reperfusion therapy with primary PCI. The role of abciximab pretreatment to facilitate primary PCI in acute STEMI is currently being tested in the FINESSE trial, which includes diabetic patients.

Antithrombin III inhibitor therapy

Bivalirudin is a direct-acting synthetic antithrombin III inhibitor. This drug has FDA approval for use as an alternative to heparin for PCI in ACS patients. The recent Acute Catheterisation and Urgent Intervention Triage Strategy (ACUITY) trial randomised 13 819 patients (28% with diabetes) and demonstrated that bivalirudin is non-inferior to the combination of heparin plus GpIIb/IIIa inhibitor therapy for the prevention of recurrent ischaemic events but reduces the risk of bleeding events (Stone *et al.*, 2006).

4.9 Revascularisation for Acute Coronary Syndromes

Revascularisation in STEMI

Invasive management of patients who have experienced an acute STEMI is with revascularisation, a superior form of reperfusion therapy (Global Use of Strategies to Open Occluded Coronary Arteries in Acute Coronary Syndromes (GUSTO IIb) Angioplasty Substudy Investigators, 1997; Grines *et al.*, 1999; Keeley *et al.*, 2003). However, STEMI patients with diabetes have a worse prognosis than those without diabetes, even when treated by primary PCI (Harjai *et al.*, 2003) Diabetic patients with cardiogenic shock have a particularly high risk of early mortality (Shindler *et al.*, 2000) (Figure 4.2).

A consistent beneficial effect on reinfarction has been observed with an interventional approach in STEMI. Since these trials were performed, the use of bare metal and drug-eluting stents, and adjunctive pharmacological therapies, including thienopyridine and GpIIb/IIIa inhibitor therapies, has become standard practice in percutaneous revascularisation. Although no trials have been performed exclusively in diabetic patients with acute MI, the outcomes of diabetic patients included in the trials described are consistent with the overall outcomes of these trials.

GUSTO IIb

The GUSTO IIb study was a larger trial of percutaneous transluminal coronary angioplasty (PTCA) vs. thrombolysis (with t-PA) (Global Use of Strategies to Open Occluded Coronary Arteries in Acute Coronary Syndromes (GUSTO IIb) Angioplasty Substudy Investigators, 1997). The GUSTO IIb study tested whether primary PCI could be superior to systemic thrombolysis with alteplase in 1138 patients with acute STEMI presenting within 12 h after the onset of symptoms. The 6-month event rates

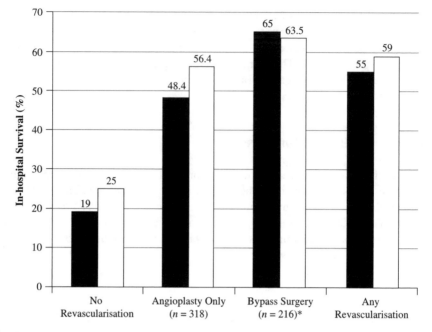

Figure 4.2 In-hospital survival in SHOCK trial registry patients according to diabetes status. Diabetic patients had a higher in-hospital mortality (59%) compared with non-diabetic patients (25%; $P = 0.007$), and diabetes status tended to predict in-hospital mortality following adjustment for other prognostic factors (odds ratio for death 1.36; 95% CI 1.00–1.84; $P = 0.051$). Notably, diabetic patients who underwent revascularisation derived a survival benefit similar to non-diabetic patients. Reproduced from Shindler *et al.* (2000). Diabetes mellitus in cardiogenic shock complicating acute myocardial infarction: A report from the SHOCK Trial Registry *Journal of the American College of Cardiology* 36: 1097–103. Figure 1, p. 1101.

for the composite outcome of death, non-fatal reinfarction and non-fatal stroke were similar for both groups; 177 of these patients were diabetic, and subgroup analysis has been published (Hasdai *et al.*, 2000). At 30 days, fewer diabetics treated with PCI experienced the composite endpoint of death, reinfarction or disabling stroke (11/99 (11%) vs. 13/78 (17%) with alteplase; absolute risk reduction 5.6%, 95% CI 4.8–15.9%). There was no difference in 30-day mortality between the two groups.

DANAMI

In the Danish Trial in Acute Myocardial Infarction (DANAMI), all patients ($n = 1008$) with an index STEMI received thrombolysis followed by stress testing (Madsen *et al.*, 1997). Of the patients randomised to revascularisation, 266 (52.9%) had a PTCA and 147 (29.2%) had a CABG (2–10 weeks after the acute MI). Of the 505 patients in the conservative treatment group, only eight (1.6%) crossed over for revascularisation. The primary endpoints were mortality, reinfarction and admission with unstable angina. At 2.4 years' follow-up (median range 1–4.5 years), mortality was 3.6% in the invasive treatment group and 4.4% in the conservative treatment group (NS).

Although the DANAMI study was not powered to detect a difference in mortality, this trial did assess the effect of revascularisation on recurrent cardiac ischaemia. Invasive treatment was associated with a lower incidence of acute MI (5.6% vs. 10.5%; $P = 0.0038$) and a lower incidence of admission for unstable angina (17.9% vs. 29.5%; $P < 0.00001$). The percentages of patients with a primary endpoint were 15.4% and 29.5% at 1 year, 23.5% and 36.6% at 2 years and 31.7% versus 44.0% at 4 years ($P < 0.00001$) in the invasive and conservative treatment groups, respectively. At 12 months, stable angina pectoris was present in 21% of patients in the invasive treatment group and 43% in the conservative treatment group. Therefore, in patients with inducible ischaemia after thrombolysis for a STEMI, an interventional approach reduces the incidence of recurrent ischaemia and MI.

DANAMI-2

The Danish Multicentre Randomised Study on Fibrinolytic Therapy versus Acute Coronary Angioplasty in Acute Myocardial Infarction (DANAMI-2) trial took place in 24 Danish hospitals between December 1997 and October 2001 (Andersen *et al.*, 2003; Kjaergard *et al.*, 2004). This trial tested whether interventional management of acute STEMI, including transfer of patients to an interventional cardiology centre where necessary, could be superior to conventional thrombolysis. A total of 1572 patients were randomised, of whom 782 were assigned fibrinolysis and 775 were assigned PCI. All patients had ST-segment elevation of ≥ 4 mm. Among patients who underwent interventional management, the primary endpoint (death/reinfarction or disabling stroke) occurred in 8%, as compared with 14% of those in the fibrinolysis group ($P = 0.0003$). Similar results were obtained at 6 months (18% and 24%, respectively; $P = 0.002$). The study was not powered for mortality: the rate of death at 6 months was 16.4% in the interventional group versus 16.0% in the thrombolytic group ($P = 0.26$).

Similarly, in DANAMI-2, although primary PCI did not reduced mortality compared to thrombolysis, there was an important reduction in the risk of recurrent myocardial ischaemia. The better outcome associated with interventional management was driven by a reduction in the rate of reinfarction (1.6% in the angioplasty group vs. 6.3% in the thrombolytic group, $P < 0.001$). These recent data, supported by meta-analyses of clinical trials of primary PCI versus thrombolysis (Grines *et al.*, 1999; Keeley *et al.*, 2003), indicate that an invasive strategy is optimal management for the prevention of reinfarction, and probably death.

PRAGUE-2

This STEMI trial enrolled patients who presented to community hospitals without invasive facilities to either thrombolysis or primary PCI following interhospital transfer. The trial took place between 1999 and 2002 in the Czech Republic and showed an early benefit in favour of primary PCI. Of 850 randomised patients ($n = 204$ (24%) with diabetes) who presented within 12 h after the onset of symptoms, 5-year follow-up data were available in 416 (98.8%) (Widimsky *et al.*, 2007). The cumulative incidence of the composite endpoint of all-cause mortality, recurrent MI, stroke or revascularisation was 53% in the medically treated group compared with 40% in the primary PCI group.

Data from registers

One recent prospective cohort study from the Register of Information and Knowledge about Swedish Heart Intensive Care Admissions (RIKS-HIA) between 1995 and 1998 included data from 61 Swedish hospitals using 1-year mortality data from the Swedish National Cause of Death Register for 21 912 individuals with an index registry-recorded acute MI who were < 80 years old and survived to day 14 (Stenestrand and Wallentin, 2002). Early coronary intervention (< 14 days post-MI) was performed in 1245 (12%) of STEMI patients, and the relative risk of death at 1 year was reduced (hazard ratio 0.65, 95% CI 0.46–0.91; $P = 0.012$) (Stenestrand and Wallentin, 2002). Diabetic patients benefited similarly from early intervention (hazard ratio 0.36, 95% CI 0.22–0.61; $P < 0.001$). Furthermore, the benefits of revascularisation were independent of treatment with other secondary prevention therapies, such as with statins or beta-blockers.

Revascularisation in NSTEMI

FRISC II

The Fragmin and Fast Revascularisation during Instability in Coronary Artery Disease (FRISC II) trial compared an early invasive strategy, which included catheterisation within 7 days and revascularisation as appropriate, to a more conservative (selectively invasive) strategy in which catheterisation was performed only if the patient had objective evidence of recurrent ischaemia or an abnormal stress test (Wallentin *et al.*, 2000). Patients were also randomised to subcutaneous administration of either LMWH (dalteparin for 3 months) or placebo. The primary endpoint was death or MI. Of 3048 eligible patients, 591 were found to be ineligible for randomisation. Of the 1222 randomised to an invasive management, 155 (13%) were diabetic, and of the 1235 randomised to non-invasive therapy, 144 (12%) were diabetic. During the first 7 days, coronary angiography was performed in 96% of the invasive group and in 7% of the non-invasive group. During the first 10 days, revascularisation was performed in 71% of the invasive group and in 9% of the non-invasive group.

Revascularisation was done within the first year in 78% and 43% of these patients, respectively. During the first year, 27 (2.2%) patients in the invasive group and 48 (3.9%) in the non-invasive group died (risk ratio 0.57, 95% CI 0.36–0.90; $P = 0.016$); 105 (8.6%) versus 143 (11.6%) had MI (0.74 (0.59–0.94); $P = 0.015$). The composite of death or MI occurred in 127 (10.4%) versus 174 (14.1%) patients (0.74 (0.60–0.92); $P = 0.005$). There were also reductions in readmission (451 (37%) vs. 704 (57%); 0.67 (0.62–0.72)) and revascularisation after the initial admission (92 (7.5%) vs. 383 (31%); 0.24 (0.20–0.30)). An interaction was observed for gender, whereby an interventional approach was associated with a reduction in death or MI in men, but not in women.

No interaction was observed with the dalteparin/placebo allocation. Of the diabetic patients, 32/154 (21%) who underwent invasive management experienced the primary endpoint, compared with 43/144 (30%) who underwent non-invasive management. The risk ratio (95% CI) was 0.7(0.47–1.04), which was largely driven by a reduction in reinfarction.

TIMI 18

In the Thrombolysis in Myocardial Infarction 18 (TIMI 18) investigation (TACTICS) of an early invasive strategy versus a conservative strategy for the management of unstable angina or NSTEMI, 2220 patients were treated with aspirin, heparin and the GpIIb/IIIa inhibitor tirofiban (Cannon *et al.*, 2001). Of these, 613 (28%) were diabetic, of whom 313 (28%) and 300 (27%) underwent invasive or conservative management, respectively. They were randomly assigned to an early invasive strategy, which included catheterisation within 4–48 h and revascularisation as appropriate, or a conservative strategy. The primary endpoint was a composite of death, non-fatal MI and rehospitalisation for an ACS at 6 months. The rate of the primary endpoint was 16% with use of the early invasive strategy and 19% with use of the conservative strategy (odds ratio 0.78, 95% CI 0.62–0.97; $P = 0.025$). The rate of death or non-fatal MI at 6 months was similarly reduced (7.3% vs. 9.5%; odds ratio 0.74, 95% CI 0.54–1.00; $P < 0.05$). Of the diabetic patients, 20% who underwent an invasive approach experienced the primary endpoint, compared with 28% who underwent a conservative approach. In this trial, interactions were observed in patients with ST-segment changes and in those with prior aspirin use.

RITA-3

The RITA-3 trial also compared whether an interventional strategy might be superior to a conservative strategy in UA-NSTEMI patients (Fox *et al.*, 2002). A total of 1810 patients with NSTEMI (mean age 62 years, 38% women) were assigned an early intervention or conservative strategy. The antithrombin agent in both groups was enoxaparin. The co-primary endpoints were a combined rate of death, non-fatal MI or refractory angina at 4 months, and a combined rate of death or non-fatal MI at 1 year. At 4 months, 86 (10%) of 895 patients in the intervention group had died or had an MI or refractory angina, compared with 133 (14%) of 915 patients in the conservative group (risk ratio 0.66, 95% CI 0.51–0.85; $P = 0.001$). This difference was mainly due to a halving of refractory angina in the intervention group. Death or MI was similar in both treatment groups at 1 year (68 (7.6%) vs. 76 (8.3%), respectively; risk ratio 0.91, 95% CI 0.67–1.25; $P = 0.58$). Symptoms of angina were improved and use of anti-anginal medications significantly reduced with the interventional strategy ($P < 0.0001$).

Thus, in FRISC II, TACTICS/TIMI-18 and RITA-3 an early, interventional approach reduced recurrent ischaemia and reinfarction, whereas a survival benefit was only observed in FRISC II.

In the Swedish registry of ACS, of those patients with an NSTEMI, 1309 (12%) underwent revascularisation management, compared with 9929 (88%) who underwent a non-interventional approach (Stenestrand and Wallentin, 2002). The 1-year mortality was 38 (3%) compared with 981 (10%) (Cox hazard ratio 0.35 (0.24–0.50); $P < 0.001$), and similar benefits were experienced in diabetic and non-diabetic patients.

Stent thrombosis

Diabetes is a predictor of subacute and late (> 12 months, postimplantation) stent thrombosis. For this reason, compliance with antiplatelet therapy, including long-term clopidogrel whenever it may be prescribed, is a key consideration in the management of diabetic patients with unstable coronary artery disease undergoing PCI (Hodgson *et al.*, 2007).

4.10   Device Therapy Post-MI

The Mulitcentre Automatic Defibrillator Implantation Trial was designed to evaluate the benefit of prophylactically implanted defibrillatory in patients who had sustained an acute Q-wave MI and who had an ejection fraction of 30% or less (Moss *et al.*, 2002). Exclusion criteria included New York Heart Association (NYHA) class IV at enrolment, recent myocardial revascularisation (< 3 months), an MI within the previous month or prognostically important concomitant health problems. A Guidant transvenous defibrillator was used in this trial, and optimal secondary prevention therapy was also encouraged. Of the 1232 patients randomised in this trial, 742 (33% diabetic) went into the defibrillator group and 490 (38% diabetic) into the conventional therapy group. Of these patients, 105 (14.2%) of the defibrillator patients and 97 (19.8%) of the conventional therapy group patients died (hazard ratio 0.69 (0.51–0.93); $P = 0.016$). The Kaplan-Meier survival curves began to diverge at 9 months. The benefit of defibrillator therapy was similar in diabetic and non-diabetic patients (Moss *et al.*, 2002).

4.11   Management of Glycaemia

The DIGAMI studies

The metabolic consequences of acute coronary syndromes include the release of epinephrine, glucagon and other counter-regulatory hormones. These antagonise the effects of insulin, and cause further worsening of insulin resistance. In the myocardium this insulin resistance favours the utilisation of free fatty acids, which may have a deleterious effect on myocardial function. In non-diabetic subjects, this may cause temporary hyperglycaemia, sometimes called 'stress hyperglycaemia', that requires further investigation at a later stage for possible impaired glucose tolerance or diabetes (Chapter 11). In patients with established diabetes this can cause significant increases in hyperglycaemia, and may be a cause of metabolic decompensation and hyperglycaemic states.

DIGAMI

The DIGAMI (Diabetes Mellitus Insulin-Glucose Infusion in Acute Myocardial Infarction) study was based on the hypothesis that the administration of a high-dose intravenous insulin infusion followed by intensive subcutaneous insulin administration would overcome the worsening insulin resistance, suppress free fatty acid release, reduce hyperglycaemia, improve glucose utilisation in the myocardium and thus reduce mortality (Malmberg *et al.*, 1994). A small pilot study was performed to establish the safety of a high-dose insulin infusion. The insulin was added to a bag of 5% dextrose and infused at 30 ml/h, which is roughly 5 units of insulin per hour (Malmberg *et al.*, 1994). The main study was perfomed in 19 Swedish Coronary Care Units (CCUs) and randomised 620 patients to either insulin infusion followed by multidose subcutaneous insulin injection (usually four times daily) ($n = 306$), or conventional treatment ($n = 314$) (Malmberg *et al.*, 1995). A further 620 subjects who were potentially eligible for inclusion in the study were seen in the CCUs during the time the study was running, but were not included either because of inability or unwillingness to comply with the study treatment protocol. Subjects were included if their random blood glucose was above 11.1 within the first 24 h. Most were previously diagnosed as having diabetes, but some were previously unknown. There was an insignificant reduction in total mortality (the primary endpoint) at hospital discharge and at 3 months, which was the initial proposed duration of follow-up. When the study was extended to 1 year of follow-up a significant absolute reduction in total mortality of 7% was observed in the intervention group compared to the conventional treatment group (Malmberg *et al.*, 1995, 1996), and this was increased to an 11% absolute reduction at a mean follow-up of 3.4 years (Malmberg, 1997) (Figure 4.3). DIGAMI also confirmed that admission blood glucose and HbA1c were predictors of short-term and long-term mortality following MI (Malmberg *et al.*, 1997, 1999).

Although the study was significantly positive, and the longer term follow-up results receved wide exposure in the medical literature, it did not lead to major changes in clinical practice for several reasons. Firstly, it was the only large study to show benefit of insulin treatment in diabetic patients, although some studies on the use of glucose–insulin–potassium therapy in non-diabetic subjects following MI had demonstrated similar benefits. Secondly, it was a complex intervention combining the use of intravenous followed by intensive subcutaneous insulin. The study intravenous insulin regimen was rather idiosyncratic and was quite difficult for nursing staff to administer in a busy CCU setting. Because the insulin was administered in a bag of dextrose, and not via a syringe pump, a lot of fluid was infused, raising worries about possible fluid overload. In routine clinical practice the education required to teach this frail group of patients to self-administer insulin was time consuming and required the involvement of the diabetes team, and as in the DIGAMI study many patients were unwilling or unable to start insulin injections following an MI. Finally, the mechanisms of possible benefit were unstudied in the original DIGAMI study.

DIGAMI-2

A second DIGAMI study was established to address some of these difficulties (Malmberg *et al.*, 2005). DIGAMI-2 contained three groups: one that received

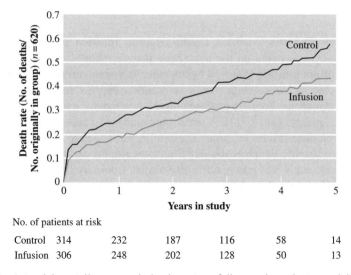

No. of patients at risk

Control	314	232	187	116	58	14
Infusion	306	248	202	128	50	13

Figure 4.3 Actuarial mortality curves during long-term follow-up in patients receiving insulin–glucose infusion and in control group among the total DIGAMI cohort. Absolute reduction in risk was 11%; relative risk 0.72 (0.55–0.92, $P = 0.011$). Reproduced from Malmberg K for the DIGAMI (Diabetes Mellitus, Insulin Glucose Infusion in Acute Myocardial Infarction) Study Group (1997). Prospective randomised study of intensive insulin treatment on long term survival after acute myocardial infarction in patients with diabetes mellitus. *British Medical Journal* **314**: 1512–15. Figure 1, p. 1514.

intravenous followed by subcutaneous insulin as in DIGAMI-1 (although most got twice-daily insulin injection); a group that got conventional treatment all the way through, as in DIGAMI-1; and a group that received intravenous insulin followed by conventional treatment. In this way it was hoped to identify if subcutaneous insulin therapy was required for benefit or whether short-term intravenous insulin alone was sufficient. It was hoped to randomise 3000 subjects but the study was halted because of slow recruitment, and less than half this number of subjects was finally included. In an attempt to improve recruitment the protocol was amended slightly so that patients with known diabetes could enter with any blood glucose concentration, whereas in DIGAMI-1 it had to be above 11.1 mol/l. Approximately half of the subjects had STEMIs and half had NSTEMIs.

The results were disappointingly negative, and if anything the total mortality at 2 years, which was the primary endpoint of the study, was lowest in the control group. Several problems can be identified with the study. As mentioned above the number of subjects recruited was low, there were baseline differences that favoured the control group, and an unexpectedly high number of non-cardiac deaths was observed in the intensive intervention group. The loosening of entry criteria to allow patients with known diabetes who had lower admission blood glucose readings meant that lower risk patients were included, as mortality is proportionate to admission blood glucose, and it also meant that there was a much smaller metabolic window for improvement with the intravenous infusion. On follow-up, blood glucose targets were not achieved, probably because of the use of a less intensive insulin regimen, and so there was no major difference in metabolic control, as measured by HbA1c, between the groups.

Other studies

A recent study from six centres examined the effects of improved glycaemic control with an insulin and dextrose infusion for at least 24 h versus conventional therapy, including subcutaneous insulin, in 240 subjects with MI and a blood glucose concentration of > 7.8 mmol/l. Half of the subjects had previously diagnosed diabetes. There was no significant effect on the primary endpoint of mortality at 3 and 6 months, but there was a significant reduction in cardiac failure and reinfarction within three months (Cheung *et al.*, 2006).

Thus, at present the evidence for reductions in mortality with intravenous insulin following acute coronary syndromes in diabetic and non-diabetic subjects is not stong. Diabetic patients should be treated with a high-dose insulin infusion to try and minimise hyperglycaemia while avoiding hypoglycaemia, and thereafter the blood glucse concentration should be controlled as tightly as possible, again avoiding hypoglycaemia, but this does not have to be insulin based (see also Chapters 9 and 11). There is a need for large, long-term studies evaluating the effects of very intensive insulin therapy in patients with diabetes and MI, preferably with a treatment goal of normalising blood glucose concentrations.

4.12 Conclusions

There are many evidence-based interventions in ACS patients that are applicable to diabetic patients with an ACS, and there are no specififc contraindications to evidence-based therapies in patients with diabetes; thrombolysis and the use of beta-blockers should be used alongside other evidence-based therapies. These therapies are now the subject of clinical guidelines that have been produced by the international cardiological societies (Bertrand *et al.*, 2002; Braunwald *et al.*, 2002; Van de Werf *et al.*, 2003; Antman *et al.*, 2004), and in the future we can anticipate the addition of new therapies as adjuncts to, or replacements of, currently recommended drugs. The role of intensive intravenous insulin for diabetic patients with acute coronary syndromes remains to be clarified.

References

Aguilar D, Solomon SD, Kober L, Rouleau JL, Skali H, McMurray JJV *et al.* (2004). Newly diagnosed and previously known diabetes mellitus and 1-year outcomes of acute myocardial infarction – The VALsartan In Acute myocardial iNfarcTion (VALIANT) trial. *Circulation* **110**: 1572–8.

Andersen HR, Nielsen TT, Rasmussen K, Thuesen L, Kelbaek H, Thayssen P *et al.* (2003). A comparison of coronary angioplasty with fibrinolytic therapy in acute myocardial infarction. *New England Journal of Medicine* **349**: 733–42.

Antman EM, Abde DT, Armstrong PW, Bates ER, Green LA, Hand M *et al.* (2004). ACC/AHA guidelines for the management of patients with ST-elevation myocardial infarction – executive summary. A report of the American College of cardiology/American Heart Association Task Force on Practice Guidelines (Writing Committee to revise the 1999 guidelines for the management of patients with acute myocardial infarction). *Journal of the American College of Cardiology* **44**: 671–719.

Aoki I, Shimoyama K, Aoki N, Homori M, Yanagisawa A, Nakahara K *et al.* (1996). Platelet-dependent thrombin generation in patients with diabetes mellitus: effects of glycemic control on coagulability in diabetes. *Journal of the American College of Cardiology* **27**: 560–6.

Aronson D, Rayfield EJ, Chesebro JH (1997). Mechanisms determining course and outcome of diabetic patients who have had acute myocardial infarction. *Annals of Internal Medicine* **126**: 296–306.

Bazzino O, Barrero C, Garre L, Sosa A, Aylward P, Slany J *et al.* (1998). Inhibition of the platelet glycoprotein IIb/IIIa receptor with tirofiban in unstable angina and non-Q-wave myocardial infarction. *New England Journal of Medicine* **338**: 1488–97.

Bertrand ME, Simoons ML, Fox KAA, Wallentin LC, Hamm CW, McFadden E *et al.* (2002). Management of acute coronary syndromes in patients presenting without persistent ST-segment elevation. *European Heart Journal* **23**: 1809–40.

Bode C, Smalling RW, Berg G, Burnett C, Lorch G, Kalbfleisch JM *et al.* (1996). Randomized comparison of coronary thrombolysis achieved with double-bolus reteplase (recombinant plasminogen activator) and front-loaded, accelerated alteplase (recombinant tissue plasminogen activator) in patients with acute myocardial infarction. *Circulation* **94**: 891–8.

Boersma E, Harrington RA, Moliterno DJ, White H, Theroux P, Van de Werf F *et al.* (2002). Platelet glycoprotein IIb/IIIa inhibitors in acute coronary syndromes: a meta-analysis of all major randomised clinical trials. *Lancet* **359**: 189–98.

Braunwald E, Neuhaus KL, Antman E, Chew P, Skene A, Wilcox R *et al.* (2000). Intravenous NPA for the treatment of infarcting myocardium early; InTIME-II, a double-blind comparison of single-bolus lanoteplase vs accelerated alteplase for the treatment of patients with acute myocardial infarction. *European Heart Journal* **21**: 2005–13.

Braunwald E, Antman EM, Beasley JW, Califf RM, Cheitlin MD, Hochman JS *et al.* (2002). ACC/AHA guideline update for the management of patients with unstable angina and non-ST-segment elevation myocardial infarction-2002: Summary article: a report of the American College of Cardiology/American Heart Association Task Force on Practice Guidelines (Committee on the Management of Patients With Unstable Angina). *Circulation* **106**: 1893–900.

Cannon CP, Weintraub WS, Demopoulos LA, Vicari R, Frey MJ, Lakkis N *et al.* (2001). Comparison of early invasive and conservative strategies in patients with unstable coronary syndromes treated with the glycoprotein IIb/IIIa inhibitor tirofiban. *New England Journal of Medicine* **344**: 1879–87.

Cheung NW, Wong VW, McLean M (2006). The Hyperglycemia:Intensive Insulin Infusion In Infarction (HI-5) study. A randomized controlled trial of insulin infusion therapy for myocardial infarction. *Diabetes Care* **29**: 765–70.

Cohen M, Theroux P, White HD (2000). Anti-thrombotic combinationusing tirofiban and enoxaparin. The ACUTE II study. Circulation **102**: II826.

COMMIT Collaborative Group (2005). Addition of clopidogrel to aspirin in 45 852 patients with acute myocardial infarction: randmised placebo-controlled trial. *Lancet* **366**: 1607–21.

Devita C, Fazzini PF, Geraci E, Tavazzi L, Tognoni G, Vecchio C *et al.* (1994). GISSI-3: effects of lisinopril and transdermal glyceryl trinitrate singly and together on 6-week mortality and ventricular function after acute myocardial-infarction. *Lancet* **343**: 1115–22.

Dickstein K, Kjekhus J (2002). Effects of losartan and captopril on mortality and morbidity in high-risk patients after acute myocardial infarction: the OPTIMAL randomised trial. *Lancet* **360**: 752–60.

Eikelboom JW, Anand SS, Malmberg K, Weitz JI, Ginsberg JS, Yusuf S (2000). Unfractionated heparin and low-molecular-weight heparin in acute coronary syndrome without ST elevation: a meta-analysis. *Lancet* **355**: 1936–42.

Fox KAA, Poole-Wilson PA, Henderson RA, Clayton TC, Chamberlain DA, Shaw TRD *et al.* (2002). Interventional versus conservative treatment for patients with unstable angina or non-ST-elevation myocardial infarction: the British Heart Foundation RITA 3 randomised trial. *Lancet* **360**: 743–51.

Global Use of Strategies to Open Occluded Coronary Arteries in Acute Coronary Syndromes (GUSTO IIb) Angioplasty Substudy Investigators (1997). A clinical trial comparing primary coronary angioplasty with tissue plasminogen activator for acute myocardial infarction. *New England Journal of Medicine* **336**: 1621–8.

Grines CL, Cox DA, Stone GW, Garcia E, Mattos LA, Giambartolomei A *et al.* (1999). Coronary angioplasty with or without stent implantation for acute myocardial infarction. Stent Primary Angioplasty in Myocardial Infarction Study Group. *New England Journal of Medicine* **341**: 1949–56.

Gruppo Italiano per lo Studio della Sprovvivenza nell'Infarto Micardico (1990). GISSI-2: a factorial randomised trial of alteplase versus streptokinase and heparin versus no heparin among 12,490 patients with acute myocardial infarction. *Lancet* **336**: 65–71.

GUSTO Angiographic Investigators (1993). The effects of tissue plasminogen activator, streptokinase, or both on cornary-artery patience, ventricular function, and survival after acute myocardial infarction. *New England Journal of Medicine* **329**: 1615–22.

GUSTO Investigators (1993). An international randomized trial comparing four thrombolytic strategies for acute myocardial infarction. *New England Journal of Medicine* **329**: 673–82.

Harjai KJ, Stone GW, Boura J, Mattos L, Chandra H, Cox D *et al.* (2003). Comparison of outcomes of diabetic and nondiabetic patients undergoing primary angioplasty for acute myocardial infarction. *American Journal of Cardiology* **91:** 1041–5.

Hasdai D, Granger CB, Srivatsa SS, Criger DA, Ellis SG, Califf RM *et al.* (2000). Diabetes mellitus and outcome after primary coronary angioplasty for acute myocardial infarction: Lessons from the GUSTO-IIb angioplasty substudy. *Journal of the American College of Cardiology* **35**: 1502–12.

Hodgson J McB, Stone GW, Lincoff MA, Klein L, Walpole H, Bottner R *et al.* (2007) *Late Stent Thrombosis: Considerations and Practical Advice for the Use of Drug-Eluting Stents: A Report From the Society for Cardiovascular Angiography and Interventions Drug-eluting Stent Task Force.* www.scai.org.

ISIS-1 Collaborative Group (1986). Randomised trial of intravenous atenolol among 16 027cases of suspected acute myocardial infarction: ISIS-1. *Lancet* **2**: 57–66.

ISIS-2 Collaborative Group (1988). Randomised trial of intravenous streptokinase, oral aspirin, both, or neither among 17187 cases of suspected acute myocardial infarction: ISIS-2. *Lancet* **2**: 349–60.

ISIS-3 Collaborative Group (1992). ISIS-3: a randomised comparison of streptokinase vs tissue plasminogen activator vs anistreplase and of aspirin plus heparin vs aspirin alone among 41,299 cases of suspected acute myocardial-infarction. *Lancet* **339**: 753–70.

ISIS-4 Collaborative Group (1995). ISIS-4: a a randomised factorial trial assessing early oral captopril, oral mononitrate, and intravenous magnesium sulfate in 58,050 patients with suspected acute myocardial-infarction. *Lancet* **345**: 669–85.

Keeley EC, Boura JA, Grines CL (2003). Primary angioplasty versus intravenous thrombolytic therapy for acute myocardial infarction: a quantitative review of 23 randomised trials. *Lancet* **361**: 13–20.

Kjaergard HK, Nielsen PH, Andreasen JJ, Steinbruchel D, Andersen LI, Rasmussen K *et al.* (2004). Coronary artery bypass grafting within 30 days after treatment of acute myocardial infarctions with angioplasty or fibrinolysis – a surgical substudy of DANAMI-2. *Scandinavian Cardiovascular Journal* **38**: 143–6.

Madsen JK, Grande P, Saunamaki K, Thayssen P, Kassis E, Eriksen U *et al.* (1997). Danish multicenter randomized study of invasive versus conservative treatment in patients with inducible ischemia after thrombolysis in acute myocardial infarction (DANAMI). *Circulation* **96**: 748–55.

Mak KH, Moliterno DJ, Granger CB, Miller DP, White HD, Wilcox RG *et al.* (1997). Influence of diabetes mellitus on clinical outcome in the thrombolytic era of acute myocardial infarction. *Journal of the American College of Cardiology* **30**: 171–9.

Malmberg K for the DIGAMI (Diabetes Mellitus, Insulin Glucose Infusion in Acute Myocardial Infarction) Study Group (1997). Prospective randomised study of intensive insulin treatment on long term survival after acute myocardial infarction in patients with diabetes mellitus. *British Medical Journal* **314**: 1512–5.

Malmberg KA, Efendic S, Ryden LE for the Multicenter Study Group (1994). Feasibility of insulin-glucose infusion in diabetic patients with acute myocardial infarction. A report from the multicenter trial: DIGAMI. *Diabetes Care* **17**: 1007–14.

Malmberg K, Ryden L, Efendic S, herlitaz J, Nicol P, Waldenstrom A *et al.* on behalf of the DIGAMI Study Group (1995). Randomized trial of insulin-glucose infusion followed by subcutaneous insulin treatment in diabetic patients with acute myocardial infarction (DIGAMI Study): effects on mortality at 1 year. *Journal of the American College of Cardiology* **26**: 57–65.

Malmberg K, Ryden L, Hamsten A, Herlitz J, Waldenstrom A, Wedel H on behalf of the DIGAMI study group (1996). Effects of insulin treatment on cause-specific one-year mortality and morbidity in diabetic patients with acute myocardial infarction. *European Heart Journal* **17**: 1337–44.

Malmberg K, Ryden L, Hamsten A, Herlitz J, Waldenstrom A, Wedel H (1997). Mortality prediction in diabetic patients with myocardial infarction: experiences from the DIGAMI study. *Cardiovascular Research* **34**: 248–53.

Malmberg K, Norhammer A, Wedel H, Ryden L (1999). Glycometabolic state at admission: important risk marker of mortality in conventionally treated patients with diabetes mellitus and acute myocardial infarction. *Circulation* **99**: 2626–32.

Malmberg K, Ryden L, Wedel H, Birkeland K, Bootsma A, Dickstein K *et al.* for the DIGAMI 2 Investigators (2005). Intense metabolic control by means of insulin in patients with diabetes mellitus and acute myocardial infarction (DIGAMI 2): effects on mortality and morbidity. *European Heart Journal* **26**: 650–61.

Mehta SR, Yusuf S, Peters RJG, Bertrand ME, Lewis BS, Natarajan MK *et al.* (2001). Effects of pretreatment with clopidogrel and aspirin followed by long-term therapy in patients undergoing percutaneous coronary intervention: the PCI-CURE study. *Lancet* **358**: 527–33.

Merlini PA, Bauer KA, Oltrona L, Ardissino D, Cattaneo M, Belli C *et al.* (1994). Persistent activation of coagulation mechanism in unstable angina and myocardia infarction. *Circulation* **90**: 61–8.

Moss AJ, Zareba W, Hall WJ, Klein H, Wilber DJ, Cannon DS *et al.* (2002). Prophylactic implantation of a defibrillator in patients with myocardial infarction and reduced ejection fraction. *New England Journal of Medicine* **346**; 877–83.

Pfeffer MA, Braunwald E, Moye LA, Basta L, Brown EJ, Cuddy TE *et al.* (1992). Effect of captopril on mortality and morbidity in patients with left-ventricular dysfunction after myocardial-infarction. Results of the Survival And Ventricular Enlargement trial. *New England Journal of Medicine* **327**: 669–77.

Pfeffer MA, McMurray J, Valquez EJ, Rouleau JL, Kober L, Maggioni AP *et al.* (2003). Valsartan, captopril, or both in myocardial infarction complicated by heart failure, left ventricular dysfunction, or both. *New England Journal of Medicine* **349**: 893–906.

PURSUIT Trial Investigators (1998). Inhibition of platelet IIb/IIIa with eptifibatide in patients with acte coronary syndromes. *New England Journal of Medicine* **339**: 436–43.

Sabatine MS, Cannon CP, Gibson CM, Lopez-Sendon JL, Montalescot G, Theroux P *et al.* (2005). Addition of clopidogrel to aspirin and fibrinolytic therapy for myocardial infarction with ST-segment elevation. *New England Journal of Medicine* **352**: 1179–89.

Schulman SP, Goldschmidt-Clermont PJ, Topol EJ, Califf RM, Navetta FI, Willerson JT *et al.* (1996). Effects of integrelin, a platelet glycoprotein IIb/IIIa receptor antagonist, in unstable angina. A randomized multicenter trial. *Circulation* **94**: 2083–9.

Shindler DM, Palmieri ST, Antonelli TA, Sleeper LA, Boland J, Cocke TP, Hochman JS (2000). Diabetes mellitus in cardiogenic shock complicating acute myocardial infarction: A report from the SHOCK Trial Registry. *Journal of the American College of Cardiology* **36**: 1097–103.

Simoons ML, Armstrong P, Califf R, Barnathan E, Hoynck M, Scherer J, Wallentin L (2001). Effect of glycoprotein IIb/IIIa receptor blocker abciximab on outcome in patients with acute coronary syndromes without early coronary revascularisation: the GUSTO IV-ACS randomised trial. *Lancet* **357**: 1915–24.

Stenestrand U, Wallentin L (2002). Early revascularisation and 1-year survival in 14-day survivors of acute myocardial infarction: a prospective cohort study. *Lancet* **359**: 1805–11.

Stone GW, McLaurin BT, Cox DA, Bertrand ME, Lincoff AM, Moses JW *et al.* (2006). Bivalirudin for patients with acute coronary syndromes. *New England Journal of Medicine* **355**: 2203–16.

Tcheng JE, O'Shea JC, Cohen EA, Pacchiana CM, Kitt MM, Lorenz TJ *et al.* (2000). Novel dosing regimen of eptifibatide in planned coronary stent implantation (ESPRIT): a randomised, placebo-controlled trial. *Lancet* **356**: 2037–44.

Theroux P, Alexander J, Pharand C, Barr E, Snapinn S, Ghannam AF, Sax FL (2000). Glycoprotein IIb/IIIa receptor blockade improves outcomes in diabetic patients presenting with unstable angina/non-ST-elevation myocardial infarction: results from the Platelet Receptor Inhibition in Ischemic Syndrome Management in Patients Limited by Unstable Signs and Symptoms (PRISM-PLUS) study. *Circulation* **102**: 2466–72.

Vaccaro O, Eberly LE, Neaton JD, Yang LF, Riccardi G, Stamler J (2004). Impact of diabetes and previous myocardial infarction on long-term survival: 25-year mortality follow-up of primary screenees of the Multiple Risk Factor Intervention Trial. *Archives of Internal Medicine* **164**: 1438–43.

Van De Werf F, Adgey J, Ardissino D, Armstrong PW, Aylward P, Barbash G *et al.* (1999). Single-bolus tenecteplase compared with front-loaded alteplase in acute myocardial infarction: the ASSENT-2 double-blind randomised trial. *Lancet* **354**: 716–22.

Van de Werf F, Armstrong PW, Granger C, Wallentin L (2001). Efficacy and safety of tenecteplase in combination with enoxaparin, abciximab, or unfractionated heparin: the ASSENT-3 randomised trial in acute myocardial infarction. *Lancet* **358**: 605–13.

Van de Werf F, Ardissino D, Bertriu A, Cokkinos DV, Falk E, Fox KAA *et al.* (2003). Management of acute myocardial infarction in patients presenting with ST elevation myocardial infarction. *European Heart Journal* **24**: 28–66.

Wallentin L, Lagerqvist B, Husted S, Kontny F, Stahle E, Swahn E (2000). Outcome at 1 year after an invasive compared with a non-invasive strategy in unstable coronary-artery disease: the FRISC II invasive randomised trial. *Lancet* **356**: 9–16.

Widimsky P, Bilkova D, Penicka M, Novak M, Lanikova M, Porizka V, Groch L, Zelizko M, Budensinsky T, Aschermann M on behalf of the PRAGUE Study Group Investigators (2007). European Heart Journal **28**: 679–684.

Woodfield SL, Lundergan CF, Reiner JS, Greenhouse SW, Thompson MA, Rohrbeck SC *et al.* (1996). Angiographic findings and outcome in diabetic patients treated with thrombolytic therapy for acute myocardial infarction: the GUSTO-I experience. *Journal of the American College of Cardiology* **28**: 1661–9.

Yusuf S, Zhou F, Mehta SR, Chrolavicius S, Togoni G, Fox KK (Clopidogrel In Unstable Angina to Prevent Recurrent Events Trial Investigators) (2001). Effects of clopidogrel in addition to aspirin in patients with acute coronary syndromes without ST-segment elevation. *New England Journal of Medicine* **345**: 494–502.

Yusuf S, Mehta SR, Bassand JP, Budaj A, Chrolavicius S, Fox KAA *et al.* (2006). Comparison of fondaparinux and enoxaparin in acute coronary syndromes. *New England Journal of Medicine* **354**: 1464–76.

Zuanetti G, Latini R, Maggioni AP, Franzosi MG, Santoro L, Tognini G for the GISSI-3 Investigators (1997). Effect of the ACE inhibitor lisinopril on mortality in diabetic patients with acute myocardial infarction. *Circulation* **94**: 4239–45.

5 Diabetes, Left Ventricular Systolic Dysfunction and Chronic Heart Failure

Michael R. MacDonald, Mark C. Petrie, Nathaniel M. Hawkins and John J. McMurray

5.1 Introduction

Chronic heart failure (CHF) and diabetes are common. Not only are they common, but they often occur in the same patients. Clinicians commonly manage either CHF (cardiologists or internists) or diabetes (diabetologists), but few are specialists in both areas, and there are difficulties managing these two conditions when they coexist, for example the management of diabetes in patients with CHF is problematic because many of the drugs used to control hyperglycaemia are relatively 'contraindicated' in CHF. In this chapter we review the pathophysiological and clinical interactions between these two conditions.

5.2 Prevalence

The prevalence of CHF in the general population is 1–4% depending on the age of the population studied (McDonagh *et al.*, 1997; Mosterd *et al.*, 1999; Davies *et al.*, 2001). The prevalence of diabetes in the general population is 4–7% (Harris *et al.*, 1998), and approximately 0.3–0.5% of the general population is estimated to suffer from both CHF and diabetes (Thrainsdottir *et al.*, 2005).

Prevalence of CHF in populations with diabetes

Approximately 12% of patients with diabetes in general population studies have CHF (Figure 5.1) (Nichols *et al.*, 2001; Thrainsdottir *et al.*, 2005), and in diabetic

Diabetic Cardiology Editors Miles Fisher and John J. McMurray
© 2007 John Wiley & Sons, Ltd.

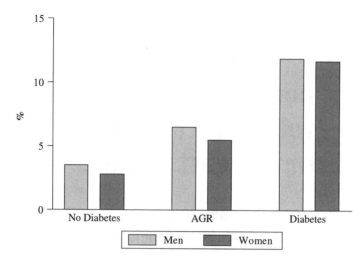

Figure 5.1 The prevalence of CHF in men and women in the Rekjavik population study. Reproduced from Thrainsdottir IS, Aspelund T, Thorgeirsson G, Gudnason V, Hardarson T, Malmberg K *et al.* (2005). The association between glucose abnormalities and heart failure in the population-based Reykjavik study. *Diabetes Care* **28:** 612–16.

patients over 64 years of age the prevalence of CHF rises to 22% (Bertoni *et al.*, 2004).

All large-scale clinical trials on glycaemia in patients with diabetes have either excluded patients with CHF by design (UK Prospective Diabetes Study (UKPDS) Group, 1998; The Diabetes Control and Complications Trial/Epidemiology of Diabetes Interventions and Complications (DCCT/EDIC) Study Research Group, 2005) or not reported CHF as a co-morbidity.

Prevalence of diabetes in populations with CHF

General population studies

The prevalence of diabetes in populations with left ventricular systolic dysfunction (LVSD) varies from 6 to 25% (Table 5.1) (McDonagh *et al.*, 1997; Morgan *et al.*, 1999; Davies *et al.*, 2001; Hedberg *et al.*, 2001; Raymond *et al.*, 2003; Redfield *et al.*, 2003; Kistorp *et al.*, 2005). In population studies of CHF, the prevalence of diabetes in patients with CHF was between 12 and 30% (Table 5.2) (Amato *et al.*, 1997; Mosterd *et al.*, 2001; Thrainsdottir *et al.*, 2005). The absolute numbers of patients with diabetes who also suffer from CHF in these epidemiological studies are small, making further groupings by age and gender inaccurate.

Hospitalised populations

In populations of patients hospitalised with CHF, the prevalence of diabetes is greater than that found in general population studies (Table 5.3). The prevalence of diabetes

Table 5.1 The prevalence of diabetes in populations with and without left ventricular systolic dysfunction (LVSD).

Study and date	Type of study	No. of participants	Age range (years)	Mean age (years)	Definition of LVSD	Prevalence of LVSD	Prevalence of symptomatic/ asymptomatic LVSD	Prevalence of diabetes in population with LVSD	Prevalence of diabetes in population without LVSD
ECHOES, England 2001 (Davies et al., 2001).	Epidemiological – primary care	3960	>45	61	LVEF < 40%	1.8% (n=72)	Symptomatic LVEF < 40% n=38(1%) Asymptomatic LVEF < 40% n=34(0.9%)	Symptomatic LVEF < 40% n=9(24%) Asymptomatic LVEF < 40% n=2(6%)	n=146(3.8%) in population with LVEF > 40%
Copenhagen 2003 (Raymond et al., 2003)	Epidemiological – primary care (stratified by age)	764	50–89	66 (Median)	LVEF ≤ 40%	n=36 (4.7%)	33% Asymptomatic	LVEF ≤ 40% n=5(7.2%)	n=43(5.9%)
Poole, England 1999 (Morgan et al., 1999)	Epidemiological – primary care	817	70–84	76	Qualitative assessment	n=61 (7.5%)	79% Asymptomatic (self-reported history)	n=6(10%)	n=43(6%)

Table 5.1 Continued

Study and date	Type of study	No. of participants	Age range (years)	Mean age (years)	Definition of LVSD	Prevalence of LVSD	Prevalence of symptomatic/asymptomatic LVSD	Prevalence of diabetes in population with LVSD	Prevalence of diabetes in population without LVSD
Glasgow 1997 (McDonagh et al., 1997)	Epidemiological	1640	25–74	50	LVEF≤ 30% LVEF≤ 35%	n = 43(2.9%) n = 113(7.7%)	77% of participants with LVEF≤ 35% were asymptomatic	n=14(12.4%)	n=34(2.5%) in population with LVEF> 35%
Vasteras, Sweden 2001 (Hedberg et al., 2001)	Epidemiological	412	75	75	LVWMI <1.7%	n=28(6.8%)	46% Asymptomatic	n = 6(22%)	n = 27(7%)
Olmsted, USA 2003 (Redfield et al., 2003)	Epidemiological	1888	> 45	63	LVEF ≤ 50% LVEF≤ 40%	n = 123(6.5%) n = 40(1.8%)	–	n = 21(17%) n = 6(15%)	n=130(6.8%)
Copenhagen 2005 (Kistorp et al., 2005)	Prospective, hospital heart failure clinic	188	–	69	LVEF< 45%	All had LVSD	All were symptomatic	n = 48(25.5%)	–

(LVEF = left ventricular ejection fraction, LVWMI = left ventricular wall motion index.)

Table 5.2 The prevalence of diabetes in general populations with and without chronic heart failure (CHF).

Study	Date	No. of participants	Age range (years)	Mean age (years)	Prevalence of CHF	Prevalence of diabetes in population with CHF	Prevalence of diabetes in population without CHF
Rotterdam (Mosterd et al., 2001)	2001	5255	55–94	69	$n=181(3.4\%)$	$n=32(17.5\%)$	$n=523(10.3\%)$
Italy (Amato et al., 1997)	1997	1339	>65	74	$n=125(9.5\%)$	$n=37(29.6\%)$	$n=160(13.2\%)$
Rekjavik (Thrainsdottir et al., 2005)	2005	19381	33–84	–	$n=733(3.8\%)$	$n=85(11.6\%)$	$n=635(3.4\%)$

Table 5.3 Prevalence of diabetes in patients hospitalised with chronic heart failure in ethnic subgroups.

Location	Year	Race	Mean age	No. of patients	Prevalence of diabetes
USA (Agoston et al., 2004)	2004	White	70	183	48%
		Black	66	144	37%
New Zealand (Bhoopatkar and Simmons, 1996)	1996	European	–	–	17%
		Maori	–	–	34%
		Pacific Isles	–	–	36%
UK (Blackledge et al., 2003)	2003	Whites	78	5057	16%
		South Asians	70	306	46%
USA (Vaccarino et al., 2002)	2002	White	75	316	45%
		African American	67	82	55%
USA (Deswal et al., 2004)	2004	White	71	17093	43%
		Black	67	4901	41%
Malaysia (Chong et al., 2003)	2003	Malay	61	45	22%
		Chinese	67	27	19%
		Indian	65	22	59%
USA (Rathore et al., 2003)	2003	White	80	26283	37%
		Black	77	3449	48%
USA (Singh et al., 2005)	2005	White	67	48	65%
		Black	65	52	33%

is approximately 40% in the larger studies of patients hospitalised with CHF (Rathore et al., 2003; Deswal et al., 2004). Whether or not the prevalence of diabetes in CHF varies according to ethnic group is uncertain (Table 5.3). Most of the studies addressing this issue include small numbers of patients, and no consistent pattern is seen.

Table 5.4 Prevalence of diabetes in clinical trials of chronic heart failure.

	Diabetes (%)		Diabetes (%)
CONSENSUS (CONSENSUS Trial Study Group, 1987)	23	CHARM-Alt (Granger et al., 2003)	27
SOLVD-T (SOLVD Investigators, 1991)	26	CHARM-Added (McMurray et al., 2003)	30
SOLVD-P (SOLVD Investigators, 1992)	15	ELITE-II (Pitt et al., 2000)	24
ATLAS (Ryden et al., 2000)	19	RESOLVD (RESOLVD Investigators, 2000)	25
MERIT-HF (MERIT-HF Study Group, 1999)	25	Val-HeFT (Cohn et al., 2001)	26
CIBIS II (Erdmann et al., 2001)	12	A-HeFT (Taylor et al., 2004)	41
COPERNICUS (Mohacsi et al., 2001)	26	DIG (Digitalis Investigation Group, 1997)	28
COMET (Poole-Wolson et al., 2003)	24	COMPANION (Bristow et al., 2004)	41
ANZ (Australia/New Zealand Heart Failure Research Collaborative Group, 1997)	19	SCD-HEFT (Bardy et al., 2005)	30

Clinical trials of CHF

The prevalence of diabetes in clinical trials of CHF ranges from 12 to 41% (Table 5.4). These trials are highly selected and not representative of the general population with CHF, as patients are typically younger, with less co-morbidity.

5.3 Incidence

Incidence of CHF in patients with diabetes

Chronic heart failure is more common in patients with diabetes than in those without diabetes. In the NHANES and Framingham studies, the incidence of CHF in patients with diabetes was two- and fourfold higher than in patients without diabetes (Kannel et al., 1974; He et al., 2001). A UK case–control study also found that both male and female patients with diabetes have a twofold greater risk of developing CHF than those without diabetes (Johansson et al., 2001).

In the USA, a retrospective study of 9951 patients with diabetes, matched with patients without diabetes, found an incidence of CHF in patients with diabetes 2.5 times that of those without diabetes (30.9 vs. 12.4 cases per 1000 person-years) (Nichols et al., 2004). In a UK population of patients with diabetes, the incidence of CHF was 21 cases per 1000 person-years (Maru et al., 2005).

Over 4 years, 39% of elderly nursing home residents with diabetes developed CHF compared to 23% of those without (Aronow and Ahn, 1999). This high incidence rate in the elderly was confirmed by a large US cohort study in 115 803 patients with diabetes over 64 years old (12.6 cases of incident CHF per 100 person-years) (Bertoni *et al.*, 2004).

Incidence of CHF in clinical trials of patients with diabetes

Clinical trial populations are very different from real-life patient cohorts. The UKPDS included patients with a mean age of 53 years with newly diagnosed diabetes (UK Prospective Diabetes Study (UKPDS) Group, 1998). The incidence of CHF was 2.3 per 1000 person-years for those with an HbA1c of < 6 and 11.9 per 1000 person-years for those with an HbA1c of > 10 (Stratton *et al.*, 2000).

Incidence of diabetes in patients with CHF

There is only one study of the incidence of diabetes in a population with CHF outwith clinical trials. In a group of elderly Italians with CHF, the 3-year incidence of new-onset diabetes was 28.8% compared to 18.3% in matched controls without CHF (Amato *et al.*, 1997).

Clinical trials of CHF

Of the patients with CHF in the placebo arm of the CHARM study, 7.4% ($n = 202$) developed diabetes over a median follow-up of 3.1 years (Yusuf *et al.*, 2005). A single-centre substudy of the SOLVD trial found an incidence of diabetes in the treatment arm of 5.9% ($n = 9$) over a mean of 2.9 years (Vermes *et al.*, 2003).

5.4   Risks of Developing CHF and Diabetes

Which patients with diabetes develop CHF?

Diabetes is an independent risk factor for the development of CHF (Kannel *et al.*, 1974; He *et al.*, 2001; Thrainsdottir *et al.*, 2005). In the Framingham study, for those between the ages of 45 and 74 years the presence of diabetes increased the risk of CHF in men by twofold and in women by fivefold (Kannel *et al.*, 1974). This effect was even more apparent in the younger age group. Under the age of 65 years, diabetes increased the risk of developing CHF by four- and eightfold for men and women, respectively. In the NHANES study, diabetes was an independent risk factor for CHF with a hazard ratio of 1.85 (1.51–2.28, $P <$ 0.001) (He *et al.*, 2001). In Iceland, the age-adjusted odds ratio for development of CHF in those with diabetes compared to those without diabetes was 2.8 (2.2–3.6) (Thrainsdottir *et al.*, 2005), and several other studies have identified diabetes as an independent risk factor for CHF (Aronow and Ahn, 1999; Chen *et al.*, 1999; Iribarren *et al.*, 2001).

In populations with diabetes there are identifiable risk factors for the development of CHF. These include increased HbA1c (Stratton *et al.*, 2000; Iribarren *et al.*, 2001; Vaur *et al.*, 2003; Nichols *et al.*, 2004) and increased body mass index (BMI). An increased BMI in patients with diabetes predicts development of CHF, and a 2.5 unit increase in BMI increases the risk of CHF by 12% (Nichols *et al.*, 2004). As noted above in the UKPDS population, the incidence of CHF increased with HbA1c. For every 1% reduction in HbA1c, the risk of CHF was seen to fall by 16% (Stratton *et al.*, 2000).

Other independent risk factors for CHF in patients with diabetes are increasing age, coronary heart disease (CHD), use of insulin, retinopathy, proteinuria, nephropathy, end-stage renal disease and duration of diabetes (Vaur *et al.*, 2003; Bertoni *et al.*, 2004; Nichols *et al.*, 2004; Wong *et al.*, 2005).

The two most important risk factors for the development of CHF are CHD and hypertension. These conditions are more prevalent in the patients with diabetes than in those without diabetes. A meta-analysis including 447 064 patients with diabetes estimated the rate of fatal CHD to be 5.4% in those with diabetes compared to 1.6% in those without (Huxley *et al.*, 2006). The prevalence of hypertension in those with diabetes is approximately double that in those without (Simonson, 1988) (see also Chapter 6).

Risk of developing diabetes in patients with CHF

Patients with advanced CHF (i.e. those in New York Heart Association (NYHA) classes III and IV) appear to have a greater risk of developing diabetes than those with milder symptoms (i.e. those in NYHA class II). In a subgroup analysis of 630 patients with CHF secondary to CHD in the Bezafibrate Infarction Prevention (BIP) study, NYHA class III was an independent risk factor for diabetes while NYHA class II was not (Tenenbaum *et al.*, 2003). In an Italian longitudinal study of 1339 elderly patients, CHF was an independent predictor of diabetes (Amato *et al.*, 1997). The association of CHF with diabetes was greater in patients in NYHA III and IV than those in NYHA I and II.

5.5   Diabetes and Mortality in Patients with CHF

Population studies

Diabetes is consistently an independent predictor of mortality in population studies of CHF:

- In Scotland, diabetes was as an independent predictor of mortality in both genders with CHF: hazard ratio 1.55 (1.41–1.70) and 1.50 (1.38–1.62) for men and women, respectively (Macintyre *et al.*, 2000).

- In Rotterdam, the presence of diabetes conferred a worse prognosis in patients with CHF: hazard ratio 3.19 (1.80–5.65) (Mosterd *et al.*, 2001).

- In the USA, diabetes was an independent predictor of mortality in 170 239 Medicare patients, with hazard ratios of 1.11 (1.06–1.16, $P < 0.05$) in Black patients and 1.22 (1.24–1.25, $P < 0.05$) in White patients (Croft *et al.*, 1999).

- In another small study of 495 patients with CHF, diabetes independently predicted mortality: odds ratio 1.71 (1.16–2.51, $P = 0.0065$) (Kamalesh and Nair, 2005).

Only one population study has considered whether or not diabetes might predict mortality according to aetiology of CHF. In 1246 French patients, diabetes was a risk factor for mortality only in patients with CHF secondary to CHD (hazard ratio 1.54 (1.13–2.09, $P=0.006$) but not for those with CHF secondary to other aetiologies (hazard ratio 0.65 (0.39–1.07, $P=0.09$) (de Groote *et al.*, 2004).

Clinical trials

In clinical trials of CHF, patients with diabetes have a consistently higher mortality rate than patients without diabetes (Ryden *et al.*, 2000; Erdmann *et al.*, 2001; Haas *et al.*, 2003; Deedwania *et al.*, 2005). Diabetes is an independent predictor of mortality in patients with CHF (Shindler *et al.*, 1996; Dries *et al.*, 2001; Domanski *et al.*, 2003; Brophy *et al.*, 2004; Gustafsson *et al.*, 2004; Pocock *et al.*, 2006).

In the SOLVD (enalapril versus placebo), BEST (bucindolol versus placebo) and DIG (digoxin versus placebo) studies, diabetes was an independent risk factor for mortality in patients with CHF. In these three trials the increased risk appeared to be confined to patients with CHF due to CHD. In the SOLVD study, the hazard ratio (HR) for those with diabetes was 1.29 (1.1–1.5). The HR was 1.37 (1.21–1.55) and 0.98 (0.76–1.32) for CHF secondary to CHD and non-CHD, respectively (Shindler *et al.*, 1996; Dries *et al.*, 2001). In the BEST study, the HR for those with diabetes and CHF secondary to CHD and non-CHD was 1.33 (1.12–1.58, $P=0.001$) and 0.98 (0.74–1.30, $P=0.89$), respectively (Domanski *et al.*, 2003). In the DIG study, the HR for those with diabetes and CHF secondary to CHD was 1.43 (1.26–1.63) (Brophy *et al.*, 2004). In DIG, no HR is available for CHF of non-CHD aetiology.

That diabetes is a predictor of mortality only in those with CHF due to CHD is not a consistent finding. Both DIAMOND-CHF (dofetilide versus placebo in CHF) and CHARM (candesartan versus placebo in CHF) reported that diabetes was an independent predictor of mortality regardless of the aetiology of CHF (Gustafsson *et al.*, 2004; Pocock *et al.*, 2006). In the CHARM study, patients with CHF and diabetes treated with insulin had an 80% increased risk of death compared to those without diabetes (HR 1.80 (1.56–2.08)). Patients with CHF and diabetes not treated with insulin had a 50% increased risk of death compared to those without diabetes (HR 1.50 (1.34–1.68)) (Pocock *et al.*, 2006).

Gender differences

Subgroup analysis of the Framingham study suggested that diabetes might be a predictor of mortality in women but not in men with CHF (HR 1.70 (1.21–2.38) and 0.99 (0.70–1.40) for women and men, respectively) (Ho *et al.*, 1993). The only clinical trial to report outcome of patients with diabetes by gender (the DIAMOND-CHF study) did not report this apparent mortality difference (Gustafsson *et al.*, 2004). The relative risk for mortality was 1.7 for women (95% CI 1.4–1.9, $P < 0.0001$) and 1.4 for men (95% CI 1.3–1.6, $P < 0.0001$).

Glycated haemoglobin (HbA1c)

One recent observational study of 123 patients with diabetes and advanced CHF compared the outcome of patients with HbA1c ≤ 7 against those with HbA1c > 7 (Eshaghian et al., 2006). Surprisingly, those with HbA1c ≤ 7 had an increased mortality rate (75% versus 50%, 2-year mortality, respectively). After multivariate adjustment HbA1c remained a significant independent predictor of mortality (HR 2.3, 95% CI 1.0–5.2). One possible explanation is that a low HbA1c reflects cachexia found in the sickest patients with CHF.

Chronic heart failure and mortality in patients with diabetes

Not surprisingly, patients with diabetes who develop CHF have a markedly increased mortality. Patients with diabetes in the DIABHYCAR study who developed CHF had a 12 times higher annual mortality than those who did not develop CHF (36.4% vs. 3.2%) (Vaur et al., 2003). In one large American cohort study of patients over the age of 64, patients with diabetes who developed CHF had a 5-year survival rate of 12.5% in comparison to an 80% 5-year survival rate of patients with diabetes who did not develop CHF (Bertoni et al., 2004).

5.6 Morbidity

Incidence of hospitalisation due to CHF in patients with diabetes

Patients with diabetes are frequently hospitalised for CHF. In a cohort of 48 000 patients with diabetes in California, those with HbA1c < 7 had an incidence of hospitalisation due to CHF of 4.5 per 1000 person-years compared to 9.2 per 1000 person-years for those with HbA1c > 10 (Iribarren et al., 2001). In the DIABHYCAR study, patients with diabetes and albuminuria had a similar incidence of hospitalisation due to CHF (10 per 1000 patient-years) (Vaur et al., 2003). Albuminuria is an independent predictor of first hospitalisation for CHF in patients with both diabetes and hypertension, with no previous history of myocardial infarction (MI) or heart failure (Hockensmith et al., 2004).

Hospitalisation due to CHF in patients with both diabetes and CHF

Patients with both diabetes and CHF are frequently hospitalised due to CHF. In the BEST trial, diabetes was an independent predictor of hospitalisation due to CHF (relative risk 1.16 (1.02–1.32), $P=0.027$) (Domanski et al., 2003). In the RESOLVD study, diabetes was again an independent predictor of CHF hospitalisation (Suskin et al., 2000).

In the placebo arm of MERIT-HF, patients with diabetes had a 76% (38–126%, $P < 0.0001$) greater risk of hospitalisation due to CHF compared to those without diabetes (Deedwania *et al.*, 2005). Patients with diabetes in the placebo group with NYHA III and IV CHF and ejection fraction < 25 had a risk of hospitalisation due to CHF that was almost four times higher than the risk for all placebo-treated patients without diabetes.

Patients with diabetes in the ATLAS CHF trial had more admissions to hospital than patients without diabetes (Ryden *et al.*, 2000). Patients with diabetes had an average of three all-cause hospitalisations with a mean of 21.4 days in hospital compared to 2.2 all-cause hospitalisations with a mean of 17.7 days in hospital for patients without diabetes.

Diabetes and severity of CHF

Patients with CHF and diabetes have more symptoms than those without diabetes. In a substudy of the RESOLVD trial, the presence of diabetes was associated with lower functional capacity and more severe heart failure symptoms (Suskin *et al.*, 2000).

5.7 Chronic Heart Failure and Abnormalities of Insulin and Glucose Metabolism

The prevalence of diabetes in populations with CHF has already been discussed. Insulin resistance, impaired fasting glucose and hyperinsulinaemia in the absence of diabetes are also common in CHF (Paolisso *et al.*, 1991, 1999; Swan *et al.*, 1994, Suskin *et al.*, 2000). Hyperinsulinaemia, impaired glucose tolerance and insulin resistance are risk factors for CHF, independent of diabetes and other established risk factors (Ingelsson *et al.*, 2005; Nielson and Lange, 2005).

A substudy of RESOLVD measured fasting glucose and insulin concentrations in 663 patients with NYHA class II–IV CHF (Suskin *et al.*, 2000). Of these patients 27% had diabetes. Of the 'non-diabetics' 11% met diagnostic criteria for diabetes, 12% had impaired fasting glucose concentrations and 34% had elevated plasma insulin concentration and insulin resistance (Figure 5.2). The presence of insulin resistance, hyperinsulinaemia or impaired fasting glucose was associated with lower functional capacity and more severe CHF symptoms.

Insulin resistance, in the absence of diabetes, is a prognostic indicator in CHF secondary to valvular heart disease (Paolisso *et al.*, 1999). Data are not available for CHF secondary to other aetiologies. Why insulin resistance is prevalent in patients with CHF is not fully understood, but the relationship is likely to be multifactorial (Coats and Anker, 2000). Hypotheses have arisen primarily from non-CHF populations. Possible contributing factors are sympathetic overactivity (Scherrer and Sartori, 1997), sedentary lifestyle, endothelial dysfunction, loss of skeletal muscle mass (Mancini *et al.*, 1992) and influence of cytokines such as TNF-α (Levine *et al.*, 1990; Miles *et al.*, 1997) and leptin (Doehner *et al.*, 2002) on peripheral insulin sensitivity.

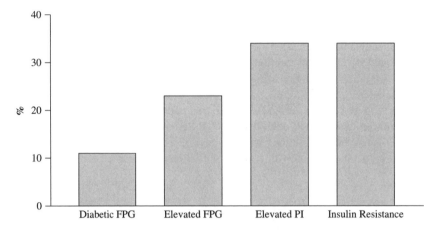

Figure 5.2 Non-diabetic patients in RESOLVD. FPG = fasting plasma glucose, PI = plasma insulin. Reproduced from Suskin N, McKelvie RS, Burns RJ, Latini R, Pericak D, Probstfield J *et al.* (2000). Glucose and insulin abnormalities relate to functional capacity in patients with congestive heart failure. *European Heart Journal* **21:** 1368–75.

The sympathetic nervous system (SNS) and insulin resistance

Patients with CHF have persistent activation of their sympathetic nervous system (SNS) (Reaven *et al.*, 1996; Scherrer and Sartori, 1997), and excessive activation of the SNS might lead to insulin resistance. In normal individuals, adrenaline infusion leads to acute insulin resistance (Scherrer and Sartori, 1997).

Skeletal muscle

Insulin increases skeletal muscle uptake of glucose. In healthy subjects, acute SNS activation decreases glucose uptake by skeletal muscles. Unloading of cardiopulmonary receptors, a manoeuvre that leads to selective reflex sympathetic activation in skeletal muscle, reduces insulin-induced stimulation of muscle glucose uptake by up to 25% (Scherrer and Sartori, 1997).

Adipose tissue

Stimulation of β-receptors in humans increases lipolysis, resulting in raised plasma free fatty acid (FFA) levels (Schiffelers *et al.*, 2001). In normal subjects infusion of norepinephrine results in increased plasma levels of FFAs (Marangou *et al.*, 1988). In patients with CHF, norepinephrine concentrations have been correlated with FFA concentrations (Paolisso *et al.*, 1991). The FFAs impair insulin-mediated glucose disposal in human skeletal muscle (Roden, 2004) and can stimulate hepatic gluconeogenesis (Lam *et al.*, 2003), further potentiating hyperglycaemia.

Norepinephrine and epinephrine also inhibit pancreatic insulin secretion in humans and stimulate hepatic gluconeogenesis and glycogenolysis, further worsening hyperglycaemia (Nonogaki, 2000).

How do abnormalities of glucose and insulin metabolism affect the SNS and renin–angiotensin–aldosterone system (RAAS)?

There is some experimental evidence suggesting that neurohormonal systems are activated by diabetes and/or insulin resistance, but this has not been demonstrated in patients with CHF. Hyperinsulinaemia increases circulating levels of norepinephrine and angiotensin II in normal volunteers (Anderson *et al.*, 1991; Reaven *et al.*, 1996; Scherrer and Sartori, 1997). Insulin resistance enhances the pressor response to angiotensin II in hypertensive patients (Gaboury *et al.*, 1994). Infusion of FFAs in rats appears to activate the SNS, increase norepinephrine levels and increase insulin resistance (Benthem *et al.*, 2000). Hyperglycaemia in normal humans and patients with diabetes causes increased SNS activity (Hoffman *et al.*, 1999; Marfella *et al.*, 2000). In experimental diabetes, although the circulating RAAS is usually normal or suppressed, there may be activation of the RAAS at the tissue level (Giacchetti *et al.*, 2005).

5.8 Why do Patients with Diabetes develop CHF?

Why are diabetes and insulin resistance associated with CHF? Several mechanisms may explain this:

- Risk factors for CHF are common in patients with diabetes (e.g. hypertension and CHD).

- Diabetes may have a direct effect on the myocardium.

- Diabetes may activate neurohormonal systems.

Effects of diabetes on the myocardium

Both systolic and diastolic abnormalities have been demonstrated in patients with diabetes without symptomatic evidence of cardiovascular disease. These abnormalities correlate with duration of diabetes and evidence of retinopathy / neuropathy (Annonu *et al.*, 2001). A full review of the molecular processes occurring in the heart of patients with diabetes is outwith the scope of this chapter and has been reviewed elsewhere (Taegtmeyer *et al.*, 2002; Young *et al.*, 2002). There are many putative metabolic mechanisms of the effect of diabetes on the myocardium, but most have been demonstrated in animals rather than in patients with CHF:

- *Hyperinsulinaemia* – In rats, insulin stimulates an increase in myocardial mass (Holmang *et al.*, 1996). Insulin may be a myocardial growth factor, increasing myocardial hypertrophy.

- *Advanced Glycosylation End-products (AGEs)* – In hyperglycaemia, glucose reacts non-enzymatically with proteins, producing AGEs (Jyothirmayi *et al.*, 1998). The AGEs are thought to be involved in a number of detrimental biochemical processes in diabetes. For example, in the myocardium of dogs with diabetes, cross-linking of collagen and subsequent deposition in the myocardium leads to increased chamber stiffness (Jyothirmayi *et al.*, 1998).

- *Reactive Oxygen Species* – Prolonged hyperglycaemia causes increased oxidative stress that leads to apoptosis in the myocardium of diabetic rats (Rosen *et al.*, 1998; Bojunga *et al.*, 2004). Increased oxidative stress has been noted in human failing myocardium (Sam *et al.*, 2005) and diabetic myocardium (Frustaci *et al.*, 2000).

- *Sarcoplasmic/ Endoplasmic-Reticulum* Ca^{2+}*-ATPase 2a (SERCA2a)* – SERCA2a replenishes intracellular calcium stores and is thought to play an important role in cardiac relaxation. AGEs cause post-translational modification of SERCA2a and result in a decrease in its activity in diabetic rats (Bidasee *et al.*, 2004). Subsequent treatment of the diabetic rats with insulin was found to decrease the modification of SERCA2a by AGEs and significantly improve cardiac function.

- *Free Fatty Acids (FFAs)* – Diabetic myocardium is more dependent on FFAs than normal myocardium. When insulin resistance is present, excess FFAs rather than glucose and lactate are metabolised by the myocardium. Patients with diabetes have increased plasma levels of FFAs, demonstrate increased utilisation and oxidation of FFAs in their myocardium and decreased myocardial glucose uptake (Herrero *et al.*, 2006). In obese rats, prolonged exposure to elevated levels of FFA causes myocardial apoptosis and contractile dysfunction (Zhou *et al.*, 2000). Increased FFA utilisation results in the uncoupling of oxidative phosphorylation, the inhibition of membrane ATPase activity and increased myocardial oxygen consumption. High levels of plasma FFAs in humans post-MI have been linked to an increase in serious arrhythmias (Gupta *et al.*, 1969; Tansey and Opie, 1983; Oliver and Opie, 1994). During myocardial ischaemia, FFAs have been shown to suppress myocardial contractility in rats (Henderson *et al.*, 1969). The partial inhibition of FFA oxidation in ischaemic swine myocardium leads to improved contractility (Chandler *et al.*, 2003). The influence of FFAs on contractility and apoptosis has not been demonstrated in patients with CHF.

- *Protein Kinase C* – Increased activation of the signal transduction pathway for protein kinase C has been demonstrated in diabetic rat hearts (Way *et al.*, 2001), and elevated levels of protein kinase C are found in failing human myocardium (Bowling *et al.*, 1999). In transgenic mice, over-expression of protein kinase C has lead to myocardial hypertrophy and dysfunction (Wakasaki *et al.*, 1997). Elevations in protein kinase C activity in response to hyperglycaemia have been demonstrated in various animal tissues and cultured endothelium (Way *et al.*, 2001). Increased protein kinase C activity leads to an increase in extracellular matrix deposition, causing thickening of the basement membrane, altered blood flow and increased vascular permeability. In rat cardiomyocytes, protein kinase C increases levels of ACE, leading to increases in angiotensin II (Zhang *et al.*, 2003).

- *Vascular Endothelial Growth Factor (VEGF)* – VEGF is expressed in response to hypoxia and may play an important role in the response to vascular injury. Following myocardial infarction, VEGF mRNA is increased in arteriolar smooth-muscle cells and infiltrating macrophages around the infarct site (Shinohara *et al.*, 1996). In patients with diabetes, there is a reduction in the amount of VEGF and its receptor found in the myocardium in comparison to patients without diabetes (Chou *et al.*, 2002). This is consistent with pathological reports of decreased collateralisation in diabetic myocardium following ischaemia (Abaci *et al.*, 1999).

In addition, there may be abnormalities of gene expression in the diabetic heart:

* In the myocardium of diabetic rats, prolonged hyperglycaemia has been shown to increase gene expression of muscle carnitine palmitoyltransferase-1 (Zhang *et al.*, 2002). This is a mitochondrial enzyme involved in the transportation of FFAs into the mitochondria, promoting myocardial use of FFAs.

* In non-ischaemic heart failure in humans, SERCA2a gene expression was decreased in those with diabetes (Razeghi *et al.*, 2002). An induction of the foetal gene programme occurs in patients with diabetes (Bristow, 1998; Razeghi *et al.*, 2001). Myosins are actin-based molecular motors. After birth β (slow)-myosin heavy chain (MHC) is down-regulated and α (fast)-MHC is up-regulated. In the diabetic rat heart there is induction of the fetal gene program and β-MHC is re-expressed whilst α-MHC is down-regulated (Depre *et al.*, 2000). This results in impaired contractility of the myocardium in diabetic animals (Dillman, 1980; Malhotra and Sanghi, 1997). A similar induction of the foetal gene programme, or down-regulation of the adult genes, is seen in the human failing heart (Bristow, 1998; Razeghi *et al.*, 2001). Diabetic patients with CHF are found to have lower levels of α-MHC gene expression than non-diabetics with CHF (Razeghi *et al.*, 2002). It may be that these changes are adaptive to reduce myocardial energy expenditure in the failing heart. Beta-blockers decrease expression of β-MHC and increase SERCA2a gene expression in patients with CHF (Young *et al.*, 2002; Yasumura *et al.*, 2003).

Pathological effects in the heart and blood vessels

Endothelial dysfunction

Endothelial dysfunction is a feature of both diabetes and CHF. In patients with diabetes and insulin-resistant individuals endothelial function is markedly impaired (Steinberg *et al.*, 1996). Hyperglycaemia has been shown to impair production of endothelium-derived nitric oxide in rabbit aorta (Tesfamariam *et al.*, 1991). Hyperglycaemia also stimulates extracellular matrix production, thickening the basement membrane in cultured human endothelial cells (Cagliero *et al.*, 1991). Both FFAs and hyperglycaemia have been shown to increase production of reactive oxygen species by cultured endothelial cells (Inoguchi *et al.*, 2000). The AGEs are involved in deactivation of nitric oxide and they impair vasodilation (Singh *et al.*, 2001).

Arterial stiffness

Diabetes increases arterial stiffness in humans (Wahlqvist *et al.*, 1988; Cockcroft *et al.*, 2005). Pulse pressure is a marker of arterial stiffness and predicts cardiovascular risk in patients with diabetes (Cockcroft *et al.*, 2005). Stiff arteries alter the haemodynamic state in such a way that afterload is increased and coronary perfusion pressure is decreased. It has been suggested that resultant myocardial ischaemia, if chronic, could lead to myocardial fibrosis and impaired systolic function (Ohtsuka et al., 1996; London and Guerin, 1999; Vinereanu et al., 2003).

Cardiac autonomic neuropathy

Patients with diabetic autonomic neuropathy have an impaired coronary vasodilatory response to sympathetic stimulation (Di Carli et al., 1999).

Diabetic microangiopathy

Microvascular disease has been suggested as a potential contributor to myocardial dysfunction in patients with diabetes (Kannel and McGee, 1979; Factor et al., 1980). The study of coronary microcirculation in vivo is particularly difficult. What is known has been derived from measurements such as coronary flow reserve. Microvascular processes can be studied in the retina but whether or not these same processes are occurring in the myocardium is unknown (Lawrenson et al., 2002). A recent study examined the relationship of retinopathy to the risk of developing CHF (Wong et al., 2005). The Atherosclerosis Risk in Community (ARIC) study is a population cohort study originally including 15 792 men and women aged 45–64 years old, of which 11 612 had retinal photography. The cumulative incidence of CHF was 5.4% over 6.2 years; 40% of those who developed CHF had diabetes and 13% of those who did not develop CHF had diabetes. After adjustment for risk factors, retinopathy remained independently related to incident CHF (relative risk 1.96 (1.51–2.54)). The pathogenesis of CHF in patients with diabetes may involve microvascular processes.

Is there a distinct 'diabetic cardiomyopathy'?

It has been proposed that diabetes has an effect on myocardial structure and function, independent of hypertension and CHD. Raised pro-insulin levels predict left ventricular systolic dysfunction independent of CHD and hypertension in the general population (Arnlov et al., 2001). Insulin resistance, glucose intolerance and diabetes are independently associated with adverse left ventricular remodelling, increased left ventricular mass and left ventricular hypertrophy in US population studies (Devereux et al., 2000; Sundstrom et al., 2000; Rutter et al., 2003). In the Framingham cohort, insulin resistance was associated with an increase in left ventricular mass in women but not in men (Rutter et al., 2003).

Over 30 years ago, Rubler et al. (1972) were the first to propose the existence of a cardiomyopathy associated specifically with diabetes. They described the pathology of four diabetic patients with dilated cardiomyopathy and significant renal disease but with no identifiable cause of their CHF. Each heart was dilated, with significant ventricular hypertrophy and areas of fibrosis. Rubler may have been describing four cases of cardiomyopathy unrelated to diabetes. Since then the existence of a distinct 'diabetic cardiomyopathy' has stimulated much debate. Studies in both animals and humans have demonstrated a number of different processes occurring in the myocardium of patients with diabetes that could influence its contractile function. These underlying processes are said to lead to a fibrosed, hypertrophied myocardium that is 'stiff' and 'poorly compliant' with impaired function.

5.9 Reducing the Risk of Diabetes in Patients with CHF

Lifestyle changes

Studies reporting that weight reduction and increased physical activity reduce the risk of progression to diabetes excluded patients with CHF by design (Diabetes Prevention Program Research Group, 2002) (see also Chapter 10).

Inhibition of the RAAS

Evidence that blocking the RAAS in patients with hypertension reduces the progression to diabetes is discussed in Chapter 6. There is a small amount of evidence that blocking the RAAS reduces the development of diabetes in patients with CHF.

- Enalapril reduced the incidence of diabetes when compared to placebo in a retrospective analysis of data from a single centre in the SOLVD study (HR 0.22 (0.10–0.46), $P < 0.0001$) (Vermes *et al.*, 2003).

- Candesartan reduced the incidence of diabetes in patients with CHF (Yusuf *et al.*, 2005). Of the 5436 patients who did not have diabetes at entry, 202 (7.4%) patients in the placebo group developed diabetes compared to 163 (6.0%) in the candesartan group (HR 0.78(0.64–0.96), $P = 0.02$).

5.10 Reducing the Development of CHF in Patients with Diabetes

Glycaemic control

Patients with diabetes and higher HbA1c concentrations are at increased risk of CHF (Iribarren *et al.*, 2001), but it is not known if improving glycaemic control in patients with diabetes reduces the incidence of CHF. For patients with type 2 diabetes the UKPDS trial did not show a significant reduction in the incidence of CHF with intensive glycaemic control (UK Prospective Diabetes Study (UKPDS) Group, 1998), and for patients with type 1 diabetes the DCCT/EDIC study did not report CHF event rates (Diabetes Control and Complications Trial / Epidemiology of Diabetes Interventions and Complications (DCCT/EDIC) Study Research Group, 2005).

Blood pressure control

Tight blood pressure control in patients with diabetes has been shown to reduce the incidence of CHF. In UKPDS 1148 hypertensive patients with diabetes without CHF were randomised to tight or less tight blood pressure control. Those patients assigned to tight blood pressure control had a decreased risk of developing CHF (HR 0.44 (0.2–0.94), $P = 0.0043$) (UK Prospective Diabetes Study Group, 1998a).

ACE Inhibitors

MICRO-HOPE was a substudy of 3577 patients with diabetes involved in the HOPE trial, and ramipril lowered the risk of developing CHF by 20% (4–34, $P = 0.019$) (Heart Outcomes Prevention Evaluation (HOPE) Study Investigators, 2000). PERSUADE was a substudy of 1502 patients with diabetes without CHF enrolled in EUROPA. Perindopril did not show a significant reduction in first hospitalisation for CHF, although the relative risk reduction was 46% (Daly *et al.*, 2005).

Angiotensin receptor blockers

In the diabetes subgroup of the LIFE study, losartan reduced the risk of first hospitalisation for CHF when compared to atenolol for the treatment of hypertension, with an HR of 0.59 (0.38–0.92, $P = 0.019$) (Lindholm *et al.*, 2002). The RENAAL study enrolled 1513 patients with diabetes and nephropathy. Patients were randomised to 50–100 mg of losartan or placebo, and a 32% reduction ($P = 0.005$) in the rate of first hospitalisation for CHF was observed with losartan (Brenner *et al.*, 2001). Similarly, in the Irbesartan Diabetic Nephropathy Trial (IDNT) 1715 patients with diabetes and nephropathy were randomised to irbesartan, amlodipine or placebo, and irbesartan reduced the incidence of CHF when compared to placebo (HR 0.72 (0.52–1.00), $P = 0.048$) (Lewis *et al.*, 2001).

5.11   Treatment of Diabetes in Patients with CHF

Screening for CHF in patients with diabetes

The presence of risk factors, particularly CHD, hypertension, proteinuria (Vaur *et al.*, 2003) and retinopathy (Wong *et al.*, 2005), should alert the physician to the increased risk of CHF. A history of symptoms of CHF should be sought. Electrocardiography, brain natriuretic peptide (BNP) and echocardiography should be investigated as potential strategies for identifying patients with diabetes who have asymptomatic LVSD or CHF.

Non-pharmacological measures

Strategies to improve glycaemic control through weight loss or increased physical activity have not been specifically studied in patients with both diabetes and CHF.

Metformin

Metformin is frequently said to be 'contraindicated' in patients with CHF. The American Diabetic Association guidelines state that metformin is contraindicated in patients with CHF (American Diabetes Association, 2006). The FDA have placed a 'black-box' warning on the metformin product packaging, stating that it is contraindicated in patients with CHF requiring pharmacological management. In the United Kingdom, neither the Scottish Intercollegiate Guideline Network nor the National Institute for Clinical Excellence, in their diabetes or CHF guidelines, state that metformin is contraindicated in CHF. There is no statement regarding metformin in the European Society of Cardiology or American Heart Association CHF guidelines.

Despite being 'contraindicated' in CHF, metformin is commonly used in patients with CHF in routine clinical practice. Of 1833 Canadians with diabetes and a new diagnosis of CHF, 11% were taking metformin alone and 47% were taking combination therapy with sulphonylurea and metformin (Eurich *et al.*, 2005). Of 16 417 Americans with diabetes admitted to hospital with CHF, 13% were discharged on metformin (Masoudi *et al.*, 2005). As metformin is commonly used in patients with diabetes and CHF, and the alternatives for treating diabetes in patients with CHF are limited, the risks of metformin in this population need to be established.

Metformin and lactic acidosis

In the 1970s phenformin, a drug from the same class (biguanides), was withdrawn after 306 cases of lactic acidosis were reported (Misbin, 1977). Metformin differs from phenformin in many ways. In contrast to phenformin, metformin does not require hepatic metabolism and is excreted unchanged by the kidney. As metformin is related to phenformin, there was much debate before its approval for use in the USA by the FDA in 1995. The FDA approved metformin but the presence of CHF was stated as a contraindication. In the first year of postmarketing surveillance in the USA, metformin was associated with a total of 47 cases of lactic acidosis and 18 of these patients had CHF (Misbin *et al.*, 1998).

Neither of the two retrospective cohort studies examining metformin use in patients with diabetes and CHF reported high rates of lactic acidosis (Eurich *et al.*, 2005; Masoudi *et al.*, 2005). The Canadian study ($n = 1833$) did not report any cases of lactic acidosis during the follow-up period (Eurich *et al.*, 2005). The American study ($n = 16417$) reported readmission rates with metabolic acidosis as 2.3% for those treated with metformin and 2.6% for those not treated with metformin ($P = 0.40$) (Masoudi *et al.*, 2005). The risk of lactic acidosis associated with metformin in patients with diabetes and CHF does not appear to be high.

Outcomes of patients with diabetes and CHF on metformin

The two retrospective, non-randomised cohort studies of patients with diabetes and CHF suggest that outcomes may, if anything, be better on metformin therapy than other therapies for diabetes. It must be stressed that these two studies were not prospective, randomised or designed to address the safety or efficacy of metformin in this population. In the Canadian patients with a new diagnosis of CHF, metformin monotherapy was associated with a reduced 1-year mortality when compared to those on sulphonylureas (adjusted HR 0.66 (0.44–0.97)) (Eurich *et al.*, 2005). One-year mortality was also reduced for patients taking metformin and sulphonylurea combination therapy when compared to those on sulphonylurea monotherapy (adjusted HR 0.54 (0.42–0.70)). In Americans admitted to hospital with CHF, metformin was associated with a reduced 1-year mortality when compared to those treated with insulin or sulphonylurea (24.7% vs. 36%, $P < 0.0001$) (Masoudi *et al.*, 2005). Patients treated with metformin had a significantly lower risk of readmission for all-causes than those not treated with an insulin-sensitising drug (68% compared to 72%, $P = 0.0003$). Patients treated with metformin had a significantly lower risk of readmission due to CHF than those not treated with an insulin-sensitising drug (59% compared to 65%, $P < 0.0001$).

There are theoretical reasons that support why metformin might not be detrimental in CHF. Metformin improves endothelial function in patients with diabetes treated with insulin (Jager *et al.*, 2005). In a canine model of diabetes, metformin decreased cross-linking of collagen by AGEs with consequent improvement in myocardial performance (Jyothirmayi *et al.*, 1998).

An argument can therefore be made that metformin should not be universally 'contraindicated' in CHF. The incidence of lactic acidosis does not appear to be high. Before definitive conclusions can be drawn, prospective randomised studies both in stable CHF and in acute decompensated CHF are necessary to determine beneficial or adverse effects.

Insulin

Insulin and the incidence of CHF in patents with diabetes

The use of insulin is an independent risk factor for the development of CHF in patients with diabetes (Nichols *et al.*, 2004). An American retrospective cohort study of 23 440 patients with diabetes but without CHF examined the effect of initiation of any single new therapy for diabetes on admission to hospital for CHF (Karter *et al.*, 2005). Patients commenced on insulin had a higher incidence of hospitalisation due to CHF than those commenced on sulphonylureas (adjusted HR 1.56 (1.00–2.45), $P = 0.05$). It seems likely that, rather than insulin causing CHF, insulin use is a marker for patients who have diabetes of longer duration and have more severe macrovascular complications. The UKPDS did not show an increase in CHF with insulin treatment (UK Prospective Diabetes Study (UKPDS) Group, 1998).

Insulin and mortality in CHF

In subgroup analyses of clinical trials in patients with diabetes and CHF, insulin has been an independent predictor of mortality. An analysis of the CHARM study demonstrated that patients with diabetes treated with insulin had a greater risk of death than patients with diabetes not treated with insulin (HR 1.80 (1.56–2.08) vs. HR 1.5 (1.34–1.68)) (Pocock *et al.*, 2006). Similarly, data from the BEST trial demonstrated that treatment with insulin was a significant independent predictor of cardiovascular mortality (HR 1.3 (1.03–1.65)) (Domanski *et al.*, 2003).

In a retrospective analysis, 132 of 554 consecutive patients referred to an advanced heart failure centre had diabetes (Smooke *et al.*, 2005). Forty-three were insulin treated. One-year survival was 89.7% in patients without diabetes, 85.8% in patients with diabetes not on insulin and 62.1% in patients with diabetes on insulin. After multivariate analysis, treatment with insulin was an independent predictor of mortality (HR 4.30 (1.69–10.94)), while for patients with diabetes on no insulin treatment it was not (HR 0.95 (0.31–2.93)). The baseline characteristics were markedly different between the three groups.

In contrast, an American retrospective cohort study of over 16 000 patients with diabetes and CHF did not identify any association between insulin and mortality (HR 0.96 (0.88–1.05)) (Masoudi *et al.*, 2005), and in the UKPDS study insulin use did not predict mortality (UK Prospective Diabetes Study (UKPDS) Group, 1998).

It is unlikely that insulin causes increased mortality in patients with CHF and diabetes. In some trials, insulin appears to be a marker for patients with diabetes of longer duration, perhaps with more extensive macrovascular disease.

Experimental evidence: effects of insulin in CHF?

There is experimental evidence that has led some to suggest that insulin is theoretically attractive in CHF. Insulin is a potent vasodilator of human skeletal muscle in patients with CHF (but without diabetes) (Parsonage *et al.*, 2001), and insulin is a positive inotrope in heart tissue (in patients with and without diabetes but without CHF) (von Lewinski *et al.*, 2005). In normal volunteers, however, insulin decreases renal excretion of sodium (DeFronzo *et al.*, 1975). Insulin also up-regulates the AT1 receptor in opossum kidney cells, which could further contribute to sodium retention (Nickenig and Bohm, 1998; Banday *et al.*, 2005), and sodium retention might unmask previous subclinical myocardial dysfunction. To determine whether insulin-based strategies for the management of CHF are beneficial or detrimental, prospective trials randomising to different treatment strategies are needed.

Sulphonylureas

Sulphonylureas are frequently used in patients with diabetes and CHF. Of 1833 Canadians with diabetes and a new diagnosis of CHF, 42% were treated with sulphonylurea monotherapy and 47% were treated with a combination of sulphonylurea and metformin (Eurich *et al.*, 2005). The mechanism of action of sulphonylureas involves increased insulin production, and sulphonylureas stimulate endogenous insulin production (see also Chapter 11). This is not the most attractive mechanism of improving glycaemic control in patients with the insulin-resistant states of diabetes and CHF. Primarily due to concerns relating to the other classes of oral hypoglycaemic agents, this class of drug is preferentially used in patients with CHF.

Sulphonylureas and mortality

An American retrospective cohort study of over 16 000 patients with diabetes and CHF did not identify any relationship between sulphonylurea use and mortality (HR 0.99 (0.91–1.08)) (Masoudi *et al.*, 2005). As previously cited, in a non-randomised cohort study of patients with diabetes and CHF, those with a new diagnosis of CHF had a better 1-year mortality on metformin when compared to those on sulphonylureas (adjusted HR 0.66 (0.44–0.97)) (Eurich *et al.*, 2005).

Sulphonylureas and the incidence of CHF in patients with diabetes

In the UKPDS study, sulphonylurea use in patients with diabetes but not CHF was not associated with the development of CHF (UK Prospective Diabetes Study (UKPDS) Group, 1998). As previously cited, an American retrospective cohort study found that patients with diabetes but without CHF commenced on insulin had a higher incidence of hospitalisation due to CHF than those commenced on sulphonylureas (adjusted HR 1.56 (1.00–2.45), $P = 0.05$) (Karter *et al.*, 2005).

To establish whether sulphonylurea-based strategies result in improved outcomes when compared to metformin or insulin-based strategies, a prospective study would be needed

Thiazolidinediones

Thiazolidinediones (glitazones) are a new group of oral anti-diabetic agents that are peroxisome proliferator-activated (PPAR-γ) receptor agonists. In clinical trials, both rosiglitazone and pioglitazone cause weight gain that averages between 1 and 3 kg (Aronoff *et al.*, 2000; Philips *et al.*, 2001; Baksi *et al.*, 2004; Tan *et al.*, 2004; Charbonnel *et al.*, 2005; Weissman *et al.*, 2005). This weight gain is thought to be multifactorial. An increase in subcutaneous fat and a decrease in visceral fat have been demonstrated in patients with diabetes treated with glitazones (Miyazaki *et al.*, 2002; Smith *et al.*, 2005). Fluid retention has been evident in many trials of glitazones, with an associated decrease in haemoglobin and haematocrit, and rosiglitazone and pioglitazone appear to cause peripheral oedema to a similar extent (Aronoff *et al.*, 2000; Philips *et al.*, 2001; Baksi *et al.*, 2004; Tan *et al.*, 2004; Charbonnel *et al.*, 2005; Weissman *et al.*, 2005). The mechanisms whereby glitazones increase plasma volume and cause peripheral oedema are not clear. In healthy volunteers, glitazones promote renal sodium retention (Zanchi *et al.*, 2004). Increased renal sodium and water retention has also been demonstrated in normal rats (Song *et al.*, 2004). Glitazones have also been shown to stimulate an increase in human endothelial permeability *in vitro* (Idris *et al.*, 2003) and to increase intestinal ion transport in humans, promoting water retention (Hosokawa *et al.*, 1999).

The rate of oedema increases markedly when glitazones are used in combination with insulin. For example, when rosiglitazone was used in combination with insulin the rate of oedema was 16.2% for those treated with 8 mg, 13.1% for those with 4 mg and 4.7% for those treated with placebo (Raskin *et al.*, 2001). When pioglitazone was combined with insulin, the rate of oedema was 15.3% for those treated with pioglitazone and insulin compared to 7.0% for those treated with insulin and placebo (Rosenstock *et al.*, 2002).

Should glitazones be used in patients with NYHA class III or IV CHF?

Glitazones cause weight gain and fluid retention, and some studies have reported an increased incidence of CHF. Very few of the clinical trials looking at glitazones as monotherapy or in combination with other oral hypoglycaemics reported cases of CHF, and CHF was an exclusion criterion for entry into the study (e.g. Baksi *et al.*, 2004; Kerenyi *et al.*, 2004; Bailey *et al.*, 2005). In the clinical trials where glitazones were used in conjunction with insulin the incidence of CHF increases (Raskin *et al.*, 2001; Rosenstock *et al.*, 2002; Davidson *et al.*, 2006). One trial of pioglitazone in combination with insulin reported an incidence of CHF of 1.1% ($n = 4$) with pioglitazone and insulin compared to 0% with placebo and insulin (Rosenstock *et al.*, 2002). The largest trial using rosiglitazone in combination with insulin reported an incidence of CHF of 1.9% ($n = 4$) with rosiglitazone and insulin compared to 1% ($n = 1$) with placebo and insulin (Raskin *et al.*, 2001).

The PROactive study randomised 5238 patients with type 2 diabetes and evidence of macrovascular disease to pioglitazone or placebo (Dormandy *et al.*, 2005): 48% had CHD. Patients on pioglitazone had a reduction in cardiovascular death, MI and strokes, which was the main secondary endpoint in the study. Oedema without CHF was reported in 21.6% of those taking pioglitazone versus 12.9% of those taking placebo. Patients with diabetes but without CHF gained an average of 3 kg on pioglitazone (those on placebo had no weight gain). Hospitalisation due to CHF occurred in 6% of those taking pioglitazone and 4% of those taking placebo.

Three cohort studies have examined the incidence of CHF in patients with diabetes (without CHF) treated with glitazones: 33 544 patients with diabetes but without CHF in a health insurance claims database were studied over 40 months (Delea *et al.*, 2003). New users of glitazones were compared to those established on other oral treatments. New onset CHF (both in- and out-patient diagnoses) was increased for those on glitazones compared to other therapies (adjusted HR 1.76 (1.43–2.18), $P < 0.001$). In absolute terms, the adjusted incidence of CHF at 40 months was 8.2% among patients on glitazones and 5.3% among those on other therapies.

An American cohort study of 23 440 patients with diabetes but without CHF examined the initiation of any single new therapy for diabetes and its impact on time to admission to hospital for CHF (Karter *et al.*, 2005). Although the incidence of CHF was higher in those patients on pioglitazone, after adjusting for confounding factors the initiation of pioglitazone, relative to sulphonylureas, did not significantly increase the incidence of hospitalisation due to CHF (adjusted HR 1.28 (0.85–1.92), $P = 0.2$).

One further retrospective case–control study examined 288 patients with diabetes hospitalised due to CHF and matched them with 1652 patients with diabetes who had not been hospitalised due to CHF (Hartung *et al.*, 2005). After adjustment, there was a non-significant trend towards an increase in hospitalisations due to CHF in those on glitazones (adjusted HR 1.37(0.98–1.92)).

Cohort studies of patients with diabetes and CHF receiving glitazones

Two studies have examined the use of glitazones in patients with CHF. The American retrospective cohort study of over 16 000 patients with diabetes and CHF demonstrated that 1-year mortality was lower for those treated with glitazones than for those not treated with an insulin-sensitiser (30.1% vs. 36%, $P < 0.0001$) (Masoudi *et al.*, 2005). Even after adjustment for patient characteristics and other medications, glitazones were still associated with a lower risk of death (HR 0.87(0.80–0.94)). Patients treated with glitazones had a significantly higher risk of readmission for all-causes than those not treated with an insulin-sensitising drug (75% compared to 72%, $P = 0.02$). Patients treated with glitazones also had a significantly higher risk of readmission due to CHF than those not treated with an insulin-sensitising drug (68% compared to 65%, $P = 0.02$). The risk of readmission due to CHF with glitazones was no different with or without concurrent insulin treatment.

A retrospective casenote review of 111 consecutive out-patients with CHF treated with glitazones included 50 patients in NYHA class III (Tang *et al.*, 2003). Mean ejection fraction was 28.6%. Nineteen (17.1%) patients developed fluid retention following glitazone initiation. Fluid retention was defined as weight gain of over 10 lb with clinical signs of fluid overload. Peripheral oedema was identified in 18 of the 19 patients. Two of the 19 patients had clinical or x-ray evidence of pulmonary congestion. Five of the 19 were hospitalised for management of the fluid retention. Fluid retention was usually quickly reversed upon drug withdrawal and an increase in diuretics.

Glitazones and cardiac structure and function

Do glitazones simply precipitate CHF through weight gain, fluid retention and peripheral oedema, or do they have detrimental effects on cardiac structure and function as well? In isolated rat hearts, trogliazone has positive inotropic actions and negative chronotropic actions (Shimoyama *et al.*, 1999). A 48-week study with troglitazone in patients with diabetes demonstrated no change in left ventricular mass or cardiac function as measured by echocardiography, but troglitazone did increase stroke volume and cardiac index (Ghazzi *et al.*, 1997). A 52-week study comparing glibencalmide with rosiglitazone demonstrated that neither drug caused a reduction in ejection fraction as measured by echocardiography (St John Sutton *et al.*, 2002).

Little is known about the effect of glitazones on cardiac function in patients with CHF. One small study in eight patients with NYHA class II and III CHF and diabetes surprisingly demonstrated an increase in stroke volume and ejection fraction after a single oral dose of troglitazone (Ogino *et al.*, 2002), and the mechanism for this is not clear.

Thus, there are no clinical data to suggest that glitazones affect cardiac structure and function but studies in patients with CHF and diabetes with more detailed cardiac imaging are required.

Should glitazones be contraindicated in patients with CHF and diabetes?

Glitazones are an effective therapy to control blood glucose in patients with diabetes. They cause weight gain, fluid retention and peripheral oedema and it is therefore appropriate that they are not recommended in patients with NYHA class III or IV CHF. Should glitazones be contraindicated in those with diabetes and NYHA class I or II as well? There are few data to guide this decision but it is likely that these agents would result in more frequent decompensations of CHF. A consensus statement published jointly by the ADA/AHA states that glitazones can be used cautiously in patients with

NYHA class I/II CHF, but should not be used in patients with NYHA class III/IV CHF (Nesto *et al.*, 2003). The FDA states that glitazones are not recommended for use in patients with NYHA class III/IV CHF.

5.12 Treatment of CHF in Patients with Diabetes

The diagnosis of diabetes in clinical trials of CHF

Various definitions of diabetes are used in clinical trials of CHF. For example, in ATLAS only those receiving medical therapy for diabetes were considered as having diabetes (Ryden *et al.*, 2000) whereas in SOLVD the diagnosis was based on self-reporting by the patient or documentation in the patient's medical records (Shindler *et al.*, 1996). The unrecognised prevalence of diabetes and impaired glucose tolerance in RESOLVD suggests that it is likely that many patients with unrecognised abnormalities of glucose metabolism are included in the major trials of CHF. The diagnostic criteria for diabetes in clinical practice are described in Chapter 11.

Pharmacological therapies

Diuretics

Diuretics are necessary for the treatment of the symptoms of fluid overload in CHF. There are few data to indicate their effects in patients with and without diabetes. In the RALES study 25% of patients have a history of diabetes at baseline (Pitt and Perez, 2000). The mortality benefit with spironolactone was seen in those with diabetes (HR 0.70 (0.52–0.94), $P = 0.019$) and without diabetes (HR 0.70 (0.60–0.82), $P < 0.001$).

Digoxin, nitrates and hydralazine

No diabetes subgroup analysis is available from DIG, V-HeFT, V-HeFT II or A-HeFT.

ACE inhibitors

Neither the CONSENSUS nor the SOLVD trials have published data analysed by the presence or absence of diabetes. In the ATLAS trial (19% with diabetes) of high-versus low-dose lisinopril, the relative risk reduction in mortality between high- and low-dose lisinopril was 14% in patients with diabetes and 6% in those without diabetes (Ryden *et al.*, 2000). The interaction P value was not significant ($P = 0.502$).

A large meta-analysis of seven ACE-inhibitor trials was not exclusively of CHF but included three trials of post-MI left ventricular dysfunction (Shekelle *et al.*, 2003). A total of 2398 patients with diabetes and 10 188 patients without diabetes were included. The relative risk of mortality for treatment with ACE inhibitors versus placebo was 0.85 (0.78–0.92) in patients without diabetes and 0.84 (0.70–1.00) in patients with diabetes.

ACE inhibitors and hypoglycaemia

ACE inhibitors may increase the risk of hypoglycaemia (see also Chapter 6, p. 148). Two case–control studies identified an association between ACE inhibitors and hypoglycaemia, albeit in a population without CHF. The first was a Dutch study of patients with diabetes treated with insulin or oral hypoglycaemics (Herings *et al.*, 1995). Hypoglycaemia was independently associated with ACE inhibitors (odds ratio 2.8(1.4–5.7)). A Scottish case–control study confirmed this finding (adjusted odds ratio 4.3 (1.2–16.0), $P = 0023$) (Morris *et al.*, 1997). A larger cohort study in patients with diabetes (the proportion with CHF was not stated), using insulin or sulphonylureas, did not identify an association between severe hypoglycaemia and ACE inhibitors after adjusting for confounding factors (Shorr *et al.*, 1997). An experimental study in normal volunteers showed that captopril did not attenuate the hormonal or symptomatic response to hypoglycaemia (Oltmanns *et al.*, 2003).

ACE inhibitors should therefore be prescribed for all patients with diabetes and CHF. The apparent small increase in hypoglycaemic episodes warrants further patient education.

Beta-blockers

Patients with CHF and diabetes are less likely to be discharged from hospital on beta-blocker treatment than patients with CHF who do not have diabetes (odds ratio 0.72 (0.55–0.94) (Wlodarczyk *et al.*, 2003). It is possible that this stems from concerns over beta-blocker use in patients with diabetes. In the 1980s, beta-blockers were thought to be 'contraindicated' in patients with diabetes. We will review the evidence of clinical benefit of beta-blockers in patients with CHF and diabetes. We will then discuss the historical issues that led to the previous concerns.

The major trials of beta-blockers in CHF that demonstrated a reduction in mortality included between 12% and 29% of patients with diabetes (Packer *et al.*, 1996; CIBIS II Investigators and Committee, 1999; MERIT-HF Study Group, 1999; Packer *et al.*, 1996, 2001). Subgroup analyses suggest that patients with and without diabetes have similar benefits (Bristow *et al.*, 1996; Erdmann *et al.*, 2001; Mohacsi *et al.*, 2001; Deedwania *et al.*, 2005).

A total of 24.6% of patients in a meta-analysis of landmark trials of beta-blockers in CHF had diabetes (Haas *et al.*, 2003). Patients with diabetes on beta-blockers had a relative risk of mortality of 0.84 (0.73–0.96, $P = 0.011$) when compared to placebo. Patients without diabetes had a relative risk of mortality of 0.72 (0.65–0.79, $P < 0.001$) when compared to placebo.

A second meta-analysis of CIBIS-II, COPERNICUS and MERIT-HF confirmed the benefit of beta-blockers in patients with CHF and diabetes (Shekelle *et al.*, 2003). Patients without diabetes on beta-blockers had a relative risk of mortality of 0.65 (0.57–0.74) compared to placebo. Patients with diabetes on beta-blockers had a relative risk of mortality of 0.77 (0.61–0.96) compared to placebo.

Beta-blockers reduce hospitalisations for CHF (Packer *et al.*, 1996, 2001; Australia/New Zealand Heart Failure Research Collaborative Group, 1997; CIBIS II Investigators and Committee, 1999; Hjalmarson *et al.*, 2000; Beta-Blocker Evaluation of Survival Trial Investigators, 2001). Patients with diabetes on subgroup analysis have similar benefits to those without diabetes (Erdmann *et al.*, 2001; Mohacsi *et al.*, 2001; Domanski *et al.*, 2003; Deedwania *et al.*, 2005). Metoprolol CR/XL significantly reduced the relative risk of hospitalisation in patients with diabetes by 37% (53–15%, $P = 0.0026$) compared to 35% (48–19%, $P = 0.0002$) in those patients without diabetes. In the BEST study, treatment with bucindolol was associated with a reduction in total hospitalisations (HR 0.85 (0.73–0.99), $P = 0.039$) and CHF hospitalisations (HR 0.72 (0.60–0.88), $P = 0.001$) in patients with diabetes (Domanski *et al.*, 2003). In patients without diabetes there was a reduction in CHF hospitalisations (HR 0.81 (0.69–0.95), $P = 0.0078$), but not total hospitalisations (HR 0.95 (0.84–1.08), $P = 0.4270$).

In the 1980s, concerns about the adverse effects of beta-blockers on patients with diabetes included increased hypoglycaemia, dyslipidaemia and decreased insulin sensitivity. Beta-blockers in hypertensive patients cause small changes in lipids, with reductions in high-density lipoprotein and raised triglycerides (Fogari *et al.*, 1990; Kostis and Sanders, 2005), but this has not been studied in patients with CHF. In hypertensive patients without CHF, first- and second-generation beta-blockers decrease insulin sensitivity and can increase the risk of developing diabetes (Kostis and Sanders, 2005).

The biological response to hypoglycaemia involves SNS activation, which leads to the symptoms of hypoglycaemia: tremor, palpitations, tachycardia and sweating. Adrenaline stimulates hepatic gluconeogenesis and glycogenolysis to restore glucose levels. There are concerns that beta-blockade may decrease hypoglycaemic awareness and blunt the compensatory increase in plasma glucose.

Frequency of hypoglycaemic episodes

One large retrospective cohort study examined the use of antihypertensive agents in 13 559 elderly patients with diabetes but without CHF prescribed insulin or sulphonylureas (Shorr *et al.*, 1997). Patients on insulin experienced a significant increase in the risk of serious hypoglycaemia with non-selective beta-blockers (relative risk 2.16 (1.15–4.02)), but not cardioselective beta-blockers (relative risk 0.86 (0.36–1.33)). No such effect was seen for those on sulphonylueas. Two smaller case–control studies of patients with diabetes did not identify a relationship between beta-blockers and hypoglycaemia (Herings *et al.*, 1995; Morris *et al.*, 1997). The proportion of patients with CHF in these studies was not stated.

The UKPDS blood pressure study examined the efficacy of atenolol versus captopril in reducing complications in 758 patients with diabetes and hypertension, and there was no difference in the rate of hypoglycaemia between the two groups (UK Prospective Diabetes Study Group, 1998b).

Hypoglycaemic awareness

Small studies in patients without CHF suggest that the response to hypoglycaemia might change with use of beta-blockers. Tremor and palpitations decrease, but sweating increases (Sawicki and Siebenhofer, 2001). In healthy volunteers, hypoglycaemic awareness was not affected by treatment with either cardioselective or non-cardioselective beta-blockers (Kerr *et al.*, 1990).

Recovery from hypoglycaemia

Hepatic glucose production is controlled in part by β_2 receptor stimulation. Blockade of this receptor could theoretically lead to prolonged recovery from hypoglycaemia. Prolonged hypoglycaemia has been described with use of a non-cardioselective beta-blocker (propanolol), but not with β_1-selective beta-blockers or carvedilol (Giugliano *et al.*, 1997; Sawicki and Siebenhofer, 2001). However, in one small study in patients with type 1 diabetes, both non-cardioselective and cardioselective beta-blockers led to prolongation of hypoglycaemia (Popp *et al.*, 1984). These studies were small studies in patients without CHF, and there is no evidence specifically addressing the frequency or severity of hypoglycaemic episodes in patients with CHF and diabetes.

The marked clinical benefits of beta-blockers in patients with diabetes and CHF outweigh a possible increased risk of hypoglycaemia and dyslipidaemia or decreased insulin sensitivity. Education of prevention, recognition and management of hypoglycaemic episodes is already established in the management of patients with diabetes.

Angiotensin receptor blockers

There have been no separate diabetes subgroup analyses published for ELITE-I, ELITE-II, VAL-HeFT, CHARM-alternative or CHARM-added. A separate analysis has been published analysing pooled data from the low ejection fraction CHARM trials (Young *et al.*, 2004): 35.7% of the patients taking candesartan experienced cardiovascular death or CHF hospitalisation compared to 41.3% in the placebo group (HR 0.82 (0.74–0.90), $P < 0.001$), and the benefit of candesartan was similar in those with and without diabetes (P value for interaction was 0.12).

Complex pacemaker therapies

Cardiac resynchronisation therapy (CRT)

Large randomised trials have demonstrated the safety and efficacy of CRT in patients with CHF with marked symptoms (Bristow *et al.*, 2004; Cleland *et al.*, 2005) The major clinical trials of these devices have not reported data for the diabetes subgroup. One small ($n = 97$) non-randomised observational study of CRT has specifically examined the effects of CRT in patients with and without diabetes (Kies *et al.*, 2005): 33% of the patients had diabetes, and there was no statistical difference in the clinical response rate between patients with and without diabetes.

Implantable cardioverter-defibrillator (ICD)

Of the patients in SCD-HeFT 30% had diabetes. For ICD therapy versus placebo the hazard ratios were 0.95 (97.5% CI 0.68–1.33) for patients with diabetes ($n = 524$) and 0.67 (97.5% CI 0.50–0.90) for patients without diabetes (Bardy *et al.*, 2005). This possible (subgroup derived) lack of efficacy in patients with diabetes may warrant further study.

Possible future therapy

Etomoxir

Etomoxir is an inhibitor of FFA metabolism and promoter of glucose metabolism. It has been shown to reverse foetal gene expression in animals, and in a single clinical study in patients with CHF it improved systolic function (Bristow, 2000).

5.13   Conclusions

Diabetes and CHF have overlapping pathophysiological processes, and commonly coexist. Patients with both diabetes and CHF should be managed by clinicians (doctors and nurses) with an interest in both diabetes and CHF, and those caring for patients with both CHF and diabetes should be aware of the issues that arise when these conditions occur together. Local discussions should focus on the management of issues raised by the concurrence of diabetes and CHF. Doctors and nurse specialists with an interest in diabetes and CHF should be aware of the issues that complicate the management of these patients and systems of care put in place to achieve optimal management. Efforts should be directed towards establishing patients with diabetes and CHF on optimal medical therapy for CHF, including the use of diuretics, ACE inhibitors and beta-blockers. Strategies for managing diabetes in patients with CHF should be prospectively compared.

References

Abaci A, Kahraman S, Eryol NK, Arinc H, Ergin A (1999). Effect of diabetes mellitus on formation of coronary collateral vessels. *Circulation* **99**: 2239–42.

Agoston I, Cameron CS, Yao D, Dela RA, Mann DL, Deswal A (2004). Comparison of outcomes of white versus black patients hospitalized with heart failure and preserved ejection fraction. *American Journal of Cardiology* **94**: 1003–7.

Amato L, Paolisso G, Cacciatore F, Ferrara N, Ferrara P, Canonico S *et al.* (1997). Congestive heart failure predicts the development of non-insulin-dependent diabetes mellitus in the elderly. The Osservatorio Geriatrico Regione Campania Group. *Diabetes and Metabolism* **23**: 213–8.

American Diabetes Association (2006). Standards of medical care in diabetes – 2006. *Diabetes Care* **29**: S4–42.

Anderson EA, Hoffman RP, Balon TW, Sinkey CA, Mark AL (1991). Hyperinsulinemia produces both sympathetic neural activation and vasodilation in normal humans. *Journal of Clinical Investigation* **87**: 2246–52.

Annonu AK, Fattah AA, Mokhtar MS, Ghareeb S, Elhendy A (2001). Left ventricular systolic and diastolic functional abnormalities in asymptomatic patients with non-insulin-dependent diabetes mellitus. *Journal of the American Society of Echocardiography* **14**: 885–91.

Arnlov J, Lind L, Zethelius B, Andren B, Hales CN, Vessby B *et al.* (2001). Several factors associated with the insulin resistance syndrome are predictors of left ventricular systolic dysfunction in a male population after 20 years of follow-up. *American Heart Journal* **142**: 720–4.

Aronoff S, Rosenblatt S, Braithwaite S, Egan JW, Mathisen AL, Schneider RL (2000). Pioglitazone hydrochloride monotherapy improves glycemic control in the treatment of patients with type 2 diabetes: a 6-month randomized placebo-controlled dose–response study. The Pioglitazone 001 Study Group. *Diabetes Care* **23**: 1605–11.

Aronow WS, Ahn C (1999). Incidence of heart failure in 2,737 older persons with and without diabetes mellitus. *Chest* **115**: 867–8.

Australia/New Zealand Heart Failure Research Collaborative Group (1997). Randomised, placebo-controlled trial of carvedilol in patients with congestive heart failure due to ischaemic heart disease. *Lancet* **349**: 375–80.

Bailey CJ, Bagdonas A, Rubes J, McMorn SO, Donaldson J, Biswas N *et al.* (2005). Rosiglitazone/metformin fixed-dose combination compared with uptitrated metformin alone in type 2 diabetes mellitus: A 24-week, multicenter, randomized, double-blind, parallel-group study. *Clinical Therapeutics* **27**: 1548–61.

Baksi A, James RE, Zhou B, Nolan JJ (2004). Comparison of uptitration of gliclazide with the addition of rosiglitazone to gliclazide in patients with type 2 diabetes inadequately controlled on half-maximal doses of a sulphonylurea. *Acta Diabetologica* **41**: 63–9.

Banday AA, Siddiqui AH, Menezes MM, Hussain T (2005). Insulin treatment enhances AT1 receptor function in OK cells. *American Journal of Physiology. Renal Physiology* **288**: F1213–9.

Bardy GH, Lee KL, Mark DB, Poole JE, Packer DL, Boineau R *et al.* (2005). Amiodarone or an implantable cardioverter-defibrillator for congestive heart failure. *New England Journal of Medicine* **352**: 225–37.

Benthem L, Keizer K, Wiegman CH, de Boer SF, Strubbe JH, Steffens AB *et al.* (2000). Excess portal venous long-chain fatty acids induce syndrome X via HPA axis and sympathetic activation. *American Journal of Physiology. Endocrinology and Metabolism* **279**: E1286–93.

Bertoni AG, Hundley WG, Massing MW, Bonds DE, Burke GL, Goff DC, Jr (2004). Heart failure prevalence, incidence, and mortality in the elderly with diabetes. *Diabetes Care* **27**: 699–703.

Beta-Blocker Evaluation of Survival Trial Investigators (2001). A trial of the beta-blocker bucindolol in patients with advanced chronic heart failure. *New England Journal of Medicine* **344**: 1659–67.

Bhoopatkar H, Simmons D (1996). Diabetes and hyperglycaemia among patients with congestive cardiac failure in a multiethnic population. *New Zealand Medical Journal* **109**: 268–70.

Bidasee KR, Zhang Y, Shao CH, Wang M, Patel KP, Dincer UD *et al.* (2004). Diabetes increases formation of advanced glycation end products on sarco(endo)plasmic reticulum Ca^{2+}-ATPase. *Diabetes* **53**: 463–73.

Blackledge HM, Newton J, Squire IB (2003). Prognosis for South Asian and white patients newly admitted to hospital with heart failure in the United Kingdom: historical cohort study. *British Medical Journal* **327**: 526–31.

Bojunga J, Nowak D, Mitrou PS, Hoelzer D, Zeuzem S, Chow KU (2004). Antioxidative treatment prevents activation of death-receptor- and mitochondrion-dependent apoptosis in the hearts of diabetic rats. *Diabetologia* **47**: 2072–80.

Bowling N, Walsh RA, Song G, Estridge T, Sandusky GE, Fouts RL *et al.* (1999). Increased protein kinase C activity and expression of Ca^{2+}-sensitive isoforms in the failing human heart. *Circulation* **99**: 384–91.

Brenner BM, Cooper ME, de Zeeuw D, Keane WF, Mitch WE, Parving HH *et al.* (2001). Effects of losartan on renal and cardiovascular outcomes in patients with type 2 diabetes and nephropathy. *New England Journal of Medicine* **345**: 861–9.

Bristow MR (1998). Why does the myocardium fail? Insights from basic science. *Lancet* **352**: SI8–SI14.

Bristow M (2000). Etomoxir: a new approach to treatment of chronic heart failure. *Lancet* **356**: 1621–2.

Bristow MR, Gilbert EM, Abraham WT, Adams KF, Fowler MB, Hershberger R *et al.* (1996). Effect of carvedilol on LV function and mortality in diabetic versus non-diabetic patients with ischaemic or nonischaemic dilated cardiomyopathy. *Circulation* **94**: I-664.

Bristow MR, Saxon LA, Boehmer J, Krueger S, Kass DA, De Marco T *et al.* (2004). Cardiac-resynchronization therapy with or without an implantable defibrillator in advanced chronic heart failure. *New England Journal of Medicine* **350**: 2140-50.

Brophy JM, Dagenais GR, McSherry F, Williford W, Yusuf S (2004). A multivariate model for predicting mortality in patients with heart failure and systolic dysfunction. *American Journal of Medicine* **116**: 300-4.

Cagliero E, Roth T, Roy S, Lorenzi M (1991). Characteristics and mechanisms of high-glucose-induced overexpression of basement membrane components in cultured human endothelial cells. *Diabetes* **40**: 102-10.

Chandler MP, Chavez PN, McElfresh TA, Huang H, Harmon CS, Stanley WC (2003). Partial inhibition of fatty acid oxidation increases regional contractile power and efficiency during demand-induced ischemia. *Cardiovascular Research* **59**: 143-51.

Charbonnel BH, Matthews DR, Schernthaner G, Hanefeld M, Brunetti P (2005). A long-term comparison of pioglitazone and gliclazide in patients with Type 2 diabetes mellitus: a randomized, double-blind, parallel-group comparison trial. *Diabetic Medicine* **22**: 399-405.

Chen YT, Vaccarino V, Williams CS, Butler J, Berkman LF, Krumholz HM (1999). Risk factors for heart failure in the elderly: a prospective community-based study. *American Journal of Medicine* **106**: 605-12.

Chong AY, Rajaratnam R, Hussein NR, Lip GY (2003). Heart failure in a multiethnic population in Kuala Lumpur, Malaysia. *European Journal of Heart Failure* **5**: 569-74.

Chou E, Suzuma I, Way KJ, Opland D, Clermont AC, Naruse K *et al.* (2002). Decreased cardiac expression of vascular endothelial growth factor and its receptors in insulin-resistant and diabetic states: a possible explanation for impaired collateral formation in cardiac tissue. *Circulation* **105**: 373-9.

CIBIS II Investigators and Committee (1999). The Cardiac Insufficiency Bisoprolol Study II (CIBIS-II): a randomised trial. *Lancet* **353**: 9-13.

Cleland JGF, Daubert JC, Erdmann E, Freemantle N, Gras D, Kappenberger L *et al.* (2005). The effect of cardiac resynchronization on morbidity and mortality in heart failure. *New England Journal of Medicine* **352**: 1539-49.

Coats AJ, Anker SD (2000). Insulin resistance in chronic heart failure. *Journal of Cardiovascular Pharmacology* **35**: S9-14.

Cockcroft JR, Wilkinson IB, Evans M, McEwan P, Peters JR, Davies S *et al.* (2005). Pulse pressure predicts cardiovascular risk in patients with type 2 diabetes mellitus. *American Journal of Hypertension* **18**: 1463-7.

Cohn JN, Tognoni G, the Valsartan Heart Failure Trial Investigators (2001). A randomized trial of the angiotensin-receptor blocker valsartan in chronic heart failure. *New England Journal of Medicine* **345**: 1667-75.

CONSENSUS Trial Study Group (1987). Effects of enalapril on mortality in severe congestive heart failure. Results of the Cooperative North Scandinavian Enalapril Survival Study (CONSENSUS). *New England Journal of Medicine* **316**: 1429-35.

Croft JB, Giles WH, Pollard RA, Keenan NL, Casper ML, Anda RF (1999). Heart failure survival among older adults in the United States: a poor prognosis for an emerging epidemic in the Medicare population. *Archives of Internal Medicine* **159**: 505-10.

Daly CA, Fox KM, Remme WJ, Bertrand ME, Ferrari R, Simoons ML on behalf of the EUROPA Investigators (2005). The effect of perindopril on cardiovascular morbidity and mortality in patients with diabetes in the EUROPA study: results from the PERSUADE substudy. *European Heart Journal* **26**: 1369-78.

Davidson JA, Perez A, Zhang J (2006). Addition of pioglitazone to stable insulin therapy in patients with poorly controlled type 2 diabetes: results of a double-blind, multicentre, randomized study. *Diabetes, Obesity and Metabolism* **8**: 164–74.

Davies M, Hobbs F, Davis R, Kenkre J, Roalfe AK, Hare R *et al.* (2001). Prevalence of left-ventricular systolic dysfunction and heart failure in the Echocardiographic Heart of England Screening study: a population based study. *Lancet* **358**: 439–44.

Deedwania PC, Giles TD, Klibaner M, Ghali JK, Herlitz J, Hildebrandt P *et al.* (2005). Efficacy, safety and tolerability of metoprolol CR/XL in patients with diabetes and chronic heart failure: experiences from MERIT-HF. *American Heart Journal* **149**: 159–67.

DeFronzo RA, Cooke CR, Andres R, Faloona GR, Davis PJ (1975). The effect of insulin on renal handling of sodium, potassium, calcium, and phosphate in man. *Journal of Clinical Investigation* **55**: 845–55.

Delea TE, Edelsberg JS, Hagiwara M, Oster G, Phillips LS (2003). Use of thiazolidinediones and risk of heart failure in people with type 2 diabetes: a retrospective cohort study. *Diabetes Care* **26**: 2983–9.

Depre C, Young ME, Ying J, Ahuja HS, Han Q, Garza N *et al.* (2000). Streptozotocin-induced changes in cardiac gene expression in the absence of severe contractile dysfunction. *Journal of Molecular and Cellular Cardiology* **32**: 985–96.

Deswal A, Petersen NJ, Souchek J, Ashton CM, Wray NP (2004). Impact of race on health care utilization and outcomes in veterans with congestive heart failure. *Journal of the American College of Cardiology* **43**: 778–84.

Devereux RB, Roman MJ, Paranicas M, O'Grady MJ, Lee ET, Welty TK *et al.* (2000). Impact of diabetes on cardiac structure and function: the Strong Heart Study. *Circulation* **101**: 2271–6.

Di Carli MF, Bianco-Batlles D, Landa ME, Kazmers A, Groehn H, Muzik O *et al.* (1999). Effects of autonomic neuropathy on coronary blood flow in patients with diabetes mellitus. *Circulation* **100**: 813–19.

Diabetes Control and Complications Trial/Epidemiology of Diabetes Interventions and Complications (DCCT/EDIC) Study Research Group (2005). Intensive diabetes treatment and cardiovascular disease in patients with type 1 diabetes. *New England Journal of Medicine* **353**: 2643–53.

Diabetes Prevention Program Research Group (2002). Reduction in the incidence of type 2 diabetes with lifestyle intervention or metformin. *New England Journal of Medicine* **346**: 393–403.

Digitalis Investigation Group (1997). The effect of digoxin on mortality and morbidity in patients with heart failure. *New England Journal of Medicine* **336**: 525–33.

Dillmann WH (1980). Diabetes mellitus induces changes in cardiac myosin of the rat. *Diabetes* **29**: 579–82.

Doehner W, Rauchhaus M, Godsland IF, Egerer K, Niebauer J, Sharma R *et al.* (2002). Insulin resistance in moderate chronic heart failure is related to hyperleptinaemia, but not to norepinephrine or TNF-alpha. *International Journal of Cardiology* **83**: 73–81.

Domanski M, Krause-Steinrauf H, Deedwania P, Follmann D, Ghali JK, Gilbert E *et al.* (2003). The effect of diabetes on outcomes of patients with advanced heart failure in the BEST trial. *Journal of the American College of Cardiology* **42**: 914–22.

Dormandy JA, Charbonnel B, Eckland DJ, Erdmann E, Massi-Benedetti M, Moules IK *et al.* (2005). Secondary prevention of macrovascular events in patients with type 2 diabetes in the PROactive Study (PROspective pioglitAzone Clinical Trial In macroVascular Events): a randomised controlled trial. *Lancet* **366**: 1279–89.

Dries DL, Sweitzer NK, Drazner MH, Stevenson LW, Gersh BJ (2001). Prognostic impact of diabetes mellitus in patients with heart failure according to the etiology of left ventricular systolic dysfunction. *Journal of the American College of Cardiology* **38**: 421–8.

Erdmann E, Lechat P, Verkenne P, Wiemann H (2001). Results from post-hoc analyses of the CIBIS II trial: effect of bisoprolol in high-risk patient groups with chronic heart failure. *European Journal of Heart Failure* **3**: 469–79.

Eshaghian S, Horwich TB, Fonarow GC (2006). An unexpected inverse relationship between HbA1c levels and mortality in patients with diabetes and advanced systolic heart failure. *American Heart Journal* **151**: 91.

Eurich DT, Majumdar SR, McAlister FA, Tsuyuki RT, Johnson JA (2005). Improved clinical outcomes associated with metformin in patients with diabetes and heart failure. *Diabetes Care* **28**: 2345–51.

Factor SM, Okun EM, Minase T (1980). Capillary microaneurysms in the human diabetic heart. *New England Journal of Medicine* **302**: 384–8.

Fogari R, Zoppi A, Tettamanti F, Poletti L, Lazzari P, Pasotti C *et al.* (1990). Beta-blocker effects on plasma lipids in antihypertensive therapy: importance of the duration of treatment and the lipid status before treatment. *Journal of Cardiovascular Pharmacology* **16** (Suppl 5): S76–S80.

Frustaci A, Kajstura J, Chimenti C, Jakoniuk I, Leri A, Maseri A *et al.* (2000). Myocardial cell death in human diabetes. *Circulation Research* **87**: 1123–32.

Gaboury CL, Simonson DC, Seely EW, Hollenberg NK, Williams GH (1994). Relation of pressor responsiveness to angiotensin II and insulin resistance in hypertension. *Journal of Clinical Investigation* **94**: 2295–300.

Ghazzi MN, Perez JE, Antonucci TK, Driscoll JH, Huang SM, Faja BW *et al.* (1997). Cardiac and glycemic benefits of troglitazone treatment in NIDDM. The Troglitazone Study Group. *Diabetes* **46**: 433–9.

Giacchetti G, Sechi LA, Rilli S, Carey RM (2005). The renin-angiotensin-aldosterone system, glucose metabolism and diabetes. *Trends in Endocrinology and Metabolism* **16**: 120–6.

Giugliano D, Acampora R, Marfella R, De Rosa N, Ziccardi P, Ragone R *et al.* (1997). Metabolic and cardiovascular effects of carvedilol and atenolol in non-insulin-dependent diabetes mellitus and hypertension: a randomized, controlled trial. *Annals of Internal Medicine* **126**: 955–9.

Granger CB, McMurray JJ, Yusuf S, Held P, Michelson EL, Olofsson B *et al.* (2003). Effects of candesartan in patients with chronic heart failure and reduced left-ventricular systolic function intolerant to angiotensin-converting-enzyme inhibitors: the CHARM-Alternative trial. *Lancet* **362**: 772–6.

de Groote P, Lamblin N, Mouquet F, Plichon D, McFadden E, Van Belle E *et al.* (2004). Impact of diabetes mellitus on long-term survival in patients with congestive heart failure. *European Heart Journal* **25**: 656–62.

Gupta DK, Jewitt DE, Young R, Hartog M, Opie LH (1969). Increased plasma-free-fatty-acid concentrations and their significance in patients with acute myocardial infarction. *Lancet* **2**: 1209–13.

Gustafsson I, Brendorp B, Seibaek M, Burchardt H, Hildebrandt P, Kober L *et al.* (2004). Influence of diabetes and diabetes–gender interaction on the risk of death in patients hospitalized with congestive heart failure. *Journal of the American College of Cardiology* **43**: 771–7.

Haas SJ, Vos T, Gilbert RE, Krum H (2003). Are beta-blockers as efficacious in patients with diabetes mellitus as in patients without diabetes mellitus who have chronic heart failure? A meta-analysis of large-scale clinical trials. *American Heart Journal* **146**: 848–53.

Harris MI, Flegal KM, Cowie CC, Eberhardt MS, Goldstein DE, Little RR *et al.* (1998). Prevalence of diabetes, impaired fasting glucose, and impaired glucose tolerance in U.S. adults. The Third National Health and Nutrition Examination Survey, 1988–1994. *Diabetes Care* **21**: 518–24.

Hartung DM, Touchette DR, Bultemeier NC, Haxby DG (2005). Risk of hospitalization for heart failure associated with thiazolidinedione therapy: a Medicaid claims-based case-control study. *Pharmacotherapy* **25**: 1329–36.

He J, Ogden LG, Bazzano LA, Vupputuri S, Loria C, Whelton PK (2001). Risk factors for congestive heart failure in US men and women: NHANES I epidemiologic follow-up study. *Archives of Internal Medicine* **161**: 996–1002.

Heart Outcomes Prevention Evaluation (HOPE) Study Investigators (2000). Effects of ramipril on cardiovascular and microvascular outcomes in people with diabetes mellitus: results of the HOPE study and MICRO-HOPE substudy. *Lancet* **355**: 253–9.

Hedberg P, Lonnberg I, Jonason T, Nilsson G, Pehrsson K, Ringqvist I (2001). Left ventricular systolic dysfunction in 75-year-old men and women; a population-based study. *European Heart Journal* **22**: 676–83.

Henderson AH, Most AS, Sonnenblick EH (1969). Depression of contractility in rat heart muscle by free fatty acids during hypoxia. *Lancet* **294**: 825–6.

Herings RMC, de Boer A, Leufkens HGM, Porsius A, Stricker BHC (1995). Hypoglycaemia associated with use of inhibitors of angiotensin converting enzyme. *Lancet* **345**: 1195–8.

Herrero P, Peterson LR, McGill JB, Matthew S, Lesniak D, Dence C *et al.* (2006). Increased myocardial fatty acid metabolism in patients with type 1 diabetes mellitus. *Journal of the American College of Cardiology* **47**: 598–604.

Hjalmarson A, Goldstein S, Fagerberg B, Wedel H, Waagstein F, Kjekshus J *et al.* (2000). Effects of controlled-release metoprolol on total mortality, hospitalizations, and well-being in patients with heart failure: the Metoprolol CR/XL Randomized Intervention Trial in congestive heart failure (MERIT-HF). MERIT-HF Study Group. *Journal of the American Medical Association* **283**: 1295–302.

Ho KK, Anderson KM, Kannel WB, Grossman W, Levy D (1993). Survival after the onset of congestive heart failure in Framingham Heart Study subjects. *Circulation* **88**: 107–15.

Hockensmith ML, Estacio RO, Mehler P, Havranek EP, Ecder ST, Lundgren RA *et al.* (2004). Albuminuria as a predictor of heart failure hospitalizations in patients with type 2 diabetes. *Journal of Cardiac Failure* **10**: 126–31.

Hoffman RP, Hausberg M, Sinkey CA, Anderson EA (1999). Hyperglycemia without hyperinsulinemia produces both sympathetic neural activation and vasodilation in normal humans. *Journal of Diabetes Complications* **13**: 17–22.

Holmang A, Yoshida N, Jennische E, Waldenstrom A, Bjorntorp P (1996). The effects of hyperinsulinaemia on myocardial mass, blood pressure regulation and central haemodynamics in rats. *European Journal of Clinical Investigation* **26**: 973–8.

Hosokawa M, Tsukada H, Fukuda K, Oya M, Onomura M, Nakamura H *et al.* (1999). Troglitazone inhibits bicarbonate secretion in rat and human duodenum. *Journal of Pharmacology and Experimental Therapies* **290**: 1080–4.

Huxley R, Barzi F, Woodward M (2006). Excess risk of fatal coronary heart disease associated with diabetes in men and women: meta-analysis of 37 prospective cohort studies. *British Medical Journal* **332**: 73–8.

Idris I, Gray S, Donnelly R (2003). Rosiglitazone and pulmonary oedema: an acute dose-dependent effect on human endothelial cell permeability. *Diabetologia* **46**: 288–90.

Ingelsson E, Sundstrom J, Arnlov J, Zethelius B, Lind L (2005). Insulin resistance and risk of congestive heart failure. *Journal of the American Medical Association* **294**: 334–41.

Inoguchi T, Li P, Umeda F, Yu HY, Kakimoto M, Imamura M *et al.* (2000). High glucose level and free fatty acid stimulate reactive oxygen species production through protein kinase C-dependent activation of NAD(P)H oxidase in cultured vascular cells. *Diabetes* **49**: 1939–45.

Iribarren C, Karter AJ, Go AS, Ferrara A, Liu JY, Sidney S *et al.* (2001). Glycemic control and heart failure among adult patients with diabetes. *Circulation* **103**: 2668–73.

Jager J, Kooy A, Lehert P, Bets D, Wulffele MG, Teerlink T *et al.* (2005). Effects of short-term treatment with metformin on markers of endothelial function and inflammatory activity in type 2 diabetes mellitus: a randomized, placebo-controlled trial. *Journal of Internal Medicine* **257**: 100–9.

Johansson S, Wallander MA, Ruigomez A, Garcia Rodriguez LA (2001). Incidence of newly diagnosed heart failure in UK general practice. *European Journal of Heart Failure* **3**: 225–31.

Jyothirmayi GN, Soni BJ, Masurekar M, Lyons M, Regan TJ (1998). Effects of metformin on collagen glycation and diastolic dysfunction in diabetic myocardium. *Journal of Cardiovascular Pharmacology and Therapeutics* **3**: 319–26.

Kamalesh M, Nair G (2005). Disproportionate increase in prevalence of diabetes among patients with congestive heart failure due to systolic dysfunction. *International Journal of Cardiology* **99**: 125–7.

Kannel WB, McGee DL (1979). Diabetes and cardiovascular disease. The Framingham study. *Journal of the American Medical Association* **241**: 2035–8.

Kannel WB, Hjortland M, Castelli WP (1974). Role of diabetes in congestive heart failure: the Framingham study. *American Journal of Cardiology* **34**: 29–34.

Karter AJ, Ahmed AT, Liu J, Moffet HH, Parker MM (2005). Pioglitazone initiation and subsequent hospitalization for congestive heart failure. *Diabetic Medicine* **22**: 986–93.

Kerenyi Z, Samer H, James R, Yan Y, Stewart M (2004). Combination therapy with rosiglitazone and glibenclamide compared with upward titration of glibenclamide alone in patients with type 2 diabetes mellitus. *Diabetes Research and Clinical Practice* **63**: 213–23.

Kerr D, Macdonald IA, Heller SR, Tattersall RB (1990). β-Adrenoceptor blockade and hypoglycaemia. A randomised, double-blind, placebo controlled comparison of metoprolol CR, atenolol and propranolol LA in normal subjects. *British Journal of Clinical Pharmacology* **29**: 685–93.

Kies P, Bax JJ, Molhoek SG, Bleeker GB, Boersma E, Steendijk P *et al.* (2005). Comparison of effectiveness of cardiac resynchronization therapy in patients with versus without diabetes mellitus. *American Journal of Cardiology* **96**: 108–11.

Kistorp C, Galatius S, Gustafsson F, Faber J, Corell P, Hildebrandt P (2005). Prevalence and characteristics of diabetic patients in a chronic heart failure population. *International Journal of Cardiology* **100**: 281–7.

Kostis JB, Sanders M (2005). The association of heart failure with insulin resistance and the development of type 2 diabetes. *American Journal of Hypertension* **18**: 731–7.

Lam TKT, Carpentier A, Lewis GF, van de Werve G, Fantus IG, Giacca A (2003). Mechanisms of the free fatty acid-induced increase in hepatic glucose production. *American Journal of Physiology. Endocrinology and Metabolism* **284**: E863–73.

Lawrenson JG, Glyn MC, Ward BJ (2002). Ultrastructural and morphometric comparison of retinal and myocardial capillaries following acute ischaemia. *Microvascular Research* **64**: 65–74.

Levine B, Kalman J, Mayer L, Fillit HM, Packer M (1990). Elevated circulating levels of tumor necrosis factor in severe chronic heart failure. *New England Journal of Medicine* **323**: 236–41.

Lewis EJ, Hunsicker LG, Clarke WR, Berl T Pohl MA, Lewis JB *et al.* for the Collaborative Study Group (2001). Renoprotective effect of the angiotensin-receptor antagonist irbesartan in patients with nephropathy due to type 2 diabetes. *New England Journal of Medicine* **345**: 851–60.

Lindholm LH, Ibsen H, Dahlof B, Devereux RB, Beevers G, de Faire U *et al.* (2002). Cardiovascular morbidity and mortality in patients with diabetes in the Losartan Intervention For Endpoint reduction in hypertension study (LIFE): a randomised trial against atenolol. *Lancet* **359**: 1004–10.

London GM, Guerin AP (1999). Influence of arterial pulse and reflected waves on blood pressure and cardiac function. *American Heart Journal* **138**: 220–4.

Macintyre K, Capewell S, Stewart S, Chalmers JWT, Boyd J, Finlayson A *et al.* (2000). Evidence of improving prognosis in heart failure : trends in case fatality in 66 547 patients hospitalized between 1986 and 1995. *Circulation* **102**: 1126–31.

Malhotra A, Sanghi V (1997). Regulation of contractile proteins in diabetic heart. *Cardiovascular Research* **34**: 34–40.

Mancini DM, Walter G, Reichek N, Lenkinski R, McCully KK, Mullen JL *et al.* (1992). Contribution of skeletal muscle atrophy to exercise intolerance and altered muscle metabolism in heart failure. *Circulation* **85**: 1364–73.

Marangou AG, Alford FP, Ward G, Liskaser F, Aitken PM, Weber KM *et al.* (1988). Hormonal effects of norepinephrine on acute glucose disposal in humans: a minimal model analysis. *Metabolism* **37**: 885–91.

Marfella R, Nappo F, De Angelis L, Paolisso G, Tagliamonte MR, Giugliano D (2000). Hemodynamic effects of acute hyperglycemia in type 2 diabetic patients. *Diabetes Care* **23**: 658–63.

Maru S, Koch GG, Stender M, Clark D, Gibowski L, Petri H *et al.* (2005). Antidiabetic drugs and heart failure risk in patients with type 2 diabetes in the U.K. primary care setting. *Diabetes Care* **28**: 20–6.

Masoudi FA, Inzucchi SE, Wang Y, Havranek EP, Foody JM, Krumholz HM (2005). Thiazolidinediones, metformin, and outcomes in older patients with diabetes and heart failure: an observational study. *Circulation* **111**: 583–90.

McDonagh TA, Morrison CE, Lawrence A, Ford I, Tunstall-Pedoe H, McMurray JJ *et al.* (1997). Symptomatic and asymptomatic left-ventricular systolic dysfunction in an urban population. *Lancet* **350**: 829–33.

McMurray JJ, Ostergren J, Swedberg K, Granger CB, Held P, Michelson EL *et al.* (2003). Effects of candesartan in patients with chronic heart failure and reduced left-ventricular systolic function taking angiotensin-converting-enzyme inhibitors: the CHARM-Added trial. *Lancet* **362**: 767–71.

MERIT-HF Study Group (1999). Effect of metoprolol CR/XL in chronic heart failure: Metoprolol CR/XL Randomised Intervention Trial in Congestive Heart Failure (MERIT-HF). *Lancet* **353**: 2001–7.

Miles PD, Romeo OM, Higo K, Cohen A, Rafaat K, Olefsky JM (1997). TNF-alpha-induced insulin resistance in vivo and its prevention by troglitazone. *Diabetes* **46**: 1678–83.

Misbin RI (1977). Phenformin-associated lactic acidosis: pathogenesis and treatment. *Annals of Internal Medicine* **87**: 591–5.

Misbin RI, Green L, Stadel BV, Gueriguian JL, Gubbi A, Fleming GA (1998). Lactic acidosis in patients with diabetes treated with metformin. *New England Journal of Medicine* **338**: 265–6.

Miyazaki Y, Mahankali A, Matsuda M, Mahankali S, Hardies J, Cusi K *et al.* (2002). Effect of pioglitazone on abdominal fat distribution and insulin sensitivity in type 2 diabetic patients. *Journal of Clinical Endocrinology and Metabolism* **87**: 2784–91.

Mohacsi P, Fowler MB, Krum H, Tendera M, Coats AJ, Rouleau JL *et al.* (2001). Should physicians avoid the use of beta-blockers in patients with heart failure who have diabetes? Results of the COPERNICUS study. *Circulation* **104**: II–754.

Morgan S, Smith H, Simpson I, Liddiard GS, Raphael H, Pickering RM *et al.* (1999). Prevalence and clinical characteristics of left ventricular dysfunction among elderly patients in general practice setting: cross sectional survey. *British Medical Journal* **318**: 368–72.

Morris AD, Boyle DI, McMahon AD, Pearce H, Evans JM, Newton RW *et al.* (1997). ACE inhibitor use is associated with hospitalization for severe hypoglycemia in patients with diabetes. DARTS/MEMO Collaboration. Diabetes Audit and Research in Tayside, Scotland. Medicines Monitoring Unit. *Diabetes Care* **20**: 1363–7.

Mosterd A, Hoes AW, de Bruyne MC, Deckers JW, Linker DT, Hofman A *et al.* (1999). Prevalence of heart failure and left ventricular dysfunction in the general population: The Rotterdam Study. *European Heart Journal* 20: 447–55.

Mosterd A, Cost B, Hoes AW, de Bruijne MC, Deckers JW, Hofman A *et al.* (2001). The prognosis of heart failure in the general population: The Rotterdam Study. *European Heart Journal* 22: 1318–27.

Nesto RW, Bell D, Bonow RO, Fonseca V, Grundy SM, Horton ES *et al.* (2003). Thiazolidinedione use, fluid retention, and congestive heart failure: a consensus statement from the American Heart Association and American Diabetes Association *Circulation* 108: 2941–8.

Nichols GA, Hillier TA, Erbey JR, Brown JB (2001). Congestive heart failure in type 2 diabetes: prevalence, incidence, and risk factors. *Diabetes Care* 24: 1614–9.

Nichols GA, Gullion CM, Koro CE, Ephross SA, Brown JB (2004). The incidence of congestive heart failure in type 2 diabetes: an update. *Diabetes Care* 27: 1879–84.

Nickenig G, Bohm M (1998). Interaction between insulin and AT1 receptor. Relevance for hypertension and arteriosclerosis. *Basic Research in Cardiology* 93 (Suppl 2): 135–9.

Nielson C, Lange T (2005). Blood glucose and heart failure in nondiabetic patients. *Diabetes Care* 28: 607–11.

Nonogaki K (2000). New insights into sympathetic regulation of glucose and fat metabolism. *Diabetologia* 43: 533–49.

Ogino K, Furuse Y, Uchida K, Shimoyama M, Kinugawa T, Osaki S *et al.* (2002). Troglitazone improves cardiac function in patients with congestive heart failure. *Cardiovascular Drugs and Therapy* 16: 215–20.

Ohtsuka S, Kakihana M, Watanabe H, Enomoto T, Ajisaka R, Sugishita Y (1996). Alterations in left ventricular wall stress and coronary circulation in patients with isolated systolic hypertension. *Journal of Hypertension* 14: 1349–55.

Oliver MF, Opie LH (1994). Effects of glucose and fatty acids on myocardial ischaemia and arrhythmias. *Lancet* 343: 155–8.

Oltmanns KM, Deininger E, Wellhoener P, Schultes B, Kern W, Marx E *et al.* (2003). Influence of captopril on symptomatic and hormonal responses to hypoglycaemia in humans. *British Journal of Clinical Pharmacology* 55: 347–53.

Packer M, Bristow MR, Cohn JN, Colucci WS, Fowler MB, Gilbert EM *et al.* (1996). The effect of carvedilol on morbidity and mortality in patients with chronic heart failure. U.S. Carvedilol Heart Failure Study Group. *New England Journal of Medicine*

Packer M, Coats AJ, Fowler MB, Katus HA, Krum H, Mohacsi P *et al.* (2001). Effect of carvedilol on survival in severe chronic heart failure. *New England Journal of Medicine* 344: 1651–8.

Paolisso G, De Riu S, Marrazzo G, Verza M, Varricchio M, D'Onofrio F (1991). Insulin resistance and hyperinsulinemia in patients with chronic congestive heart failure. *Metabolism* 40: 972–7.

Paolisso G, Tagliamonte MR, Rizzo MR, Gambardella A, Gualdiero P, Lama D *et al.* (1999). Prognostic importance of insulin-mediated glucose uptake in aged patients with congestive heart failure secondary to mitral and/or aortic valve disease. *American Journal of Cardiology* 83: 1338–44.

Parsonage WA, Hetmanski D, Cowley AJ (2001). Beneficial haemodynamic effects of insulin in chronic heart failure. *Heart* 85: 508–13.

Phillips LS, Grunberger G, Miller E, Patwardhan R, Rappaport EB, Salzman A (2001). Once- and twice-daily dosing with rosiglitazone improves glycemic control in patients with type 2 diabetes. *Diabetes Care* 24: 308–15.

Pitt B, Perez A for the Randomized Aldactone Evaluation Study Investigators (2000). Spironolactone in patients with heart failure. *New England Journal of Medicine* 342: 132–4.

Pitt B, Poole-Wilson PA, Segal R, Martinez FA, Dickstein K, Camm AJ *et al.* (2000). Effect of losartan compared with captopril on mortality in patients with symptomatic heart failure: randomised trial – the Losartan Heart Failure Survival Study ELITE II. *Lancet* **355**: 1582–7.

Pocock SJ, Wang D, Pfeffer MA, Yusuf S, McMurray JJ, Swedberg KB *et al.* (2006). Predictors of mortality and morbidity in patients with chronic heart failure. *European Heart Journal* **27**: 65–75.

Poole-Wilson PA, Swedberg K, Cleland JG, Di Lenarda A, Hanrath P, Komajda M *et al.* (2003). Comparison of carvedilol and metoprolol on clinical outcomes in patients with chronic heart failure in the Carvedilol Or Metoprolol European Trial (COMET): randomised controlled trial. *Lancet* **362**: 7–13.

Popp DA, Tse TF, Shah SD, Clutter WE, Cryer PE (1984). Oral propranolol and metoprolol both impair glucose recovery from insulin-induced hypoglycemia in insulin-dependent diabetes mellitus. *Diabetes Care* **7**: 243–7.

Raskin P, Rendell M, Riddle MC, Dole JF, Freed MI, Rosenstock J (2001). A randomized trial of rosiglitazone therapy in patients with inadequately controlled insulin-treated type 2 diabetes. *Diabetes Care* **24**: 1226–32.

Rathore SS, Foody JM, Wang Y, Smith GL, Herrin J, Masoudi FA *et al.* (2003). Race, quality of care, and outcomes of elderly patients hospitalized with heart failure. *Journal of the American Medical Association* **289**: 2517–24.

Raymond I, Groenning BA, Hildebrandt PR, Nilsson JC, Baumann M, Trawinski J *et al.* (2003). The influence of age, sex and other variables on the plasma level of N-terminal pro brain natriuretic peptide in a large sample of the general population. *Heart* **89**: 745–51.

Razeghi P, Young ME, Alcorn JL, Moravec CS, Frazier OH, Taegtmeyer H (2001). Metabolic gene expression in fetal and failing human heart. *Circulation* **104**: 2923–31.

Razeghi P, Young ME, Cockrill TC, Frazier OH, Taegtmeyer H (2002). Downregulation of myocardial myocyte enhancer factor 2C and myocyte enhancer factor 2C-regulated gene expression in diabetic patients with nonischemic heart failure. *Circulation* **106**: 407–11.

Reaven GM, Lithell H, Landsberg L (1996). Hypertension and associated metabolic abnormalities–the role of insulin resistance and the sympathoadrenal system. *New England Journal of Medicine* **334**: 374–81.

Redfield MM, Jacobsen SJ, Burnett JC, Jr., Mahoney DW, Bailey KR, Rodeheffer RJ (2003). Burden of systolic and diastolic ventricular dysfunction in the community: appreciating the scope of the heart failure epidemic. *Journal of the American Medical Association* **289**: 194–202.

RESOLVD Investigators (2000). Effects of metoprolol CR in patients with ischemic and dilated cardiomyopathy: the randomized evaluation of strategies for left ventricular dysfunction pilot study. *Circulation* **101**: 378–84.

Roden M (2004). How free fatty acids inhibit glucose utilization in human skeletal muscle. *News in Physiological Sciences* **19**: 92–6.

Rosen P, Du X, Tschope D (1998). Role of oxygen derived radicals for vascular dysfunction in the diabetic heart: prevention by alpha-tocopherol? *Molecular and Cellular Biochemistry* **188**: 103–11.

Rosenstock J, Einhorn D, Hershon K, Glazer NB, Yu S (2002). Efficacy and safety of pioglitazone in type 2 diabetes: a randomised, placebo-controlled study in patients receiving stable insulin therapy. *International Journal of Clinical Practice* **56**: 251–7.

Rubler S, Dlugash J, Yuceoglu YZ, Kumral T, Branwood AW, Grishman A (1972). New type of cardiomyopathy associated with diabetic glomerulosclerosis. *American Journal of Cardiology* **30**: 595–602.

Rutter MK, Parise H, Benjamin EJ, Levy D, Larson MG, Meigs JB *et al.* (2003). Impact of glucose intolerance and insulin resistance on cardiac structure and function: sex-related differences in the Framingham Heart Study. *Circulation* **107**: 448–54.

Ryden L, Armstrong PW, Cleland JG, Horowitz JD, Massie BM, Packer M *et al.* (2000). Efficacy and safety of high-dose lisinopril in chronic heart failure patients at high cardiovascular risk, including those with diabetes mellitus. Results from the ATLAS trial. *European Heart Journal* **21**: 1967–78.

Sam F, Kerstetter DL, Pimental DR, Mulukutla S, Tabaee A, Bristow MR *et al.* (2005). Increased reactive oxygen species production and functional alterations in antioxidant enzymes in human failing myocardium. *Journal of Cardiac Failure* **11**: 473–80.

Sawicki PT, Siebenhofer A (2001). Betablocker treatment in diabetes mellitus. *Journal of Internal Medicine* **250**: 11–7.

Scherrer U, Sartori C (1997). Insulin as a vascular and sympathoexcitatory hormone: implications for blood pressure regulation, insulin sensitivity, and cardiovascular morbidity. *Circulation* **96**: 4104–13.

Schiffelers SLH, Saris WHM, Boomsma F, van Baak MA (2001). β1- and β2-Adrenoceptor-mediated thermogenesis and lipid utilization in obese and lean men. *Journal of Clinical Endocrinology and Metabolism* **86**: 2191–9.

Shekelle PG, Rich MW, Morton SC, Atkinson C, Tu W, Maglione M *et al.* (2003). Efficacy of angiotensin-converting enzyme inhibitors and beta-blockers in the management of left ventricular systolic dysfunction according to race, gender, and diabetic status: A meta-analysis of major clinical trials. *Journal of the American College of Cardiology* **41**: 1529–38.

Shimoyama M, Ogino K, Tanaka Y, Ikeda T, Hisatome I (1999). Hemodynamic basis for the acute cardiac effects of troglitazone in isolated perfused rat hearts. *Diabetes* **48**: 609–15.

Shindler DM, Kostis JB, Yusuf S, Quinones MA, Pitt B, Stewart D *et al.* (1996). Diabetes mellitus, a predictor of morbidity and mortality in the Studies of Left Ventricular Dysfunction (SOLVD) Trials and Registry. *American Journal of Cardiology* **77**: 1017–20.

Shinohara K, Shinohara T, Mochizuki N, Mochizuki Y, Sawa H, Kohya T *et al.* (1996). Expression of vascular endothelial growth factor in human myocardial infarction. *Heart Vessels* **11**: 113–22.

Shorr RI, Ray WA, Daugherty JR, Griffin MR (1997). Antihypertensives and the risk of serious hypoglycemia in older persons using insulin or sulfonylureas. *Journal of the American Medical Association* **278**: 40–3.

Simonson DC (1988). Etiology and prevalence of hypertension in diabetic patients. *Diabetes Care* **11**: 821–7.

Singh R, Barden A, Mori T, Beilin L (2001). Advanced glycation end-products: a review. *Diabetologia* **44**: 129–46.

Singh H, Gordon HS, Deswal A (2005). Variation by race in factors contributing to heart failure hospitalizations. *Journal of Cardiac Failure* **11**: 23–9.

Smith SR, De Jonge L, Volaufova J, Li Y, Xie H, Bray GA (2005). Effect of pioglitazone on body composition and energy expenditure: a randomized controlled trial. *Metabolism* **54**: 24–32.

Smooke S, Horwich TB, Fonarow GC (2005). Insulin-treated diabetes is associated with a marked increase in mortality in patients with advanced heart failure. *American Heart Journal* **149**: 168–74.

SOLVD Investigators (1991). Effect of enalapril on survival in patients with reduced left ventricular ejection fractions and congestive heart failure. *New England Journal of Medicine* **325**: 293–302.

SOLVD Investigators (1992). Effect of enalapril on mortality and the development of heart failure in asymptomatic patients with reduced left ventricular ejection fractions. *New England Journal of Medicine* **327**: 685–91.

Song J, Knepper MA, Hu X, Verbalis JG, Ecelbarger CA (2004). Rosiglitazone activates renal sodium- and water-reabsorptive pathways and lowers blood pressure in normal rats. *Journal of Pharmacology and Experimental Therapeutics* **308**: 426–33.

St John Sutton M, Rendell M, Dandona P, Dole JF, Murphy K, Patwardhan R *et al.* (2002). A comparison of the effects of rosiglitazone and glyburide on cardiovascular function and glycemic control in patients with type 2 diabetes. *Diabetes Care* **25**: 2058–64.

Steinberg HO, Chaker H, Leaming R, Johnson A, Brechtel G, Baron AD (1996). Obesity/insulin resistance is associated with endothelial dysfunction. Implications for the syndrome of insulin resistance. *Journal of Clinical Investigation* **97**: 2601–10.

Stratton IM, Adler AI, Neil HA, Matthews DR, Manley SE, Cull CA *et al.* (2000). Association of glycaemia with macrovascular and microvascular complications of type 2 diabetes (UKPDS 35): prospective observational study. *British Medical Journal* **321**: 405–12.

Sundstrom J, Lind L, Nystrom N, Zethelius B, Andren B, Hales CN *et al.* (2000). Left ventricular concentric remodeling rather than left ventricular hypertrophy is related to the insulin resistance syndrome in elderly men. *Circulation* **101**: 2595–600.

Suskin N, McKelvie RS, Burns RJ, Latini R, Pericak D, Probstfield J *et al.* (2000). Glucose and insulin abnormalities relate to functional capacity in patients with congestive heart failure. *European Heart Journal* **21**: 1368–75.

Swan JW, Walton C, Godsland IF, Clark AL, Coat AJS, Oliver MF (1994). Insulin resistance in chronic heart failure. *European Heart Journal* **15**: 1528–32.

Swan JW, Anker SD, Walton C, Godsland IF, Clark AL, Leyva F *et al.* (1997). Insulin resistance in chronic heart failure: relation to severity and etiology of heart failure. *Journal of the American College of Cardiology* **30**: 527–32.

Taegtmeyer H, McNulty P, Young ME (2002). Adaptation and maladaptation of the heart in diabetes: Part I: general concepts. *Circulation* **105**: 1727–33.

Tan M, Johns D, Gonzalez Galvez G, Antunez O, Fabian G, Flores-Lozano F *et al.* (2004). Effects of pioglitazone and glimepiride on glycemic control and insulin sensitivity in Mexican patients with type 2 diabetes mellitus: a multicenter, randomized, double-blind, parallel-group trial. *Clinical Therapeutics* **26**: 680–93.

Tang WH, Francis GS, Hoogwerf BJ, Young JB (2003). Fluid retention after initiation of thiazolidinedione therapy in diabetic patients with established chronic heart failure. *Journal of the American College of Cardiology* **41**: 1394–8.

Tansey MJ, Opie LH (1983). Relation between plasma free fatty acids and arrhythmias within the first twelve hours of acute myocardial infarction. *Lancet* **2**: 419–22.

Taylor AL, Ziesche S, Yancy C, Carson P, D'Agostino R, Jr., Ferdinand K *et al.* (2004). Combination of isosorbide dinitrate and hydralazine in blacks with heart failure. *New England Journal of Medicine* **351**: 2049–57.

Tenenbaum A, Motro M, Fisman EZ, Leor J, Freimark D, Boyko V *et al.* (2003). Functional class in patients with heart failure is associated with the development of diabetes. *American Journal of Medicine* **114**: 271–5.

Tesfamariam B, Brown ML, Cohen RA (1991). Elevated glucose impairs endothelium-dependent relaxation by activating protein kinase C. *Journal of Clinical Investigation* **87**: 1643–8.

Thrainsdottir IS, Aspelund T, Thorgeirsson G, Gudnason V, Hardarson T, Malmberg K *et al.* (2005). The association between glucose abnormalities and heart failure in the population-based Reykjavik study. *Diabetes Care* **28**: 612–6.

UK Prospective Diabetes Study Group (1998a). Tight blood pressure control and risk of macrovascular and microvascular complications in type 2 diabetes: UKPDS 38. *British Medical Journal* **317**: 703–13.

UK Prospective Diabetes Study Group (1998b). Efficacy of atenolol and captopril in reducing risk of macrovascular and microvascular complications in type 2 diabetes: UKPDS 39. *British Medical Journal* **317**: 713–20.

UK Prospective Diabetes Study (UKPDS) Group (1998). Intensive blood-glucose control with sulphonylureas or insulin compared with conventional treatment and risk of complications in patients with type 2 diabetes (UKPDS 33). *Lancet* **352**: 837–53.

Vaccarino V, Gahbauer E, Kasl SV, Charpentier PA, Acampora D, Krumholz HM (2002). Differences between African Americans and whites in the outcome of heart failure: evidence for a greater functional decline in African Americans. *American Heart Journal* **143**: 1058–67.

Vaur L, Gueret P, Lievre M, Chabaud S, Passa P for the DIABHYCAR Group (2003). Development of congestive heart failure in type 2 diabetic patients with microalbuminuria or proteinuria: observations from the DIABHYCAR (type 2 DIABetes, Hypertension, CArdiovascular Events and Ramipril) study. *Diabetes Care* **26**: 855–60.

Vermes E, Ducharme A, Bourassa MG, Lessard M, White M, Tardif JC (2003). Enalapril reduces the incidence of diabetes in patients with chronic heart failure: insight from the Studies Of Left Ventricular Dysfunction (SOLVD). *Circulation* **107**: 1291–6.

Vinereanu D, Nicolaides E, Boden L, Payne N, Jones CJH, Fraser AG (2003). Conduit arterial stiffness is associated with impaired left ventricular subendocardial function. *Heart* **89**: 449–50.

von Lewinski D, Bruns S, Walther S, Kogler H, Pieske B (2005). Insulin causes [Ca^{2+}]i-dependent and [Ca^{2+}]i-independent positive inotropic effects in failing human myocardium. *Circulation* **111**: 2588–95.

Wahlqvist ML, Lo CS, Myers KA, Simpson RW, Simpson JM (1988). Putative determinants of arterial wall compliance in NIDDM. *Diabetes Care* **11**: 787–90.

Wakasaki H, Koya D, Schoen FJ, Jirousek MR, Ways DK, Hoit BD *et al.* (1997). Targeted overexpression of protein kinase C beta 2 isoform in myocardium causesácardiomyopathy. *Proceedings of the National Academy of Sciences of the United States of America* **94**: 9320–5.

Way KJ, Katai N, King GL (2001). Protein kinase C and the development of diabetic vascular complications. *Diabetic Medicine* **18**: 945–59.

Weissman P, Goldstein BJ, Rosenstock J, Waterhouse B, Cobitz AR, Wooddell MJ *et al.* (2005). Effects of rosiglitazone added to submaximal doses of metformin compared with dose escalation of metformin in type 2 diabetes: the EMPIRE Study. *Current Medical Research and Opinion* **21**: 2029–35.

Wlodarczyk JH, Keogh A, Smith K, McCosker C (2003). CHART: Congestive cardiac failure in hospitals, an Australian review of treatment. *Hear, Lung and Circulation* **12**: 94–102.

Wong TY, Rosamond W, Chang PP, Couper DJ, Sharrett AR, Hubbard LD *et al.* (2005). Retinopathy and risk of congestive heart failure. *Journal of the American Medical Association* **293**: 63–9.

Yasumura Y, Takemura K, Sakamoto A, Kitakaze M, Miyatake K (2003). Changes in myocardial gene expression associated with β-blocker therapy in patients with chronic heart failure. *Journal of Cardiac Failure* **9**: 469–74.

Young ME, McNulty P, Taegtmeyer H (2002). Adaptation and maladaptation of the heart in diabetes: Part II: Potential mechanisms. *Circulation* **105**: 1861–70.

Young JB, Dunlap ME, Pfeffer MA, Probstfield JL, Cohen-Solal A, Dietz R *et al.* (2004). Mortality and morbidity reduction with candesartan in patients with chronic heart failure and left ventricular systolic dysfunction: results of the CHARM low-left ventricular ejection fraction trials. *Circulation* **110**: 2618–26.

Yusuf S, Ostergren JB, Gerstein HC, Pfeffer MA, Swedberg K, Granger CB *et al.* (2005). Effects of candesartan on the development of a new diagnosis of diabetes mellitus in patients with heart failure. *Circulation* **112**: 48–53.

Zanchi A, Chiolero A, Maillard M, Nussberger J, Brunner HR, Burnier M (2004). Effects of the peroxisomal proliferator-activated receptor-γ agonist pioglitazone on renal and hormonal responses to salt in healthy men. *Journal of Clinical Endocrinology and Metabolism* **89**: 1140–5.

Zhang F, Li G, Ding W, Liu Y, Xie C, Zhang D *et al.* (2002). Screening and analysis of early cardiopathology-related gene in type 2 diabetes mellitus. *Zhonghua Nei Ke Za Zhi* **41**: 530–3.

Zhang Y, Bloem LJ, Yu L, Estridge TB, Iversen PW, McDonald CE *et al.* (2003). Protein kinase C betaII activation induces angiotensin converting enzyme expression in neonatal rat cardiomyocytes. *Cardiovasclar Research* **57**: 139–46.

Zhou YT, Grayburn P, Karim A, Shimabukuro M, Higa M, Baetens D *et al.* (2000). Lipotoxic heart disease in obese rats: Implications for human obesity. *Proceedings of the National Academy of Sciences of the United States of America* **97**: 1784–9.

6 Diabetes and Hypertension

Gordon T. McInnes

6.1 Introduction

Clustering analysis indicates that risk factors for cardiovascular disease and diabetes are more likely to occur simultaneously than would be expected by chance, suggesting that a common metabolic disorder underlies the expression of these conditions (Betteridge, 2004). In particular, the concordance of hypertension and diabetes is increased in westernised populations (Chobanian *et al.*, 2003). Male screenees for the Multiple Risk Factor Intervention Trial (MRFIT) with type 2 diabetes had increased prevalence of systolic hypertension, as well as total cholesterol and cigarette smoking, compared with non-diabetic controls (Stamler *et al.*, 1993).

The prevalence rate of hypertension is increased in patients with diabetes (Simonson 1988; Sowers and Haffner, 2002). In type 2 diabetes, hypertension is very common. In the United Kingdom Prospective Diabetes Study (UKPDS), the prevalence of hypertension (systolic blood pressure $\geq$ 160 mmHg and/or diastolic blood pressure $\geq$ 90 mmHg, or antihypertensive drugs) was 39% (UK Prospective Diabetes Study Group, 1998a). Using more contemporary definitions of hypertension (blood pressure $\geq$ 140/90 mmHg), the prevalence rates reach 70–80% in many European countries (Williams 1999; Sowers *et al.*, 2001). Some 75% of patients with type 2 diabetes have blood pressure $\geq$ 130/80 mmHg or use antihypertensive treatment.

Hypertension in diabetes is characterised by an earlier onset of systolic hypertension and higher prevalence of isolated systolic hypertension at any age compared with people without diabetes. In type 2 diabetes, hypertension is more common in women than in men and the age-related increase in systolic blood pressure is steeper in women (Williams *et al.*, 2004). The risk of hypertension is positively associated with obesity (Hypertension in Diabetes Study (HDS), 1993).

In type 1 diabetes, hypertension often reflects the onset of diabetic nephropathy (Epstein and Sowers, 1992) whereas most hypertensives do not have albuminuria at the time of diagnosis of type 2 diabetes (Hypertension in Diabetes Study (HDS), 1993).

Diabetic Cardiology   Editors Miles Fisher and John J. McMurray
© 2007 John Wiley & Sons, Ltd.

The prevalence of hypertension (blood pressure $\geq 140/90\,\text{mm Hg}$) in type 2 diabetes and normoalbuminuria is very high (79%) and increases even further (to 90%) in the presence of microalbuminuria (Tarnow et al., 1994). Hypertension approaches 100% of those with end-stage renal disease. In 55% of these subjects blood pressure is above $140/90\,\text{mmHg}$ and only 12% have blood pressure $< 130/85\,\text{mmHg}$, with very few with blood pressure $< 130/80\,\text{mmHg}$ (Harris, 2000).

In westernised populations, the prevalence of hypertension is around 24% in adults (Burt et al., 1995) and the age-adjusted prevalence is increasing. Hypertensive individuals have a greater risk of developing type 2 diabetes than non-hypertensive people (Medalie et al., 1975; Skarfors et al., 1991; Morales et al., 1993). Hypertension is an independent risk factor for the development of diabetes (Medalie et al., 1975; Skarfors et al., 1991; Morales et al., 1993). People with elevated blood pressure are 2.5 times more likely to develop diabetes within five years (Gress et al., 2000; Sowers and Bakris, 2000). Hypertension and microalbuminuria independent of blood pressure level (Hypertension in Diabetes Study (HDS), 1993; Mykkanen et al., 1994) may precede the development of diabetes by several years.

There is a strong association between elevated blood pressure and insulin resistance (Modan et al., 1985; Ferrannini et al., 1987; Swislocki et al., 1989; Bühler et al., 1990; Ferrari and Weidmann, 1990). The prevalence of insulin resistance in hypertension has been estimated at 50% (Reaven, 1999). Several possible mechanisms have been proposed (Scheen, 2004). Impaired fasting blood glucose is associated with increased cardiovascular risk (Coutinho et al., 1999), particularly if accompanied by hypertension (Henry et al., 2002).

In people with diabetes, cardiovascular disease risk is increased two- to fourfold compared with those with normal glucose tolerance (Laakso and Lehto, 1997; Alderberth et al., 1998; Haffner et al., 1998). Diabetic people without history of previous myocardial infarction may have as high a risk of myocardial infarction as non-diabetic patients with a history of prior myocardial infarction (Haffner et al., 1998). However, this finding is controversial since it has not been confirmed in some other population-based studies (Cho et al., 2002; Lee et al., 2004) (see also Chapter 1).

The absolute risk of cardiovascular disease associated with any level of glycaemia is determined by the presence of other risk factors (Stamler et al., 1993). In both type 1 and type 2 diabetes, hypertension is a major predictor of macrovascular complications including coronary heart disease, stroke and peripheral vascular disease. Hypertension is also a risk factor for microvascular complication (retinopathy, neuropathy and nephropathy). Patients with hypertension and type 2 diabetes constitute a high-risk population (Williams, 1999).

In type 2 diabetes, cardiovascular risk factors are additive and, in some cases, multiplicative (Stamler et al., 1993). The coexistence of hypertension and diabetes is particularly pernicious because of the strong linkage of each with cardiovascular disease (Fagan and Sowers, 1999), stroke (Hansson et al., 1998; Davis et al., 1999; Fagan and Sowers, 1999; Adler et al., 2000; Goldstein et al., 2001), progression of renal disease (Maki et al., 1995; Nelson et al., 1996; Bakris et al., 2000) and diabetic retinopathy (Kohner et al., 1998). The combination of hypertension and diabetes doubles the risk of developing microvascular and macrovascular complications and the risk of mortality compared with hypertension alone (Hansson et al., 1998;

Tuomilehto *et al.*, 1999). The coexistence of diabetes (type 1 and type 2) and hypertension is associated with a twofold risk of macrovascular complications including stroke and coronary heart disease and is responsible for excess cardiovascular mortality (Pell and D'Alonzo, 1967; Jarrett *et al.*, 1982; Gerber *et al.*, 1983; Epstein and Sowers, 1992; Grossman and Messerli, 1996; Alderman *et al.*, 1999; Sowers *et al.*, 2001).

In westernised countries, diabetes and hypertension are the leading causes of end-stage renal disease with a prevalence that has increased steadily over the last two decades, while other causes have remained constant (UK Prospective Diabetes Study Group, 1998a). Renal function declines with time in both type 1 and type 2 diabetes. The rate of decline is accelerated significantly when hypertension coexists. Systolic blood pressure correlates better than diastolic blood pressure with renal disease progression in diabetes (Parving *et al.*, 1987; Maki *et al.*, 1995; Mogensen *et al.*, 1995; Nelson *et al.*, 1996; Sowers and Haffner, 2002). The rate of decline in renal function in diabetic nephropathy is a continuous function of arterial pressure down to systolic blood pressure of approximately 125–130 mmHg and diastolic blood pressure of 70–75 mmHg (Parving *et al.*, 1987; Dillon, 1993; Walker, 1993; Maki *et al.*, 1995; Mogensen *et al.*, 1995; Nelson *et al.*, 1996).

6.2 Metabolic Syndrome (see also Chapter 2)

Hypertension is frequently associated with insulin resistance (and concomitant hyperinsulinaemia), central obesity and a characteristic pattern of dislipidaemia (high triglycerides and low HDL-cholesterol) (Reaven *et al.*, 1996; Reaven, 2002). The relation between insulin resistance and hypertension is well established (Modan *et al.*, 1985; Ferrannini *et al.*, 1987; Swislocki *et al.*, 1989; Bühler *et al.*, 1990; Ferrari and Weidmann, 1990) but, despite this association, insulin resistance contributes only modestly to the prevalence of hypertension (Hanley *et al.*, 2002). This constellation of risk factors is known as the (cardiovascular) metabolic syndrome. There are various definitions but all agree on the essential components – glucose intolerance, obesity, hypertension and dyslipidaemia.

Almost one-quarter of adults in the USA has the metabolic syndrome (Ford *et al.*, 2002). This is likely to rise in the next several years primarily because of the rapid increase in obesity. People with the metabolic syndrome are at particularly high risk of cardiovascular disease because it envelopes several interrelated risk factors (Reaven, 1988; Liese *et al.*, 1998; Isomaa *et al.*, 2001; Laaksonen *et al.*, 2002; Lakka *et al.*, 2002; Hsia *et al.*, 2003). Such individuals are also predisposed to the development of chronic kidney disease (Chen *et al.*, 2004) and type 2 diabetes (Haffner, 1997).

Since people with the metabolic syndrome have increased risk of cardiovascular disease prior to the development of diabetes, the syndrome has become the focus for the primary prevention of cardiovascular disease. By broadening the clinical focus to include impaired glucose regulation outside the diabetic range, the scope and yield of cardiovascular disease prevention are increased. Management of underlying risk factors should be independent of risk status (Table 6.1).

Table 6.1 Clinical management of the metabolic syndrome: targets, goals and recommendations. Modified from Eckel RH, Grundy SM, Zimmet PZ (2005). The metabolic syndrome. *Lancet* **365**: 1415–28.

Abdominal obesity	Goal: 10% weight loss first year, thereafter continued weight loss or maintain weight Recommendation: caloric restriction; regular exercise
Physical inactivity	Goal: regular moderate-intensity physical activity Recommendation: 30–60 min moderate-intensity exercise daily
Atherogenic diet	Goals: reduced intakes of saturated fats, trans-fats and cholesterol Recommendations: saturated fat, 7% of total calories; dietary cholesterol < 200 mg daily; total fat 25–35% of total calories
Cigarette smoking	Goal and recommendation: complete smoking cessation
LDL-cholesterol	Goals: High-risk patients[a] – LDL-cholesterol < 2.6 mmol/l Therapeutics option – LDL-cholesterol < 1.8 mmol/l Moderately high-risk patients[b] – LDL-cholesterol < 3.4 mmol/l Therapeutic option – LDL-cholesterol < 2.6 mmol/l Moderate-risk patients[c] – LDL-cholesterol < 3.4 mmol/l Recommandations: High-risk patients – lifestyle therapies[d] and LDL-cholesterol-lowering drug to achieve recommended goal Moderately high-risk patients – lifestyle therapies; add LDL-cholesterol-lowering drug if necessary to achieve recommended goal when baseline LDL-cholesterol ≥ 3.4 mmol/l Moderate risk patients – lifestyle therapies; add LDL-cholesterol-lowering drug if necessary to achieve recommended goal when baseline LDL-cholesterol ≥ 4.1 mmol/l
High triglyceride or low HDL-cholesterol	Goal: insufficient data to establish goal Recommendation: high-risk patients – consider adding fibrate (preferably fenofibrate) or nicotinic acid to LDL-lowering drug therapy
Elevated blood pressure	Goals: blood pressure < 135/ < 85 mmHg. For diabetes or chronic kidney disease: blood pressure < 130/80 mmHg Recommendations: lifestyle therapies; add antihypertensive drug(s) when necessary to achieve goals of therapy
Elevated glucose	Goals: maintenance or reduction in fasting glucose if > 5.5 mmol/l, haemoglobin < 7.0% for diabetes Recommendations: lifestyle therapies; add hypoglycaemic agents as necessary to achieve goal of fasting glucose or haemoglobin A_{1C}
Pro-thrombotic state	Goal: reduction of pro-thrombotic state Recommendation: high-risk patients – initiate low-dose aspirin therapy; consider clopidogrel if aspirin is contraindicated Moderately high-risk patients – consider low-dose aspirin therapy
Pro-inflammatory state	Recommendations: no specific therapies

[a]High-risk patients: those with established atherosclerotic cardiovascular disease, diabetes or 10-year risk for coronary heart disease > 20%.
[b]Moderately high-risk patients: those with 10-year risk for coronary heart disease 10 – 20%.
[c]Moderate risk patients: those with metabolic syndrome but 10-year risk for coronary heart disease < 10%.
[d]Lifestyle therapies include weight reduction, regular exercise and antiatherogenic diet.
Modified from Eckel RH, Grundy SM, Zimmet PZ (2005). The metabolic syndrome. *Lancet* **365**: 1415–28.

6.3 Risk Stratification

Presence of one component of the metabolic syndrome places individuals at higher risk of clustering with other components. The result is an additive or a more than additive effect on cardiovascular and renal outcomes. All those with the metabolic syndrome must be stratified in the highest risk category for cardiovascular and renal disease.

For asymptomatic individuals with no history of cardiovascular disease or diabetes, the blood glucose level should be viewed in the context of total cardiovascular disease risk based on the Framingham risk algorithm (Williams *et al.*, 2004). Apparently healthy individuals with cardiovascular disease risk $\geq 20\%$ over 10 years should receive appropriate risk factor intervention. Risk assessment is not appropriate in those with type 2 diabetes because the vast majority (i.e. those aged over 50 years or diagnosed for at least 10 years) probably have a risk of cardiovascular disease equivalent to people who have had a myocardial infarction and therefore should be considered as for secondary prevention (Expert Panel on Detection, Evaluation, and Treatment of High Blood Cholesterol in Adults, 2001).

Obesity

Insulin resistance, hyperinsulinaemia, diabetes, hypertension and dyslipidaemia are much more prevalent in people with central obesity than in non-obese subjects. Obesity causes cardiac and vascular disease through hypertension, type 2 diabetes and hyperlipidaemia; obesity is an independent predictor of cardiovascular risk factors, morbidity and mortality (Stevens *et al.*, 1998; Calle *et al.*, 1999; Seidell *et al.*, 1999; Katzmarzyk *et al.*, 2001). Obesity is also a cause of abnormal renal function.

Hypertension

There is a clear relationship between higher levels of blood pressure and increased cardiovascular morbidity and mortality in the general population (National High Blood Pressure Education Program Working Group, 1994; Franklin *et al.*, 1997, 1999; Vasan *et al.*, 2001; Prospective Studies Collaboration, 2002). Epidemiological studies demonstrate that increasing systolic and diastolic blood pressure correlates with increasing risk with no evidence of 'threshold' below which lower levels are not associated with lower risks of stroke and coronary heart disease. The relationship between blood pressure and cardiovascular events is graded and extends below the traditional hypertensive threshold (Vasan *et al.*, 2001). Persons with systolic blood pressure < 120 mmHg have fewer cardiovascular events than their counterparts with systolic blood pressure 120–129 mmHg or 130–139 mmHg.

Hypertension is both a cause and a consequence of renal disease. Blood pressure is a strong independent risk factor for end-stage renal disease (Klag *et al.*, 1996; Hunsicker *et al.*, 1997). Results from MRFIT showed that the increased risk of end-stage renal disease associated with higher blood pressure was graded and continuous throughout the distribution of blood pressure above the optimal level (Klag *et al.*, 1996).

In the diabetic population, hypertension increases the risk and accelerates the progression of coronary heart disease, left ventricular hypertrophy, congestive heart failure, cardiovascular disease, peripheral vascular disease and kidney disease. Population-based observational data suggest that, when compared with the non-diabetic population cardiovascular disease risk is elevated in people with diabetes at every level of blood pressure well into the conventional normotensive range (Stamler *et al.*, 1993; Adler *et al.*, 2000). Moreover, there appears to be no threshold below which risk declines substantially. From a pathophysiological perspective, people with diabetes exhibit disturbances of blood pressure regulation and vascular function that increase vulnerability to hypertensive injury (Williams, 1999). In people with diabetes, antihypertensive therapy should be initiated if systolic blood pressure is sustained at ≥ 140 mmHg and/or diastolic blood pressure is sustained at ≥ 90 mmHg (Williams *et al.*, 2004).

6.4 Strategies to Reduce Cardiovascular Risk

Since all patients with diabetes and the metabolic syndrome are at the highest risk of cardiovascular and renal events, it is imperative to devise preventive and therapeutic strategies to reduce such events and disease progression.

Non-pharmacological interventions

Lifestyle intervention inspires a sense of well-being, may be less expensive than pharmacological interventions and has no known harmful effects. In impaired glucose tolerance, progression to diabetes can be prevented or postponed by lifestyle modifications, such as dietary manipulation and physical activity (Pan *et al.*, 1997; Tuomilehto *et al.*, 2001) (see also Chapter 10).

A variety of lifestyle modifications reduce blood pressure and the incidence of hypertension (Ebrahim and Smith, 1998; He *et al.*, 2000; Sacks *et al.*, 2001; Whelton *et al.*, 2002). Non-pharmacological interventions include weight loss in the overweight (He *et al.*, 2000, Whelton *et al.*, 2001), exercise programmes (Whelton *et al.*, 2002), moderation of alcohol intake (Xin *et al.*, 2001) and a diet with increased fruit and vegetables and reduced saturated fat content (Sacks *et al.*, 2001), reduction in dietary sodium intake (Whelton *et al.*, 1998; Sacks *et al.*, 2001) and increased dietary potassium intake (He and Whelton, 1999) (Table 6.2). When adherence is optimal, systolic blood pressure is reduced by > 10 mmHg (Sacks *et al.*, 2001). Reductions are more modest in clinical practice (Ebrahim and Smith, 1998) and studies were not designed or powered to evaluate changes in overall or cardiac mortality. However, in long-term, large-scale population studies, even small reductions in blood pressure are associated with reduced cardiovascular disease risk (Cook *et al.*, 1995).

Lifestyle modification should be provided for all people with high blood pressure and those with borderline or high-normal blood pressure. Such interventions are recommended even when antihypertensive drugs are prescribed as the blood pressure effects of drugs are complemented and thus the dose or number of drugs required to control blood pressure is reduced.

Table 6.2 Lifestyle measures recommended in management of Hypertension. Modified from Williams B, Poulter NR, Brown MJ *et al.* (2004). Guidelines for management of hypertension: report of the fourth working party of the British Hypertension Society, 2004 – BHS IV. *Journal of Human Hypertension* **18**: 139–85.

- Maintain normal weight for adults (body mass index 20–25 kg/m^2)
- Reduce salt intake to < 100 mmol/day (< 6 g NaCl or < 2.5 g sodium/day)
- Limit alcohol consumption to ≤ 3 units/day for men or ≤ 2 units/day for women
- Engage in regular aerobic physical exercise (brisk walking rather than weightlifting) for ≥ 30 minutes/day, ideally on most days of the week but at least on three days/week
- Consume at least five portions/day of fresh fruit and vegetables
- Reduce intake of total and saturated fat

Dietary modification

Weight gain is a critical factor in the progression to type 2 diabetes (Colditz *et al.*, 1995). A key component of management is to avoid overweight, particularly by calorie restriction and decrease of sodium intake because of the strong relationship between obesity, hypertension, sodium sensitivity and insulin resistance (Rocchini, 2000).

Physical activity and weight loss

The increasingly sedentary lifestyle of the general population has contributed to an epidemic of obesity and the metabolic syndrome. A graded exercise programme is strongly recommended (Wasserman and Zinman, 1994; Whelton *et al.*, 2002).

Tobacco cessation

The combination of smoking and diabetes enhances the risk of microvascular and macrovascular disease as well as premature mortality. Patients with diabetes should be counselled about smoking cessation, the enhanced risks of smoking and diabetes for morbidity and mortality, and the proven efficacy and cost-effectiveness of cessation strategies (Kawachi *et al.*, 1994; Haire-Joshu *et al.*, 1999).

Pharmacological interventions

Several drug therapies are of proven value in reducing cardiovascular risk in people with diabetes and hypertension.

Aspirin therapy

Concerns about the safety of aspirin in diabetes appear to be unfounded (Antithrombotic Trialists' Collaboration, 2002). Low-dose aspirin is recommended in diabetes whether or not there is evidence of large vessel disease. The British Hypertension Society recommends 75 mg of aspirin for all with hypertension and diabetes, unless contraindicated (Williams *et al.*, 2004); blood pressure should be controlled to audit standards ($< 150/90$ mmHg) for the general hypertension population.

Glycaemic control

Improved glycaemic control is probably associated with reduced cardiovascular events as well as microvascular complications in type 1 and type 2 diabetes (Chapter 9). Neither the Diabetes Control and Complications Trial (DCCT) (Diabetes Control and Complications Trial Research Group, 1993) nor the UKPDS (UK Prospective Diabetes Study (UKPDS) Group, 1998) proved definitively that intensive therapy to lower blood glucose levels reduced the risk of cardiovascular complications compared with less-intensive therapy, although the DCCT was under-powered for cardiovascular disease. Subsequent follow-up of DCCT patients in the Epidemiology of Diabetes Interventions and Complications (EDIC) study demonstrated a significant reduction in cardiovascular events (Diabetes Control and Complications Trial/Epidemiology of Diabetes Interventions and Complications (DCCT/EDIC) Study Research Group, 2005). Choice of treatment in type 2 diabetes with hypertension may be critical. Rosiglitazone improves glucose and blood pressure in type 2 diabetes probably by attenuation of hyperinsulinaemia and sympathetic activity, while glibenclamide, for the same plasma glucose control, worsens blood pressure control, possibly by elevation of insulin levels and activation of the sympathetic system (Yosefy et al., 2004). This area requires long-term follow-up studies (Chapter 11).

Blood pressure control

Effective blood pressure control has considerable and immediate benefit in patients with diabetes (Heart Outcomes Prevention Evaluation (HOPE) Study Investigators, 2000; Brenner et al., 2001; Lewis et al., 2001; Parving et al., 2001a). In trials that included patients with diabetes, blood pressure lowering reduced or prevented an aggregate of major cardiovascular events including heart failure, cardiovascular death and total mortality. Antihypertensive therapy diminishes the risk of macrovascular complications by around 20%. Reducing blood pressure also reduces progression of retinopathy, albuminuria and progression to nephropathy. Clinical trials with diuretics, beta-blockers, ACE inhibitors, angiotensin receptor blockers and calcium channel blockers have demonstrated benefit of treatment of hypertension in type 2 diabetes (Staessen et al., 1997; Hansson et al., 1998; UK Prospective Diabetes Study Group, 1998a; Tuomilehto et al., 1999; Brown et al., 2000; ALLHAT Officers and Coordinators for the ALLHAT Collaborative Research Group, 2002; Black et al., 2003). Although no major trial has assessed the effect of blood pressure lowering on cardiovascular morbidity and mortality exclusively in hypertensive patients with type 1 diabetes, these patients are generally managed in a similar manner.

In 492 type 2 diabetes patients with isolated systolic hypertension in the Systolic Hypertension in Europe (SYST-EUR) trials (Tuomilehto et al., 1999), all-cause mortality, all cardiovascular endpoints, fatal and non-fatal stroke and fatal and non-fatal cardiac endpoints were all reduced by antihypertensive therapy. The reduction in relative hazard ratios was greater for all outcomes in diabetics compared with non-diabetics ($n = 4213$) and, for most, these were significant treatment × diabetes interactions. A blood pressure reduction of 8.6/3.9 mmHg was associated with a 69% reduction in cardiovascular disease in the type 2 diabetes subgroup compared with a

26% reduction in non-diabetics (Figure 6.1). Similar benefits were seen in the diabetes subgroup in the Systolic Hypertension in the Elderly Programme (SHEP) (Curb *et al.*, 1996); the 5-year cardiovascular disease event rate was reduced by 34% compared with the overall reduction.

Randomised controlled trials that have included large diabetes populations have demonstrated impressive improvements in cardiovascular disease outcomes, especially stroke, and microvascular complications when rigorous blood pressure targets are achieved (Hansson *et al.*, 1998; UK Prospective Diabetes Study Group, 1998a; Tuomilehto *et al.*, 1999; Heart Outcomes Prevention Evaluation (HOPE) Study Investigators, 2000; Mann *et al.*, 2001; ALLHAT Officers and Coordinators for the ALLHAT Collaborative Research Group, 2002; Schrier *et al.*, 2002). The importance of tight blood pressure control in diabetes was illustrated in the UKPDS (UK Prospective Diabetes Study Group, 1998a). Tight blood pressure control ($< 150/85$ mmHg) was associated with an outcome benefit greater than that with less tight control ($< 180/105$ mmHg). Lowering blood pressure to a mean of $144/82$ mmHg significantly reduced stroke, diabetic-related deaths and heart failure. A $10/15$ mmHg difference over 8.4 years resulted in a 21% reduction in myocardial infarction (non-significant) and a significant reduction in stroke (44%), all macrovascular endpoints (35%) and microvascular disease (25%). There was a continuous relationship between the risk of these outcomes and systolic blood pressure, with no evidence of a threshold for these complications down to systolic blood pressure 130 mmHg. The

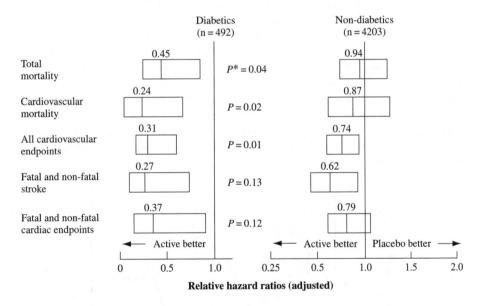

P value for treatment – diabetes interaction

Figure 6.1 The Systolic Hypertension in Europe (SYST-EUR) relative hazard ratios for active treatment versus placebo. Reproduced from Tuomilehto *et al.* for the Systolic Hypertension in Europe Trial Investigators (1999) Effects of calcium channel blockers in older patients with diabetic and systolic hypertension. New England Journal of Medicine **340**: 677–84. Copyright © 1999 Massachusetts Medical Society. All rights reserved.

lowest risk was in those with systolic blood pressure < 120 mmHg. The relative risk reductions with tight blood pressure control were greater in magnitude than those for intensive glucose control in the prevention of stroke, any type 2 diabetes endpoint, any type 2 diabetes-related death and microvascular complications (Hypertension in Diabetes Study (HDS), 1993; UK Prospective Diabetes Study Group, 1998a).

The exquisite sensitivity of patients with type 2 diabetes and hypertension to tight blood pressure control was confirmed in the Hypertension Optimal Treatment (HOT) trial (Hansson *et al.*, 1998). In 1501 patients with hypertension and type 2 diabetes, there was a stepwise reduction in cardiovascular events in those randomised to diastolic blood pressure targets ≤ 90 mmHg, ≤ 85 mmHg and ≤ 80 mmHg (Figure 6.2). The relative risk reduction for major cardiovascular events (non-fatal myocardial infarction, non-fatal stroke and cardiovascular deaths) from ≤ 90 mmmHg to ≤ 80 mmHg was 51%. Since achieved blood pressure was 85 mmHg and 81 mmHg in those randomised to ≤ 90 mmHg and ≤ 80 mmHg, respectively, the reduction resulted from a difference in diastolic blood pressure of only 4 mmHg.

In hypertensive patients with diabetes, the greater the blood pressure lowering, the greater the benefit for cardiovascular events, with no blood pressure threshold level below which risk no longer declines (Schrier *et al.*, 2002). Several trials have shown that in diabetes the reduction of diastolic blood pressure to about 80 mmHg and systolic blood pressure to about 130 mmHg is associated with further reduction in cardiovascular events and diabetes mellitus-related microvascular complications compared with less stringent blood pressure control (UK Prospective Diabetes Study Group, 1998a; Adler *et al.*, 2000; Zanchetti and Ruilope, 2002).

The blood pressure target for those with diabetes is lower than that for individuals without diabetes. Evidence from intervention trials in people with diabetes and extrapolation from epidemiological studies support a 'lower the better' policy for optimal blood pressure (Hansson *et al.*, 1998; Heart Outcomes Prevention Evaluation (HOPE) Study Investigators, 2000) with a target of < 130/80 mmHg (European Society of Hypertension–European Society of Cardiology Guidelines Committee, 2003; World Health Organization International Society of Hypertension Working Group, 2003; Williams *et al.*, 2004; American Diabetes Association, 2006). The optimal blood pressure is the lowest tolerated.

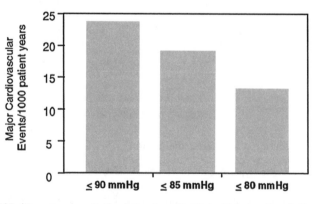

Figure 6.2 HOT (Hypertension Optimal Treatment) Trial: Diabetes Population. Reproduced from Hansson *et al.* (1998). Effects of intensive blood-pressure lowering and low-dose aspirin in patients with hypertension: principal results of the Hypertension Optimal Treatment (HOT) randomised trial. Hot Study Group. *Lancet* **351**: 1755–62.

Despite best practice, the blood pressure target of < 130/80 mmHg is difficult to achieve, particularly in an older population (Mancia and Grassi, 2002; Zanchetti and Ruilope, 2002; Williams *et al.*, 2004). Control of diastolic blood pressure is less problematic and the focus should be on systolic blood pressure control since many (especially those with type 2 diabetes) have isolated systolic hypertension. An audit standard of < 140/80 mmHg is suggested (Williams *et al.*, 2004). Thereafter, further cardiovascular benefits can be expected if blood pressure is lowered to the optimal target of < 130/80 mmHg, especially in diabetic nephropathy or retinopathy.

All patients with grade 1 hypertension (sustained systolic blood pressure 140–159 mmHg or diastolic blood pressure 90–99 mmHg, or both) or higher and diabetes should be offered treatment with antihypertensive drugs (Williams *et al.*, 2004). The composition of the treatment regimen has been an area of great controversy, myths and misconceptions (Zanchetti and Ruilope, 2002). The evidence for superiority or inferiority of different drug classes is vague and contradictory. Most comparisons come from relatively small studies or substudies of larger trials with inadequate power to test for the small difference to be expected. There is controversy about the safety and efficacy of calcium channel blockers (Estacio *et al.*, 1998) and reluctance to use thiazides and thiazide-like diuretics because of perceived effects on insulin sensitivity and metabolic indices. Many of these concerns have been allayed by the results of recent clinical trials (Curb *et al.*, 1996; Hansson *et al.*, 1998; Tuomilehto *et al.*, 1999; Brown *et al.*, 2000; ALLHAT Officers and Coordinators for the ALLHAT Collaborative Research Group, 2002; Schrier *et al.*, 2002; Black *et al.*, 2003; Bakris *et al.*, 2004).

Choice of agents

Calcium channel blockers

Calcium channel blocker-based therapy appears equivalent to conventional therapy (based on diuretics or beta-blockers) in cardiovascular risk reduction (ALLHAT Officers and Coordinators for the ALLHAT Collaborative Research Group, 2002; Black *et al.*, 2003; Bakris *et al.*, 2004). In the International Verapamil SR/Trandolapril (INVEST) study (Bakris *et al.*, 2004), there was no difference between verapamil and atenolol for the primary outcome (all-cause mortality plus non-fatal myocardial infarction plus non-fatal stroke) in the diabetes subgroup (6400 of 22 576 participants). Similar results were achieved in the diabetic subgroup of the Controlled Onset Verapamil Investigation of Cardiovascular Endpoints (CONVINCE) trial (Black *et al.*, 2003).

In the diabetes subgroup of the Antihypertensive and Lipid-lowering Treatment to Prevent Heart Attack Trial (ALLHAT), the dihydropyridine amlodipine was equivalent to chlorthalidone in reducing the primary endpoint of fatal coronary heart disease and myocardial infarction, although the calcium channel blocker was significantly inferior in protection against heart failure (ALLHAT Officers and Coordinators for the ALLHAT Collaborative Research Group, 2002). The Appropriate Blood Pressure Control in Diabetes (ABCD) study was stopped prematurely because nisoldipine was inferior to lisinopril in reducing the incidence of ischaemic cardiac events (Estacio *et al.*, 1998). However, in normotensive diabetes in the second ABCD study (ABCD2), nitrendipine was equivalent to lisinopril in stroke prevention and in retardation of the development of albuminuria (Schrier et al., 2002).

ACE inhibitors

In the UKPDS, ACE inhibitor (captopril)- and beta-blocker (atenolol)-based therapies were equally effective for all outcome measures, including diabetes-related death, myocardial infarction and all microvascular endpoints (UK Prospective Diabetes Study Group, 1998b). However, patients randomised to atenolol had slightly better blood pressure control (1 mmHg systolic and 2 mmHg diastolic).

In a subgroup analysis of the Captopril Prevention Project (CAPPP), captopril was superior to a diuretic/beta-blocker regimen in preventing cardiovascular events in hypertensive diabetic patients (Niskanen et al., 2001). In the Fosinopril versus Amlodipine Cardiovascular Events Randomised Trial (FACET), fosinopril and amlodipine reduced fasting blood sugar, serum insulin and microalbuminuria by similar magnitudes (Tatti et al., 1998) but, despite greater blood pressure reduction on amlodipine, fosinopril was associated with a 51% lower incidence of the combination of death, myocardial infarction, hospitalised angina and stroke. The combined results of ABCD, CAPPP and FACET showed a significant benefit of ACE inhibition compared with alternative treatments on the outcomes of acute myocardial infarction (63%), cardiovascular events (51%) and all-cause mortality (62%). None of these differences was explained by differences in blood pressure (Pahor et al., 2000).

The Heart Outcomes Prevention Evaluation (HOPE) provided further support for the use of ACE inhibitors. In the hypertensive and normotensive diabetes subpopulation (Heart Outcomes Prevention Evaluation (HOPE) Study Investigators, 2000), treatment with ramipril added to standard therapy reduced combined myocardial infarction, stroke and cardiovascular death by about 25% and stroke by 33% compared with placebo plus conventional therapy. Combined microvascular events were reduced by 16%. To what extent this was independent of the 2.2/1.4 mmHg difference in blood pressure remains controversial.

Despite these findings, the evidence for ACE inhibitors as first-line therapy is limited. In the ALLHAT, an ACE inhibitor did not show superiority over a thiazide-like diuretic in over 12 000 individuals with type 2 diabetes (ALLHAT Officers and Coordinators for the ALLHAT Collaborative Research Group, 2002). Indeed, the ACE inhibitor showed a trend for elevated risk of cardiovascular disease. However, the ALLHAT has been much criticised because of flaws in design and the comparability of the groups (McInnes, 2003).

The superiority of ACE inhibitors rests largely in two comparisons, with diuretics/beta-blockers (Niskanen et al., 2001) or calcium channel blockers (Estacio et al., 1998), or on analysis of cause-specific events for which the trial power is low. In type 1 diabetes mellitus, there is evidence for renoprotection with ACE inhibitors but no substantive data confirming cardioprotection with ACE inhibitor beyond the impact of blood pressure control (Lewis et al., 1993).

Angiotensin receptor blockers

In the diabetic subpopulation ($n = 1195$) of the Losartan Intervention For Endpoint (LIFE) reduction study of hypertensive patients with ECG evidence of left ventricular hypertrophy (Lindholm *et al.*, 2002a), therapy based on losartan was superior to atenolol-based therapy for the primary composite endpoint (25% reduction) and all-cause mortality (39% reduction). There was also significant reduction in cardiovascular mortality (37%), heart failure (41%) and stroke. Regression of left ventricular hypertrophy was twice as great with losartan compared with atenolol (Kjeldsen *et al.*, 2002; Okin *et al.*, 2003).

Similar results were seen in the Reduction of Endpoints in NIDDM with the Angiotensin II Antagonist Losartan (RENAAL) study, which included 1513 type 2 diabetes mellitus patients with early renal insufficiency and microalbuminuria (Brenner *et al.*, 2001). Compared with conventional therapy, losartan reduced new onset congestive heart failure with a trend to reduced myocardial infarction.

The use of renin–angiotensin system blockade in type 2 diabetes is well supported (Lindholm *et al.*, 2002a). The evidence for cardiovascular protection with angiotensin receptor blockers is more substantial than for ACE inhibitors.

Treatment strategies

Almost all patients with hypertension and diabetes require combinations of blood pressure-lowering drugs to achieve the recommended blood pressure targets (Sowers and Haffner, 2002). Three or more drugs may be needed (Mancia and Grassi, 2002; Zanchetti and Ruilope, 2002; American Diabetes Association, 2006). Clinical trial data support the combined use of a renin–angiotensin system-blocking drug and a thiazide diuretic to reduce cardiovascular events (Sowers and Bakris, 2000; Brenner *et al.*, 2001; Lewis *et al.*, 2001; Parving *et al.*, 2001a; Lindholm *et al.*, 2002a). Many patients will gain additional benefits from both beta-blockers and calcium channel blocker therapy to achieve lower blood pressure goals. For example, when combined with an ACE inhibitor, the calcium channel blocker amlodipine reduced blood pressure and also morbidity and mortality in type 2 diabetes with hypertension (Tatti *et al.*, 1998). However, alpha-blockers are probably less effective than other antihypertensive agents in reducing blood pressure in type 2 diabetes (Beckman *et al.*, 2002).

Combination therapy is likely to include a thiazide or thiazide-like diuretic (ALLHAT Officers and Coordinators for the ALLHAT Collaborative Research Group, 2002). In patients with renal impairment, a loop diuretic may be required as an alternative, or in addition, to a thiazide or a thiazide-like diuretic (Williams *et al.*, 2004). When there are no cost disadvantages, the combined drugs should be used as a fixed-dose combination to reduce the number of medications.

Role of renin–angiotensin system in diabetes mellitus and vascular complications

Local formation of angiotensin II by tissue-based renin–angiotensin systems in cardiac, renal and vascular tissues represents an important pathophysiological mechanism that is upregulated in diabetes. Short-term moderate hyperglycaemia without glycosuria during the early stages of diabetes is linked with increased plasma renin activity, mean arterial pressure and renal vascular resistance (Miller *et al.*, 1996) with activation of circulating and local renin–angiotensin systems. In animal models of diabetes, inhibition of the renin–angiotensin system with ACE inhibitor (Candido et al., 2002) or angiotensin receptor blocker (Candido et al., 2004) has been shown to prevent atherosclerosis independent of blood pressure reduction.

Improvement in insulin sensitivity follows ACE inhibition (Pollare et al., 1989; Berne et al., 1991; Donnelly, 1992; Ferrannini et al., 1994), particularly in hypertensives with type 2 diabetes (Torlone et al., 1991, 1993). Many of the initial reports were based on uncontrolled studies or flawed study design, indirect measures of insulin sensitivity or studies in patients receiving potentially confounding medications (Petrie et al., 2000). Nevertheless, data suggest that treatment of type 2 diabetes with ACE inhibition may improve glycaemic control (Heart Outcomes Prevention Evaluation (HOPE) Study Investigators, 2000) or even induce hypoglycaemia when used with insulin (Herings et al., 1995) or oral hypoglycaemic agents (Morris et al., 1997; Thamer et al., 1999).

Blockade of the renin–angiotensin system may be more effective than other antihypertensives for the same blood pressure reduction in regression of left ventricular mass (Kjeldsen et al., 2002; Okin et al., 2003). Renin–angiotensin system blockade may also reverse endothelial dysfunction in patients with coronary heart disease, hypertension and diabetes, and may favourably affect fibrinolytic balance possibly by attenuation of angiotensin II and enhancement of bradykinin (Mancini et al., 1996; Hornig et al., 1997).

More specific outcome trials in diabetes are needed to dispel the myths that seem to limit widespread use of drugs that block the renin–angiotensin system in diabetes (Lim et al., 2004). These include: fear of precipitating azotaemia with or without pre-existing renal disease; fear of haemodynamic instability, particularly in patients with suspected autonomic neuropathy; fear of hyperkalaemia; and fear of precipitating renal failure due to exacerbation of bilateral renal artery stenosis, which is more common in diabetes.

Microalbuminuria and macroalbuminuria

Microalbuminuria is one of the most important factors in predicting progression to macroalbuminuria or overt nephropathy in type 1 and type 2 diabetes (Mogensen, 1984; Mogensen et al., 1995). Microalbuminuria is also predictive of cardiovascular mortality in both diabetic and non-diabetic populations (Mogensen, 1984; Agrawal et al., 1996; Mann et al., 2001). The presence of microalbuminuria indicates widespread disturbance of endothelial function, resulting in enhanced risk of atherosclerosis (Ruilope and Rodicio, 1995). Thus, it may serve as a useful biomarker for systemic vascular disease.

In microalbuminuria, a lower blood pressure target should be considered. Subgroup analyses of type 2 diabetes in major outcome trials indicate that more intensive blood pressure control (systolic blood pressure < 130 mmHg) with blockade of the renin–angiotensin–aldosterone system as part of the regimen provides the optimal strategy for both cardiovascular risk reduction (Tatti et al., 1998; Niskanen et al., 2001) and prevention of progression from microalbuminuria to macroalbuminuria, and from macroalbuminuria to overt nephropathy (Heart Outcomes Prevention Evaluation (HOPE) Study Investigators, 2000). Normalisation of urine albumin excretion may serve as a clinical clue to optimal blood pressure control.

Correction of dyslipidaemia

The evidence for cholesterol reduction in diabetes comes predominantly from subgroup analyses of clinical trials that included people with diabetes. In those with established cardiovascular disease, gemfibrozil and statins have shown significant reduction in coronary heart disease and cardiovascular events (Frick *et al.*, 1987; Pyorala *et al.*, 1997; Goldberg *et al.*, 1998; Long-Term Intervention with Pravastatin in Ischaemic Disease (LIPID) Study Group, 1998; Rubins *et al.*, 1999; Heart Protection Study Group, 2002). In primary prevention, benefits have been shown with gemfibrozil (Frick *et al.*, 1987; Koskinen *et al.*, 1992) and a statin in a hypertensive population (Sever *et al.*, 2003). In the only trial of primary prevention exclusively in diabetes, there was reduction in acute coronary events and strokes with atorvastatin (Colhoun *et al.*, 2004).

The primary target is lowering LDL-cholesterol and recent evidence supports rigorous goals (Heart Protection Study Group, 2002; Sever *et al.*, 2003; Colhoun *et al.*, 2004). Statins are the preferred pharmacological agents (Williams *et al.*, 2004). Reduction in LDL-cholesterol should take primacy. Once LDL-cholesterol levels have been lowered, attention should be given to treatment of residual hypertriglyceridaemia and low HDL-cholesterol (Haffner, 1998).

British and European guidelines are consistent (European Society of Hypertension–European Society of Cardiology Guidelines Committee, 2003; Williams *et al.*, 2004). All hypertensive patients up to 80 years of age with type 2 diabetes should be considered for lipid lowering with a threshold total cholesterol ≥ 3.5 mmol/l. Target lipid concentrations are total cholesterol < 4.0 mmol/l (or 25% reduction) and LDL-cholesterol < 2.0 mmol/l (or 30% reduction), whichever is greater. Type 2 diabetes patients benefit from statin therapy irrespective of baseline total cholesterol (Sever *et al.*, 2003; Colhoun *et al.*, 2004). Use of statins in type 2 diabetes with hypertension should be routine (Williams et al, 2004). There is less evidence in type 1 diabetes but treatment should be as for type 2 diabetes.

Multifactorial intervention

There is limited evidence from a small study in patients with type 2 diabetes (Gaede *et al.*, 2003) that more intensive intervention incorporating modifications in lifestyle, glycaemia, blood pressure, dyslipidaemia and microalbuminuria (ACE inhibitor or angiotensin receptor blocker) is superior to conventional therapy. Cardiovascular events were reduced by 53%, stroke by 85%, amputations by 50%, nephropathy by 61%, retinopathy by 56% and autonomic neuropathy by 67% (all significant) (see also Chapter 9, p. 233). This approach is similar to current guidelines for the management of people with diabetes and hypertension.

6.5   Strategies to Reduce Kidney Disease Risk

Non-pharmacological interventions

Lifestyle intervention should focus on dietary modification, including low saturated fat and low salt diets, weight reduction and increased physical activity, cessation of tobacco use and moderation of alcohol consumption. Because the majority of patients with type 2 diabetes have hypertension, non-pharmacological interventions to assist reduction in blood pressure will help to preserve kidney function.

Increasing salt intake attenuates the antihypertensive and antiproteinuria effects of ACE inhibitors and angiotensin receptor blockers (Heeg *et al.*, 1989). Thus, salt restriction should be encouraged in hypertensive diabetic patients although clinical trials are needed to inform guidelines.

Moderate protein restriction reduces albuminuria and progression of renal disease and improves outcome in type 1 and type 2 diabetes. This benefit is additive to those of antihypertensive treatment (Pedrini *et al.*, 1996).

Pharmacological interventions

Glycaemic control

Meticulous control of glycaemia preserves kidney function and delays development of renal damage in diabetes mellitus (Gaede *et al.*, 2003). Thus, strict glycaemic control should accompany optimal blood pressure control (European Diabetes Policy Group, 1999).

Blood pressure control

Strict control of blood pressure is the most important factor in preventing the development of diabetic nephropathy and end-stage renal disease, and the progression of diabetic nephropathy to end-stage renal disease (Maki *et al.*, 1995; Mogensen *et al.*, 1995; Nelson *et al.*, 1996). Multiple placebo-controlled trials have shown significant reductions in proteinuria and slowing of progression of renal damage in type 1 and type 2 diabetes (Lewis *et al.*, 1993, 2001; Brenner *et al.*, 2001).

Compared with lesser control, more intensive blood pressure lowering significantly reduces the progression of retinopathy, albuminuria and progression of nephropathy (Curb *et al.*, 1996; UK Prospective Diabetes Study Group, 1998a; Tuomilehto *et al.*, 1999; Heart Outcomes Prevention Evaluation (HOPE) Study Investigators, 2000; Schrier *et al.*, 2002). A modest 4/2 mmHg reduction in blood pressure in type 1 and type 2 diabetes mellitus with baseline blood pressure 124/77 mmHg resulted in 50% reduction in progression from microalbuminuria to clinical proteinuria (Viberti *et al.*, 1994). In the UKPDS, lowering blood pressure by 10/5 mmHg to a mean of 144/82 mmHg significantly reduced microvascular complications compared with less aggressive treatment (UK Prospective Diabetes Study Group, 1998a). There was a continuous relation between microvascular outcomes and systolic blood pressure with no evidence of a threshold above a systolic blood pressure of 130 mmHg.

These clinical data support the advantage of lower blood pressure goals in prevention of renal disease progression in diabetes mellitus. Blood pressure control to levels lower than those necessary for the general population is a major therapeutic initiative in diabetic nephropathy (Lewis *et al.*, 1993, 2001; Viberti *et al.*, 1994; Brenner *et al.*, 2001; Parving *et al.*, 2001a). Current guidelines recommend a blood pressure goal for diabetes with any evidence of kidney damage of < 130/80 mmHg (Chobanian *et al.*,

2003; European Society of Hypertension–European Society of Cardiology Guidelines Committee, 2003; World Health Organization International Society of Hypertension Writing Group, 2003; Williams *et al.*, 2004) and lower if there is proteinuria ≥ 1 g per 24 h.

The average number of drugs required to achieve optimal blood pressure control in patients with chronic kidney disease is estimated to be 2.6–3.4 (Bakris, 1999). If initial blood pressure is more than 20/10 mmHg above goal, it may be best to consider initiating therapy with two agents.

A meta-analysis of 100 studies comprising 2494 patients with both type 1 and type 2 diabetes with proteinuria indicated that antihypertensive agents reduced urine albumin excretion compared with placebo with a rank order of benefit: ACE inhibitor > calcium channel blocker > diuretic (Kasiske *et al.*, 1993). Angiotensin receptor blockers also reduce the incidence of new proteinuria better than other agents (Lindholm *et al.*, 2002a). The finding of even microalbuminuria in type 1 and type 2 diabetes is an indication for antihypertensive therapy, which should include a blocker of the renin–angiotensin system irrespective of blood pressure level (European Society of Hypertension–European Society of Cardiology Guidelines Committee, 2003). In patients with high normal blood pressure, who may sometimes achieve blood pressure goal by monotherapy, an angiotensin receptor blocker (or ACE inhibitor) should be the first drug used. Aldosterone receptor antagonists might also have a role but need to be studied in more detail (Sato *et al.*, 2003).

Thiazides, or loop diuretics if there is renal insufficiency, facilitate the antihypertensive effects of ACE inhibitors and angiotensin receptor blockers. Likewise, calcium channel blockers have robust antihypertensive effects. Dihydropyridine calcium channel blockers increase or do not change proteinuria, and do not reduce progression of renal disease compared with angiotensin receptor blockade (Lewis *et al.*, 2001), while non-dihydropyridines may be as effective as ACE inhibitors in reducing albuminuria (Bakris *et al.*, 1996). However, in the Bergamo Nephrologic Diabetes Complications Trial (BENEDICT), despite equivalent blood pressure and glycaemic control, verapamil was less effective than trandolapril in attenuation of urinary albumin extraction (Ruggenenenti *et al.*, 2004), although the combination was highly effective in blood pressure control and reducing albuminuria.

In the UKPDS, there was no difference between atenolol and captopril in microalbuminuria, or for conversion of microalbuminuria to macroalbuminuria (UK Prospective Diabetes Study Group, 1998b). However, the low prevalence of nephropathy in the population makes it unclear whether either drug was protective in the progression of nephropathy.

Microalbuminuria

Microalbuminuria (incipient nephropathy) is highly predictive of diabetic nephropathy and worsening renal function. Approximately 30% of people with type 2 diabetes have microalbuminuria, especially those with hypertension and other features of the metabolic syndrome.

A series of studies in microalbuminuric patients provides clear evidence of an advantage of lower blood pressure goals combined with renin–angiotensin system blockade. In normotensive individuals with type 1 and type 2 diabetes, captopril-based therapy significantly reduced progression to clinical proteinuria compared with placebo (Viberti *et al.*, 1994). In 94 patients with mean post-treatment blood pressure of 130/80 mmHg, enalapril for 7 years was associated with 42% reduction in nephropathy compared with placebo (Ravid *et al.*, 1993). Similarly, angiotensin receptor blocker therapy provoked a 70% reduction in progression of microalbuminuria to clinical proteinuria compared with placebo in hypertensive patients with type 2 diabetes (Parving *et al.*, 2001a). In type 2 diabetes, a comparison of valsartan and amlodipine demonstrated a blood pressure-independent antimicroalbuminuric effect of the angiotensin receptor blocker (Viberti *et al.*, 2002).

Type 1 diabetes

In type 1 diabetes, blood pressure reduction with ACE inhibition slows the rate of decline of renal function in overt diabetic nephropathy (Lewis *et al.*, 1993) and delays progression from microalbuminuria to overt nephropathy (Mogensen *et al.*, 1995; Parving, 1996; Cooper, 1998). Smaller studies have confirmed that even among patients with initial blood pressure < 130/80 mmHg, addition of an ACE inhibitor reduces proteinuria (Viberti *et al.*, 1994; Parving *et al.*, 2001b). ACE inhibition also slows progression of diabetic retinopathy in normotensive patients (Chaturvedi *et al.*,1998).

ACE inhibitors are recommended as initial therapy in incipient and overt diabetic nephropathy. If there is ACE inhibitor cough, an angiotensin receptor blocker is the recommended alternative. ACE inhibitor dose should be titrated to the maximum recommended and tolerated. Add-on drugs include low-dose thiazide/thiazide-like diuretics, calcium channel blockers and beta-blockers (Williams *et al.*, 2004). A similar approach is recommended in persistent microalbuminuria (Lewis *et al.*, 1993; EUCLID Study Group, 1997; Cooper, 1998). It is unclear whether the benefit accrues from blockade of the renin–angiotensin system *per se* or the associated blood pressure reduction.

Type 2 diabetes

In type 2 diabetes, hypertension accelerates the decline of renal function (Gall *et al.*, 1997; Cooper, 1998). Antihypertensive therapy slows the progression of nephropathy (Cooper, 1998). ACE inhibitors have an antiproteinuric action and delay progression from microalbuminuria to overt nephropathy (Parving, 1996; Ravid *et al.*, 1996; Cooper, 1998). It is less clear whether there is a specific renoprotective action beyond blood pressure reduction.

There is good evidence that angiotensin receptor blocker-based therapy can delay progression of microalbuminuria to overt nephropathy (proteinuria) (Parving *et al.*, 2001a) and progression of overt nephropathy to end-stage renal disease (Brenner *et al.*, 2001; Lewis *et al.*, 2001). Several studies have confirmed the renoprotective effect of angiotensin receptor blockers in nephropathy associated with type 2 diabetes. The RENAAL study (Brenner *et al.*, 2001) included type 2 diabetes patients with early renal insufficiency and microalbuminuria; compared with conventional therapy, losartan-based therapy reduced proteinuria and end-stage renal disease (Figure 6.3). The

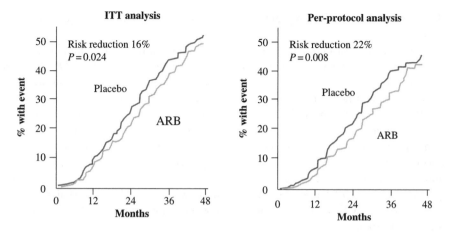

Figure 6.3 RENAAL Time to composite endpoint (doubling of serum creatinine, end stage renal disease or death). Reproduced from Brenner BM, Cooper ME, De Zeeuw D, Keane WF, Mitch WE, Parving H-H *et al.* for the RENAAL Study Investigators (2001). Effects of losartan on renal and cardiovascular outcomes in patients with type 2 diabetes and nephropathy. *New England Journal of Medicine* **345**: 861–9. Copyright © 2001 Massachusetts Medical Society. All rights reserved.

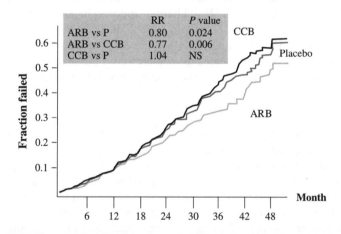

Figure 6.4 IDNT Time to doubling of serum creatinine, ESRD (End Stage Renal Disease) or death. Reproduced from Lewis EJ, Hunsicker LG, Clarke WR, Berl T Pohl MA, Lewis JB *et al.* for the Collaborative Study Group (2001). Renoprotective effect of the angiotensin-receptor antagonist irbesartan in patients with nephropathy due to type 2 diabetes. *New England Journal of Medicine* **345**: 851–60. Copyright © 2001 Massachusetts Medical Society. All rights reserved.

Irbesartan Diabetic Nephropathy Trial (IDNT) (Lewis *et al.*, 2001) also demonstrated a significant benefit of a multidrug regimen including irbesartan compared with conventional multidrug therapy or an amlodipine-based regimen in reducing the composite endpoint of a doubling in serum creatinine, end-stage renal disease or death in patients with type 2 diabetes, clinical proteinuria and early renal insufficiency (Figure 6.4). The benefit of angiotensin receptor blocker-based therapy in delaying progression of diabetic nephropathy is complementary to the more substantial benefits achieved by improved blood pressure control.

Blockade of the renin–angiotensin system in diabetic nephropathy

At least in type 2 diabetes, there is evidence for activation of the intrarenal renin–angiotensin system despite low levels of circulating renin (Price et al., 1999). Blockade of the renin–angiotensin system results in selective dilation of the efferent arterioles in the kidney and hence reduced glomerular pressure and reduced albumin excretion rate (Sharma, 2004). In addition, blockade of growth-promoting, profibrotic, non-haemodynamic actions of angiotensin may contribute to renal protection.

In a relatively small study of 409 patients with type 1 diabetes and nephropathy, most with hypertension, captopril-based therapy was superior to placebo-based therapy (with other antihypertensive agents added as needed) in reducing measures of renal dysfunction over a 5-year period of follow-up (Lewis et al., 1993). To what extent this benefit reflects ACE inhibition or better blood pressure control in the captopril arm remains uncertain.

ACE inhibitors are effective in reducing albumin excretion rate and blood pressure in type 2 diabetes and nephropathy (Kasiske et al., 1993) and in reducing microalbuminuria in normotensive non-obese type 2 diabetes (Ravid et al., 1998). ACE inhibition even confers long-term renal protection in hypertensive and non-hypertensive patients with type 2 diabetes who have not yet developed microalbuminuria (Ravid et al., 1998). The extent of ACE inhibition appears important since very-low-dose ramipril had no outcome benefit in type 2 diabetes mellitus with persistent microalbuminuria or proteinuria despite blood pressure reduction (Marre et al., 2004).

A series of trials have demonstrated the renoprotective effect of angiotensin receptor blockers in patients with type 2 diabetes, hypertension and nephropathy.

- RENAAL was a comparison of losartan plus other antihypertensives and placebo plus other antihypertensives (Brenner et al., 2001). The endpoint was doubling of serum creatinine, end-stage renal disease or death. In 1512 patients followed up for 4 years, the time to the composite endpoint was improved significantly in the losartan arm. Risk reduction was 16% in the intention-to-treat analysis and 22% in the per-protocol analysis. End-stage renal disease was reduced 28% on losartan but there was no advantage for two predefined secondary cardiovascular endpoints. The design of RENAAL ensured better blood pressure control in the losartan arm.

- IDNT was a comparison of irbesartan plus other antihypertensives, placebo plus other antihypertensives and amlodipine plus other antihypertensives. The endpoint was doubling of serum creatinine, end-stage renal disease or death (Lewis et al., 2001). In 1554 patients followed-up for 4 years, time to doubling serum creatinine, end-stage renal disease or death was improved significantly in the irbesartan arm compared with the 'placebo' or the amlodipine arm. Relative risks were 0.80 for angiotensin receptor blocker compared with 'placebo', 0.77 compared with amlodipine and 1.04 for the calcium channel blocker versus 'placebo'. Blood pressure over time was lower in the angiotensin receptor blocker group than in the 'placebo' group but there was no difference between the irbesartan and amlodipine arms. The angiotensin receptor blocker exhibited no advantages for secondary cardiovascular endpoints.

- IRMA2 (Irbesartan Microalbuminuria Type 2 Diabetes in Hypertensive Patients) compared irbesartan and placebo in 590 type 2 diabetes patients with microalbuminuria (Parving *et al.*, 2001a). The endpoint was overt proteinuria. Over a 2-year follow-up, the population with progression to overt nephropathy (overt proteinuria) was reduced in a dose-dependent manner by 150–300 mg of irbesartan daily compared with placebo. Irbesartan treatment led to 68% reduction in progression to nephropathy, 54% reduction in urine albumin excretion and 1.7 times greater regression to normoalbuminuria. Glomerular filtration rate was preserved on irbesartan. The importance of blood pressure control on these outcomes is unclear.

- The smaller Microalbuminuria Reduction with Valsartan (MARVAL) study compared treatment based on valsartan and treatment based on amlodipine in type 2 diabetes with microalbuminuria (Viberti *et al.*, 2002). Valsartan was associated with 44% reduction in albumin excretion rate compared with 8.5% reduction on amlodipine despite equivalent blood pressure reduction.

Thus angiotensin receptor blocker therapy prevents progression of microalbuminuria to overt nephropathy (IRMA2/MARVAL) and of overt nephropathy to end-stage renal disease (IDNT/RENAAL).

Angiotensin receptor blockers and ACE inhibitors reduce urinary albumin excretion (Lacourciere *et al.*, 2000). Until recently, there was no direct comparison of ACE inhibitors and angiotensin receptor blockers in diabetes. The Diabetics Exposed to Telmisartan and Enalapril (DETAIL) study (Barnett *et al.*, 2004) was a prospective, double-blind study in 250 patients with type 2 diabetes and early nephropathy, mostly with hypertension, randomised to 80 mg of telmisartan or 20 mg of enalapril daily. After 5 years, the decrement in glomerular filtration rate did not differ significantly between the groups. The findings satisfied the non-inferiority criteria although there was a trend in favour of enalapril. Although blood pressure changes were similar, these favoured telmisartan. There were no differences for secondary endpoints including serum creatinine, urinary albumin excretion, end-stage renal disease, cardiovascular deaths or deaths from all-causes. This study supports equivalence of angiotensin receptor blockers and ACE inhibitors in renoprotection in type 2 diabetes but was under-powered to detect small differences.

In patients with type 2 diabetes and nephropathy, dual blockade of the renin–angiotensin system with ACE inhibition plus angiotensin receptor blockade significantly reduces albuminuria and may be renoprotective even when the doses of the agents are reduced by half (Fujisawa *et al.*, 2005). In the Candesartan and Lisinopril Microalbuminuria (CALM) study, combination treatment with 20 mg of lisinopril plus 16 mg of candesartan daily reduced blood pressure and the urinary albumin excretion rate to a greater extent than either drug alone (Mogensen *et al.*, 2000). The combination was well tolerated with only a small increase in serum potassium (0.3 mmol/l).

The mechanism of action of the two classes appears complementary (Fujisawa *et al.*, 2005) and several studies suggest a beneficial effect of the combination in diabetic kidney disease, including a reduction in albuminuria of 16–43% (Mogensen *et al.*, 2000; Jacobsen *et al.*, 2003; Fujisawa *et al.*, 2005). However, it is uncertain whether the combination *per se* is superior to full-dose monotherapy. The combination resulted in greater blood pressure reduction in most studies (Mogensen *et al.*, 2000; Jacobsen *et al.*, 2003) and this may explain the benefit. The answer may be provided by the results of the Ongoing Telmisartan Alone and in Combination with Ramipril Global Endpoint Trial (ONTARGET), which compares ACE inhibitor, angiotensin receptor blocker and their combination in a population that includes type 2 diabetes (Zimmermann and Unger, 2004).

Preventing (or delaying) the development of microalbuminuria is a key treatment goal for renoprotection (Diabetes Control and Complications Trial Research Group, 1993; UK Prospective Diabetes Study Group, 1998a). ACE inhibitors and angiotensin receptor blockers appear to be the most effective agents (Lewis *et al.*, 1993, 2001; Brenner *et al.*, 2001, Parving *et al.*, 2001a). There is continued doubt and uncertainty about whether the small differences in blood pressure in several major outcome trials fully or only partly explain the observed reductions in renal outcomes.

Much of the evidence relating to ACE inhibition in diabetic nephropathy was obtained in type 1 diabetes. Type 2 diabetic nephropathy is a very different problem. Blockade of the renin–angiotensin system by whatever means is highly effective. ACE inhibitors are less expensive but the evidence base is less strong. It has been suggested that, while ACE inhibitors and angiotensin receptor blockers have similar effects on renal outcomes, the latter class may be associated with increased risk of myocardial infarction (Verma and Strauss, 2004) and all-cause mortality (Strippoli *et al.*, 2004). The value of angiotensin receptor blockers for renoprotection in overt type 2 diabetics nephropathy is well documented. These agents should be the standard of care. The citation of incomplete or misleading data (Strippoli *et al.*, 2004; Verma and Strauss, 2004) in support of an alarmist position should not alter this therapeutic approach.

Correction of dyslipidaemia

Lipid lowering has a moderately favourable effect (Fried *et al.*, 2001; Sica and Gehr, 2002). Treatment with atorvastatin in addition to a regimen including ACE inhibitor or angiotensin receptor blocker reduces proteinuria and the rate of progression of kidney disease in patients with chronic kidney disease, proteinuria and hypercholesterolaemia (Bianchi *et al.*, 2003). Although not all patients had diabetes, the benefit might be extrapolated to that population. Intensive strategies to control blood pressure, lipids and glucose demonstrated benefit for the development of nephropathy, autonomic neuropathy and cardiovascular deaths (Gaede *et al.*, 2003) (Figure 6.5).

6.6   Risk of Diabetes Mellitus with Antihypertensive Drugs

Individuals with hypertension, whether treated or untreated, are at increased risk of developing type 2 diabetes. In treated hypertensive subjects, compared with those who received no antihypertensive therapy, the risk of development of diabetes was not significantly altered with ACE inhibitors, calcium channel blockers or thiazide diuretics. Only those treated with beta-blockers were of increased risk of developing diabetes (Gress *et al.*, 2000).

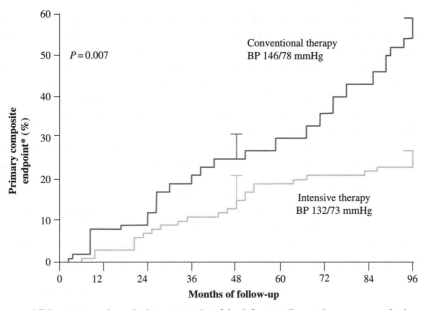

* Primary composite endpoint = composite of death from cardiovascular causes, non-fatal myocardial infarction, non-fatal stroke, revascularisation and amputation.

Figure 6.5 Intensive strategies to control blood pressure, lipids and glucose. Kaplin–Maier estimates for the composite endpoint of nephropathy, retinopathy, neuropathy and death from cardiovascular causes. Reproduced from Gaede P, Vedel P, Larsen N *et al.* (2003). Multifactorial intervention and cardiovascular disease in patients with type 2 diabetes. *New England Journal of Medicine* **348:** 383–93. Copyright © Massachusetts Medical Society. All rights reserved.

Epidemiological studies and clinical trials support the causal link between use of beta-blockers and type 2 diabetes (Padwal and Laupacis, 2004). Beta-blockers can adversely affect glucose homeostasis, including worsening of insulin sensitivity. The diabetic potential of beta-blockers may be partly related to weight gain (Scheen, 2004).

Thiazide and thiazide-like diuretics are also cited frequently as predisposing to diabetes (Lithell, 1991; Opie and Schall, 2004). Short-term metabolic studies raised concerns about the metabolic potential of these agents (Shapiro *et al.*, 1961). Subsequently, epidemiological studies and clinical trials suggested a causal link between use of thiazides and type 2 diabetes (Padwal and Laupacis, 2004). However, the studies that have suggested an increased risk of new-onset diabetes with thiazides have limitations: small numbers of patients; short follow-up; suboptimal definition of new-onset diabetes; lack of adequate comparison group; highly selected patients; and failure to allow for confounders (Gress *et al.*, 2000). In the ALLHAT, there was a tendency for chlorthalidone to increase hyperglycaemia but the effect was small and not associated with increased cardiovascular events (ALLHAT Officers and Coordinators for the ALLHAT Collaborative Research Group, 2002).

Calcium channel blockers are generally considered to be metabolically neutral (Brown *et al.*, 2000; Hansson *et al.*, 2000; ALLHAT Officers and Coordinators for the ALLHAT Collaborative Research Group , 2002). In the INVEST study, verapamil-based therapy reduced new-onset diabetes compared with atenolol-based therapy but the effect was modest compared with that of inhibitors of the renin–angiotensin system (Pepine *et al.*, 2003).

Early experience with ACE inhibitors suggested no detrimental effect on fasting blood glucose after long-term administration (Neaton *et al.*, 1993). The Swedish Trial in Old Patients with Hypertension 2 (STOP-2) study failed to show a protective effect of ACE inhibition against type 2 diabetes mellitus (Hansson *et al.*, 1999a). The study population was elderly (average age 76 years) and the criteria for definition of diabetes were not specified. In the CAPPP study there was significant reduction in new-onset diabetes in the captopril group compared with conventional therapy (Hansson *et al.*, 1999b). It is not clear whether this represented a protective effect of the ACE inhibitor or an adverse effect of beta-blockade or thiazide. The scientific value of the CAPPP study is reduced by a flaw in the randomisation procedure that resulted in an imbalance of baseline blood pressure and the prevalence of diabetes (Peto, 1999): this may have influenced the incidence of new-onset diabetes. In the HOPE study there was significant reduction in new-onset diabetes with ramipril compared with standard therapy (Heart Outcomes Prevention Evaluation Study Investigators, 2000). However, while the data on new-onset diabetes were prospective, new-onset diabetes was not a primary or even a secondary endpoint, and the analysis was *post hoc*, so the findings should be interpreted with caution.

The same investigators performed a prospective 2×2 study in 5269 subjects who were overweight with impaired glucose tolerance and/or impaired fasting glucose and were followed for 3 years (DREAM Trial Investigators, 2006). Approximately half of the subjects had treated hypertension. Treatment with rosiglitazone reduced the progression to diabetes by 60%, but ramipril treatment did not significantly effect the progression to diabetes. Regression to normoglycaemia, which was a secondary endpoint, was significantly increased with ramipril.

In the ALLHAT, lisinopril-based therapy was associated with 30% reduced new-onset diabetes compared with therapy based on chlorthalidone and 17% compared with amlodipine-based therapy (ALLHAT Officers and Coordinators for the ALLHAT Collaborative Research Group, 2002). This study provides the best evidence for an anti-diabetaginic effect of ACE inhibitors in hypertension.

In the LIFE study, losartan-based therapy was associated with a significant 25% reduction in new-onset diabetes compared with therapy based on atenolol; 70% of the time each group received concomitant thiazide therapy (Dahlöf *et al.*, 2002; Lindholm *et al.*, 2002b). Whether this finding is due to improved insulin resistance with the angiotensin receptor blocker or a decrease in insulin sensitivity with atenolol, or both, remains uncertain. A similar reduction in new-onset diabetes has been seen with candesartan (Lithell *et al.*, 2003; Pfeffer *et al.*, 2003). In the Study on Cognition and Prognosis in the Elderly (SCOPE) (Lithell *et al.*, 2003), the reduction in new-onset diabetes with candesartan was not significant but of a similar magnitude to that with losartan in the LIFE study. In the Valsartan Antihypertensive Long-term Use Evaluation (VALUE), valsartan-based therapy was associated with a 23% reduction in new-onset diabetes compared with amlodipine (Julius *et al.*, 2004). Although the results of VALUE do not establish that angiotensin receptor blockade *per se* reduces or delays the onset of type 2 diabetes, the lower incidence of new-onset diabetes in valsartan-treated subjects might well reflect an anti-diabetic effect of angiotensin receptor blockers. The Antihypertensive Treatment and Lipid Profile in a North of Sweden Efficacy Evaluation (ALPINE) (Lindholm *et al.*, 2003) confirmed the results of larger trials demonstrating a more favourable metabolic profile and lower risk of new-onset diabetes in hypertensive patients treated with an angiotensin receptor blocker compared with thiazides. Costs are greater in the short term but favourable health benefits in the long term are possible.

Recent outcome studies have reported an increased incidence of diabetes in patients treated with beta-blockers or diuretics compared with angiotensin receptor blockers, ACE inhibitors or calcium channel blockers, especially when beta-blockers and diuretics are combined. Beta-blocker/diuretic combination therapy has been associated with around 20% increase in diabetes over trial periods of approximately 5 years in comparison with therapy based on ACE inhibitors or angiotensin receptor blockers (Mason *et al.*, 2005).

The shortcomings of the evidence must be considered. Although the major antihypertensive classes appear to exert differential effects on diabetes mellitus incidence, the data are far from conclusive (Padwal and Laupacis, 2004). Only one had diabetes mellitus as a primary endpoint, and the evidence from randomised trials is limited by sources of bias, including treatment contamination and the bias of *post hoc* analysis. The data from the highest quality studies suggest that diabetes is unchanged or increased by thiazides and beta-blockers, and unchanged or decreased by ACE inhibitors, calcium channel blockers or angiotensin receptor blockers.

Both diuretics and beta-blockers may exert detrimental metabolic effects leading to increased incidence of type 2 diabetes (Padwal and Laupacis, 2004). Glucose intolerance with thiazides has been attributed to potassium depletion (Helderman *et al.*, 1983). Hypokalaemia can impair glucose tolerance by interfering with insulin release by the pancreas. *In vitro* studies and studies in animals and humans have suggested a possible relationship between the renin–angiotensin system and the pathogenesis of insulin resistance (Kurtz and Pravenec, 2004). Both animal and human studies have shown improvement in insulin resistance by inhibition of angiotensin II (Hovens *et al.*, 2005). Almost half of the studies of ACE inhibitors in hypertensive non-diabetic individuals demonstrated a slight but significant increase in insulin sensitivity as assessed by insulin-stimulated glucose disposal during englycaemic hyperinsulinaemic clamp studies, while the other half failed to reveal any significant changes (Julius *et al.*, 1991). Several clinical trials suggest that angiotensin receptor blockers have a protective effect on glucose metabolism (Dahlöf *et al.*, 2002; Lindholm *et al.*, 2002b; Lithell *et al.*, 2003; Pfeffer *et al.*, 2003; Julius *et al.*, 2004; Kurtz and Pravenec, 2004; Scheen, 2004). However, most placebo-controlled trials failed to show an anti-diabetic effect (Kurtz and Pravenec, 2004). The effects of angiotensin receptor blockers on insulin sensitivity are neutral in most studies (Scheen, 2004).

The potential mechanisms of improvement of glucose tolerance and insulin sensitivity through inhibition of the renin–angiotensin system are complex (Scheen, 2004) (Table 6.3). These may include improved blood flow and microcirculation in skeletal muscle and thereby enhancement of insulin and glucose delivery to insulin-sensitive tissue (Julius *et al.*, 1991), facilitation of insulin signally at the cellular level (Kurtz and Pravenec, 2004) and improvement of insulin secretion by the beta cells via a direct effect in blood flow to the endocrine pancreas (Carlsson *et al.*, 1998). Blockade of the renin–angiotensin system may promote recruitment and differentiation of adipocytes, which would counteract the ectopic deposition of lipid in other tissues (liver, muscle, pancreas) thereby improving insulin sensitivity (Sharma *et al.*, 2002).

Table 6.3 Potential antidiabetic mechanisms mediated by inhibitors of the Renin-Angiotensin system. Modified from Hovens MMC, Tamsma JK, Beishuizen ED, Huisman MV (2005). Pharmacological strategies to reduce cardiovascular risk in type 2 diabetes mellitus. An update. *Drugs* **65**: 433–45.

Adverse effects of angiotensin II blocked by ACE inhibitors and angiotensin receptor blockers:

- insulin signalling
- tissue blood flow
- oxidative stress
- sympathetic activity
- adipogenesis

Beyond effects on the renin–angiotensin system:

- enhanced glucose metabolism by activation of bradykinin/nitric oxide pathways (ACE inhibitors)
- improved glucose and lipid metabolism by activation of PPAR − r[a]

[a]PPAR − r = peroxisome proliferator-activated receptor gamma.

The availability of drugs that have anti-diabetic as well as antihypertensive properties should be of considerable clinical value. In ALLHAT, less new-onset diabetes did not translate into fewer cardiovascular events in the lisinopril group (ALLHAT Officers and Coordinators for the ALLHAT Collaborative Research Group, 2002). However, the complications of diabetes were reduced significantly in the ramipril group compared with conventional therapy in HOPE (Heart Outcomes Prevention Evaluation (HOPE) Study Investigators, 2000). In long-term observational studies, new-onset diabetes has the same high cardiovascular risk as that in patients with diabetes at the outset, but some years of follow-up are needed before the prognostic curves separate (Dunder *et al.*, 2003; Eberly *et al.*, 2003; Bartnik *et al.*, 2004; Verdecchia *et al*, 2004; Kostis *et al.*, 2005). In treated hypertensives, the risk of subsequent cardiovascular events was not dissimilar from that in previously known diabetes (Verdecchia *et al.*, 2004); risk was almost three times that in those who did not develop diabetes, although only 63 events were recorded in this study. The average time to an event was 6 years. Since typical outcome trials in hypertension have an average follow-up of 5 years, the average duration of new-onset diabetes is only 2.5 years, leading to underestimation of the implications for cardiovascular risk.

Patients with increased fasting glucose are more likely to develop diabetes when exposed to drugs that worsen glucose tolerance (Von Eckardstein *et al.*, 2000). The British Hypertension Society (Williams *et al.*, 2004) recommends caution when using the combination of beta-blockers and thiazide diuretics in patients at high risk of developing diabetes: impaired glucose tolerance, strong family history of diabetes mellitus, obesity, metabolic syndrome and those of South Asian or Afro-Caribbean descent.

6.7 Conclusions

Adults with diabetes have experienced a 50% reduction in the rate of incident cardiovascular disease, although persons with diabetes have remained at a consistent twofold increased risk for cardiovascular events compared with those without diabetes

(Fox *et al.*, 2004). Patients with diabetes have benefited in a similar manner to those without diabetes during the decline in cardiovascular disease rates over the last several decades. When comparing cardiovascular risk factors from earlier and later periods, there are significant declines for important cardiovascular disease risk factors, including systolic blood pressure. Ongoing efforts remain necessary to promote rigorous cardiovascular disease risk reduction among adults with diabetes. In the USA (Saadine *et al.*, 2002), 18% have poor glycaemic control, 34% have blood pressure over 140/90 mmHg and 58% have elevated LDL-cholesterol. Given the increasing prevalence of diabetes (Fox *et al.*, 2004), it is critical to make efforts to implement the findings from clinical trials to promote cardiovascular disease risk factor reduction.

Most patients with diabetes and the metabolic syndrome are diagnosed late, creating substantial difficulties in managing the cardiovascular disease burden. This often requires multiple medications and complex medical care. Better screening tests are needed to recognise higher risk patients sooner so that prevention strategies can be optimised. It is likely that this approach will be the most cost-effective.

The strategy for patients with diabetes or the metabolic syndrome should combine early detection of combined risk factors and target organ damage, and preventive approaches including lifestyle modification and multitargeted pharmacological intervention. All such patients should have assessment of obesity, tobacco use, blood pressure, lipid status and urine albumin excretion.

The risk of premature cardiovascular disease is even higher in type 1 diabetes than in type 2 diabetes. Therefore, cardiovascular risk reduction should be integral to the management of type 1 diabetes. This should include attention to lifestyle in childhood, and antihypertensive drugs and lipid-lowering therapy in adulthood.

Prevention strategies in all people with diabetes should target lifestyle. These include a well-designed exercise programme, weight loss, salt reduction, low-carbohydrate and low-fat diet, moderate protein restriction, moderation of alcohol consumption and tobacco cessation.

Pharmacological interventions should include low-dose aspirin, glycaemic control, blood pressure control to a goal of $< 130/80$ mmHg and normalisation of urine albumin excretion with a multidrug regimen including an ACE inhibitor in type 1 diabetes mellitus or an angiotensin receptor blocker in type 2 diabetes mellitus, and correction of dyslipidaemia with a statin to achieve target LDL-cholesterol and thereafter a reduction in triglycerides and an increase in HDL-cholesterol. Diabetic patients will derive greater cardiovascular and renal risk reduction benefits from these approaches if these are instituted early. This requires multiple medications, good compliance and a multidisciplinary effort.

The challenging task for patient and doctor is to achieve the defined goals of therapy. Poor adherence with guidelines and inability to reach defined targets are common (Saadine *et al.*, 2002). Nevertheless, the use of a comprehensive multifactorial cardiovascular and renal risk approach tailored to expected risk benefits in the individual patients is bound to reduce the risk of cardiovascular and renal disease in diabetes. The criteria are: attention to all risk factors, including blood pressure; a low threshold for intervention; rigorous targets; and multiple antihypertensive agents, including the use of agents to block the renin–angiotensin system. Effective cardiovascular and renal disease care requires a multiprofessional approach, involvement of the individual, integration with the management of other diabetes complications and other therapies, including aspirin and lipid-lowering drugs, particularly statins.

References

Adler AI, Stratton IM, Neil HA *et al.* (2000). Association of systolic blood pressure with macrovascular and microvascular complications of type 2 diabetes (UKPDS 36): prospective observational study. *British Medical Journal* **321**: 412–9.

Agrawal B, Berger A, Wolf K *et al.* (1996). Microalbuminuria screening by reagent predicts cardiovascular risk in hypertension. *Journal of Hypertension* **14**: 223–8.

Alderberth AM, Rosengren A, Wilhelmsen L (1998). Diabetes and long-term risk of mortality from coronary and other causes in middle-aged Swedish men. A general population study. *Diabetes Care* **21**: 539–45.

Alderman MH, Cohen H, Madhaven S (1999). Diabetes and cardiovascular events in hypertensive patients. *Hypertension* **33**: 1130–4.

ALLHAT Officers and Coordinators for the ALLHAT Collaborative Research Group (2002). Major outcomes in high-risk hypertensive patients randomized to angiotensin-converting enzyme inhibitor or calcium channel blocker vs diuretic. The Antihypertensive and Lipid-Lowering Treatment to Prevent Heart Attack Trial (ALLHAT). *Journal of the American Medical Association* **288**: 2981–97.

American Diabetes Association (2006). Standards of medical care in diabetes – 2006. *Diabetes Care* **29**: S4–S42.

Antithrombotic Trialists' Collaboration (2002). Collaborative meta-analysis of randomised trials of antiplatelet therapy for prevention of death, myocardial infarction and stroke in high risk patients. *British Medical Journal* **324**: 71–86.

Bakris GL (1999). Maximising cardiorenal benefits in the management of hypertension: Achieve blood pressure goals. *Journal of Clinical Hypertension* **1**: 141–7.

Bakris GL, Copley JB, Vicknair N, Sadler R, Leurgans S (1996). Calcium channel blockers versus other antihypertensive, therapies on progression of NIDDM associated nephropathy. *Kidney International* **50**: 1641–50.

Bakris GL, Williams M, Dworkin L *et al.* (2000). Preserving renal function in adults with hypertension and diabetes: a consensus approach. National Kidney Foundation Hypertension and Diabetes Executive Committees Working Group. *American Journal of Kidney Diseases* **36**: 646–61.

Bakris GL, Gaxiola E, Messerli FH *et al.* (2004). Clinical outcomes in the diabetes cohort of the International Verapamil SR-Trandolapril Study. *Hypertension* **44**: 637–42.

Barnett AH, Bain SC, Bouter P *et al.* for the Diabetics Exposed to Telmisartan and Enalapril Study Group (2004). Angiotensin-receptor blockade versus converting-enzyme inhibition in type 2 diabetes and nephropathy. *New England Journal of Medicine* **351**: 1952–61.

Bartnik M, Malmberg K, Norhammar A, Tenerz Å, Öhrvik J, Rydén L (2004). Newly detected abnormal glucose tolerance: an important predictor of long-term outcome after myocardial infarction. *European Heart Journal* **25**: 1990–7.

Beckman JA, Creager MA, Libby P (2002). Diabetes and atherosclerosis: epidemiology, pathophysiology and management. *Journal of the American Medical Association* **287**: 2570–81.

Berne C, Pollare T, Lithell H (1991). Effects of antihypertensive treatment on insulin sensitivity with special reference to ACE inhibitors. *Diabetes Care* **14**: 39–47.

Betteridge DJ (2004). The interplay of cardiovascular risk factor in the metabolic syndrome and type 2 diabetes. *European Heart Journal Supplements* **6** (Suppl G): G3–G7.

Bianchi S, Bigazzi R, Caiazza A *et al*. (2003). A controlled, prospective study of the effects of atorvastatin in proteinuria and prognosis of kidney disease. *American Journal of Kidney Disease* **41**: 565–70.

Black HR, Elliott WJ, Grandits G *et al*. (2003). Principal results of the Controlled Onset Verapamil Investigation of Cardiovascular End Points (CONVINCE) trial. *Journal of the American Medical Association* **289**: 2073–82.

Brenner BM, Cooper ME, De Zeeuw D, Keane WF, Mitch WE, Parving H-H *et al*. for the RENAAL Study Investigators (2001). Effects of losartan on renal and cardiovascular outcomes in patients with type 2 diabetes and nephropathy. *New England Journal of Medicine* **345**: 861–9.

Brown MJ, Palmer CR, Castaigne A, de Leeuw PW, Mancia G, Rosenthal T, Ruilope LM (2000). Morbidity and mortality in patients randomised to double-blind treatment with a long-acting calcium channel blocker or diuretic in the International Nifedipine GITS Study: Intervention as a Goal in Hypertension Treatment (INSIGHT). *Lancet* **356**: 366–77.

Bühler FR, Julius S, Reaven GM *et al*. (1990). A dimension in hypertension: role of insulin resistance. *Journal of Cardiovascular Pharmacology* **15** (Suppl 5): S1–S3.

Burt VL, Whelton P, Roccella EJ, Brown C, Cutler JA, Higgins M *et al*. (1995). Prevalence of hypertension in the US adult population. Results from the Third National Health and Nutrition Examination Survey, 1988–1991. *Hypertension* **25**: 305–13.

Calle EE, Thun MJ, Petrelli JM *et al*. (1999). Body-mass index and mortality in a prospective cohort of US adults. *New England Journal of Medicine* **341**: 1097–105.

Candido R, Jandeleit-Dahm KA, Cao Z *et al*. (2002). Prevention of accelerated atherosclerosis by angiotensin-converting enzyme inhibition in diabetic apolipoportein C-deficient mice. *Circulation* **106**: 246–53.

Candido R, Allen TJ, Lassila M, *et al*. (2004). Irbesartan but not amlodipine suppresses diabetes-associated atherosclerosis. *Circulation* **109**: 1536–42.

Carlsson P-O, Berne C, Jansson L (1998). Angiotensin II and the endocrine pancreas: effects on islet blood flow and insulin secretion in rats. *Diabetologia* **41**: 127–33.

Chaturvedi N, Sjolie A-K, Stephenson JM, *et al*. and the EUCLID Study Group (1998). Effect of lisinopril on progression of retinopathy in normotensive people with type 1 diabetes. *Lancet* **351**: 28–31.

Chen J, Muntner P, Hamon LL *et al*. (2004). The metabolic syndrome and chronic kidney disease in US adults. *Annals of Internal Medicine* **140**: 167–74.

Cho E, Rinn EB, Stampfer MJ *et al*. (2002). The impact of diabetes mellitus and prior myocardial infarction on mortality from all causes and from coronary heart disease in men. *Journal of the American College of Cardiology* **40**: 954–60.

Chobanian AV, Bakris GL, Black HL *et al*. (2003). Seventh report of the Joint National Committee on prevention, detection, evaluation, and treatment of high blood pressure. *Hypertension* **42**: 1206–52.

Colditz GA, Willett WC, Rotnitzky A, Manson JE (1995). Weight gain as a risk factor for clinical diabetes mellitus in women. *Annals of Internal Medicine* **122**: 481–6.

Colhoun H, Betteridge D, Durrington P *et al*. on behalf of the CARDS Investigators (2004). Primary prevention of cardiovascular disease with atorvastatin in type 2 diabetes in the Collaborative Atorvastatin Diabetes Study (CARDS): multicentre randomised placebo-controlled trial. *Lancet* **364**: 685–96.

Cook NR, Cohen J, Hebert PR, Taylor JO, Hennekens CH (1995). Implications of small reductions in diastolic blood pressure for primary prevention. *Archives of Internal Medicine* **155**: 701–9.

Cooper ME (1998). Pathogenesis, prevention and treatment of diabetic nephopathy. *Lancet* **352**: 213–9.

Coutinho M, Gerstein HC, Wang Y, Yusuf S (1999). The relationship between glucose and incident cardiovascular events. A metaregression analysis of published data from 20 studies of 95,783 individual followed for 12.4 years. *Diabetes Care* **22**: 233–40.

Curb JD, Pressel SL, Cutler JA, Savage PJ, Appelgate WB, Black H, Camel G, Davis BR, Frost PH, Gonzalez N, Guthrie G, Oberman A, Rutan GH, Stamler J (1996). Effect of diuretic-based antihypertensive treatment on cardiovascular disease risk in older diabetic patients with isolated systolic hypertension. *Journal of the American Medical Association* **276**: 1886–92.

Dahlöf B, Devereux RB, Kjeldson SE *et al.* for the LIFE Study Group (2002). Cardiovascular morbidity and mortality in the Losartan Intervention For Endpoint reduction in hypertension study (LIFE): a randomised trial against atenolol. *Lancet* **359**: 995–1003.

Davis TM, Millns H, Stratton IM, Holman RR, Turner RC (1999). Risk factors for stroke in type 2 diabetes mellitus. United Kingdom Prospective Diabetes Study (UKPDS) 29. *Archives of Internal Medicine* **159**: 1097–103.

Diabetes Control and Complications Trial Research Group (1993). The effect of intensive treatment of diabetes on the development and progression of long-term complications in insulin-dependent diabetes mellitus. *New England Journal of Medicine* **329**: 977–86.

Diabetes Control and Complications Trial/Epidemiology of Diabetes Interventions and Complications (DCCT/EDIC) Study Research Group (2005). Intensive diabetes treatment and cardiovascular disease in patients with type 1 diabetes. *New England Journal of Medicine* **353**: 2643–53.

Dillon JJ (1993). The quantitative relationship between treated blood pressure and progression of diabetic renal disease. *American Journal of Kidney Diseases* **22**: 798–802.

Donnelly R (1992). Angiotensin-converting enzyme inhibitors and insulin sensitivity: metabolic effects in hypertension, diabetes and heart failure. *Journal of Cardiovascular Pharmacology* **20** (Suppl 11): S38–44.

DREAM Trial Investigators (2006). Effect of ramipril on the incidence of diabetes. *New England Journal of Medicine* **355**: 1551–62.

Dunder K, Lind L, Zethelius B, Berglund L, Lithell H (2003). Increase in blood glucose concentration during antihypertensive treatment as a predictor of myocardial infarction: population based cohort study. *British Medical Journal* **326**: 681–4.

Eberly LE, Cohen JD, Prineas RP, Yang L for the MRFIT Research Group (2003). Impact of incident diabetes and incident non fatal cardiovascular disease on 18-year mortality. *Diabetes Care* **26**: 848–54.

Ebrahim S, Smith GD (1998). Lowering blood pressure: A systematic review of sustained effects of non-pharmacological interventions. *Journal of Public Health Medicine* **20**: 4441–8.

Epstein M, Sowers JR (1992). Diabetes mellitus and hypertension. *Hypertension* **19**: 403–18.

Estacio RO, Jeffers BW, Hiatt WR *et al.* (1998). The effect of nisoldipine as compared with enalapril on cardiovascular outcomes in patients with non-insulin-dependent diabetes and hypertension. *New England Journal of Medicine* **338**: 645–52.

EUCLID Study Group (1997). Randomised placebo-controlled trial of lisinopril in normotensive patients with insulin-dependent diabetes and normoalbuminuria or microalbuminuria. *Lancet* **349**: 1787–92.

European Diabetes Policy Group (1999). A desktop guide to type 2 diabetes mellitus. *Diabetic Medicine* **16**: 716–30.

European Society of Hypertension–European Society of Cardiology Guidelines Committee (2003). 2003 European Society of Hypertension–European Society of Cardiology guidelines for the management of arterial hypertension. *Journal of Hypertension* **21**: 1011–53.

Expert Panel on Detection, Evaluation, and Treatment of High Blood Cholesterol in Adults (2001). Executive summary of the third report of the National Cholesterol Education Program (NCEP) Expert Panel on Detection, Evaluation, and Treatment of High Blood Cholesterol in Adults (Adult Treatment Panel III). *Journal of the American Medical Association* **285**: 2486–97.

Fagan TC, Sowers J (1999). Type 2 diabetes mellitus: greater cardiovascular risks and greater benefits of therapy. *Archives of Internal Medicine* **159**: 1033–4.

Ferrannini E, Buzzigoli C, Bonadonna R *et al.* (1987). Insulin resistance in essential hypertension. *New England Journal of Medicine* **317**: 350–7.

Ferrannini E, Seghieri G, Muscelli E (1994). Insulin and the renin-angiotensin-aldosterone system: influence of ACE inhibitors. *Journal of Cardiovascular Pharmacology* **24** (Suppl 3): S61–9.

Ferrari P, Weidmann P (1990). Insulin, insulin sensitivity and hypertension. *Journal of Hypertension* **8**: 491–500.

Ford ES, Giles WH, Dietz WH (2002). Prevalence of the metabolic syndrome among US adults: findings from the third National Health and Nutrition Examination Survey. *Journal of the American Medical Association* **287**: 356–9.

Fox CS, Coady S, Sorlie PD *et al.* (2004). Trends in cardiovascular complications of diabetes. *Journal of the American Medical Association* **292**: 2495–9.

Franklin S, Gustin W, Wong N *et al.* (1997). Hemodynamic patterns of age-related changes in blood pressure: The Framingham Heart Study. *Circulation* **96**: 308–15.

Franklin S, Shehzad A, Khan B *et al.* (1999). Is pulse pressure useful in predicting risk for coronary heart disease? The Framingham Heart Study. *Circulation* **100**: 354–60.

Frick MH, Elo O, Haapa K *et al.* (1987). Helsinki Heart Study: a primary-prevention trial with gemfibrozil in middle-aged men with dyslipidemia. Safety of treatment, changes in risk factors and incidence of coronary heart disease. *New England Journal of Medicine* **317**: 1237–45.

Fried LF, Orchard TJ, Kasiske BL (2001). Effect of lipid reduction on the progression of renal disease: a meta-analyses. *Kidney International* **59**: 260–9.

Fujisawa T, Ikegami H, Ono M *et al.* (2005). Combination of half doses of angiotensin type 1 receptor antagonist and angiotensin-converting enzyme inhibitor in diabetic nephropathy. *American Journal of Hypertension* **18**: 13–17.

Gaede P, Vedel P, Larsen N *et al.* (2003). Multifactorial intervention and cardiovascular disease in patients with type 2 diabetes. *New England Journal of Medicine* **348**: 383–93.

Gall MA, Houguard P, Borch-Johnsen K, Parving HH (1997). Risk factors for development of incipient and overt diabetic nephropathy in patients with non-insulin dependent diabetes mellitus: prospective observational study. *British Medical Journal* **314**: 783–8.

Gerber LM, Madhaven S, Alderman MH (1983). Coincident hypertension: deleterious effects on patients with hyperglycaemia. *New York State Journal of Medicine* **83**: 693–6.

Goldberg RB, Mellies MJ, Sacks FM *et al.* (1998). Cardiovascular events and their reduction with pravastatin in diabetic and glucose-intolerant myocardial infarction survivors with average cholesterol levels: Subgroup analyses in the Cholesterol And Recurrent Events (CARE) trial. The Care Investigators. *Circulation* **98**: 2513–19.

Goldstein LB, Adams R, Becker K *et al.* (2001). Primary prevention of ischemic stroke: a statement for health professionals from the Stroke Council of the American Heart Association. *Circulation* **103**: 163–82.

Gress TW, Nieto FJ, Shahar E, Wofford MR, Brancati FL (2000). Hypertension and antihypertensive therapy as risk factors for type 2 diabetes mellitus. Atherosclerosis Risk in Communities Study. *New England Journal of Medicine* **342**: 905–12.

Grossman E, Messerli FH (1996). Diabetes and hypertensive heart disease. *Annals of Internal Medicine* **125**: 304–10.

Haffner SM (1997). The prediabetic problem: development of non-insulin-dependent diabetes mellitus and related abnormalities. *Journal of Diabetic Complications* **11**: 69–76.

Haffner SM (1998). Management of dyslipidemia in adults with diabetes. *Diabetes Care* **21**: 160–78.

Haffner SM, Lehto S, Ronnemaa T, Pyorala K, Kaakso M (1998). Mortality from coronary heart disease in subjects with type 2 diabetes and in non diabetic subjects with and without prior myocardial infarction. *New England Journal of Medicine* **339**: 229–34.

Haire-Joshu D, Glasgow RE, Tibbs TL (1999). Smoking and diabetes. *Diabetes Care* **22**: 1887–98.

Hanley AJ, Karter AJ, Festa A *et al.* (2002). Factor analysis of metabolic syndrome using directly measured insulin sensitivity. The Insulin Resistance Atherosclerosis Study. *Diabetes* **51**: 2642–7.

Hansson L, Zanchetti A, Carruthers SG, Dahlof B, Elmfeldt D, Julius S *et al.* (1998). Effects of intensive blood-pressure lowering and low-dose aspirin in patients with hypertension: principal results of the Hypertension Optimal Treatment (HOT) randomised trial. HOT Study Group. *Lancet* **351**: 1755–62.

Hansson L, Lindholm LH, Ekbom T, Dahlof B, Lanke J, Schersten B *et al.* (1999a). Randomised trial of old and new antihypertensive drugs in elderly patients: cardiovascular mortality and morbidity the Swedish Trial in Old Patients with Hypertension-2 study. *Lancet* **354**: 1751–6.

Hansson L, Lindholm LH, Niskanen L *et al.* (1999b). Effect of angiotensin-converting enzyme inhibition compared with conventional therapy on cardiovascular morbidity and mortality in hypertension: the Captopril Prevention Project (CAPPP) randomised trial. *Lancet* **353**: 611–16.

Hansson L, Hedner T, Lund-Johannsen P, Kjeldsen SE, Lindholm L, Syvertsen JO, Lanke J, de Faire H, Dahlöf B, Karlberg BE for the NORDIL Study Group (2000). Randomised trial of efforts of calcium antagonists compared with diuretics and ß-blockers on cardiovascular morbidity and mortality in hypertension: the Nordic Diltiazem (NORDIL) Study. *Lancet* **356**: 359–65.

Harris M (2000). Health care and health status and outcomes for patients with type 2 diabetes. *Diabetes Care* **23**: 754–8.

He J, Whelton PK (1999). What is the role of dietary sodium and potassium in hypertension and target organ injury? *American Journal of Medical Science* **317**: 152–9.

He J, Whelton PK, Appel LJ, Charleston J, Klag MJ (2000). Long-term effects of weight loss and dietary sodium restriction on incidence of hypertension. *Hypertension* **35**: 544–9.

Heart Outcomes Prevention Evaluation (HOPE) Study Investigators (2000). Effect of ramipril on cardiovascular and microvascular outcomes in people with diabetes mellitus: results of the HOPE study and MICRO-HOPE substudy. *Lancet* **355**: 253–9.

Heart Outcomes Prevention Evaluation Study Investigators (2000). Effects of an angiotensin-converting-enzyme inhibitor, ramipril, on cardiovascular events in high-risk patients. *New England Journal of Medicine* **342**: 145–53.

Heart Protection Study Group (2002). MRC/BHF Heart Protection study of cholesterol lowering with simvastatin in 20,536 high-risk individuals: a randomised placebo-controlled trial. *Lancet* **360**: 7–22.

Heeg J, de Jony P, Van der Hem G *et al.* (1989). Efficacy and variability of the antiproteinuric effect of ACE inhibition by lisinopril. *Kidney International* **36**: 272–9.

Helderman JH, Elahi D, Anderson DK, Raizes GS, Tobin JD, Shocken D, Andres R (1983). Prevention of the glucose intolerance of thiazide diuretics by maintenance of body potassium. *Diabetes* **32**: 106–11.

Henry P, Thomas F, Benetos A, Guize L (2002). Impaired fasting glucose, blood pressure and cardiovascular disease mortality. *Hypertension* **40**: 458–63.

Herings RMC, de Boer A, Stricker BHC *et al.* (1995). Hypoglycemia associated with use of inhibitors of angiotensin converting enzyme. *Lancet* **345**: 1195–8.

Hornig B, Kohler C, Drexler H (1997). Role of bradykinin in mediating vascular effects of angiotensin-converting enzyme inhibitors in humans. *Circulation* **95**: 1115–18.

Hovens MMC, Tamsma JK, Beishuizen ED, Huisman MV (2005). Pharmacological strategies to reduce cardiovascular risk in type 2 diabetes mellitus. An update. *Drugs* **65**: 433–45.

Hsia J, Bittner V, Tripputi M, Howard BV (2003). Metabolic syndrome and coronary angiographic disease progression: The Women's Angiographic Vitamin and Estrogen trial. *American Heart Journal* **146**: 439–45.

Hunsicker LG, Adler S, Esler A *et al.* (1997). Predictors of the progression of renal disease in the Modification of Diet in Renal Disease Study. *Kidney International* **51**: 1908–19.

Hypertension in Diabetes Study (HDS) (1993). I: Prevalence of hypertension in newly presenting type 2 diabetic patients and the association with risk factors for cardiovascular and diabetic complications. *Journal of Hypertension* **11**: 309–17.

Isomaa B, Almgren P, Tuomi T *et al.* (2001). Cardiovascular morbidity and mortality associated with the metabolic syndrome. *Diabetes Care* **24**: 683–9.

Jacobsen P, Andersen S, Rossing K *et al.* (2003). Dual blockade of the renin-angiotensin system versus maximal recommended dose of ACE inhibition in diabetic nephropathy. *Kidney International* **63**: 1874–80.

Jarrett RJ, McCartney P, Keen H (1982). The Bedford survey: 10-year mortality rates in newly diagnosed diabetics and hyperglycaemic controls and risk indices for coronary heart disease in borderline diabetics. *Diabetologia* **22**: 79–84.

Julius S, Gudbrandsson T, Jamerson KA, Tariq SS, Andersson O (1991). The haemodynamic link between insulin resistance and hypertension. *Journal of Hypertension* **9**: 983–6.

Julius S, Kjeldsen SE, Weber M *et al.* for the VALUE trial group (2004). Outcomes in hypertensive patients at high cardiovascular risk treated with regimens based on valsartan or amlodipine: the VALUE randomised trial. *Lancet* **363**: 2022–31.

Kasiske BL, Kalil RS, Ma JZ, Liao M, Keane WF (1993). Effect of antihypertensive therapy on the kidney in patients with diabetes: a meta-regression analysis. *Annals of Internal Medicine* **118**: 129–38.

Katzmarzyk PT, Craig CL, Bruchard C (2001). Underweight, overweight and obesity: Relationships with mortality in the 13-year follow-up of the Canada Fitness Survey. *Journal of Clinical Epidemiology* **54**: 916–20.

Kawachi I, Colditz GA, Stampfer MJ *et al.* (1994). Smoking cessation and time course of increased risks of coronary heart disease in middle aged women. *Archives of Internal Medicine* **154**: 169–75.

Kjeldsen SE, Dahlöf B, Devereux RB *et al.*, for the LIFE Study Group (2002). Effects of losartan on cardiovascular morbidity and mortality in patients with isolated systolic hypertension and left ventricular hypertrophy: A Losartan Intervention for Endpoint Reduction (LIFE) substudy. *Journal of the American Medical Association* **288**: 1491–8.

Klag MK, Whelton PK, Randall BL, *et al.* (1996). A prospective study of blood pressure and incidence of end-stage renal disease in 332,544 men. *New England Journal of Medicine* **334**: 13–18.

Kohner EM, Eldington SJ, Stratton IM *et al.* (1998). United Kingdom Prospective Diabetes Study, 30: diabetic retinopathy at diagnosis of non-insulin-dependent diabetes mellitus and associated risk factors. *Archives of Ophthalmology* **116**: 297–303.

Koskinen P, Manttari M, Manninen V *et al.* (1992). Coronary heart disease incidence in NIDDM patients in the Helsinki Heart Study. *Diabetes Care* **15**: 820–5.

Kostis JB, Wilson AC, Freudenberger RS, Cosgrove NM, Pressel SL, Davis BR for the SHEP Collaborative Research Group (2005). Long-term effect of diuretic-based therapy on fatal outcomes in subjects with isolated systolic hypertension with and without diabetes. *American Journal of Cardiology* **45**: 29–35.

Kurtz TW, Pravenec M (2004). Antidiabetic mechanisms of angiotensin-converting enzyme inhibitors and angiotensin II receptor antagonists: beyond the renin-angiotensin system. *Journal of Hypertension* **22**: 2253–61.

Laakso M, Lehto S (1997). Epidemiology of macrovascular diseases in diabetes. *Diabetes Reviews* **5**: 294–315.

Laaksonen DE, Lakka HM, Niskanen LK, Kaplan GA, Salonen JT, Lakka TA (2002). Metabolic syndrome and development of diabetes mellitus: application and validation of recently suggested definitions of the metabolic syndrome in a prospective cohort study. *American Journal of Epidemiology* **15**: 1070–7.

Lacourciere Y, Belanger A, Godin C *et al.* (2000). Long-term comparison of losartan and enalapril on kidney function in hypertensive type 2 diabetes with early nephropathy. *Kidney International* **58**: 762–9.

Lakka HM, Laaksonen DE, Lakka TA *et al.* (2002). The metabolic syndrome and cardiovascular disease mortality in middle-aged men. *Journal of the American Medical Association* 2709–16.

Lee CD, Folsom AR, Pankow JS *et al.* (2004). Cardiovascular events in diabetic and nondiabetic adults with or without history of myocardial infarction. *Circulation* **109**: 855–60.

Lewis EJ, Hunsicker LG, Blain RP, Rohde ED and the Collaborative Study Group (1993). The effect of angiotensin-converting enzyme inhibition on diabetic nephropathy. *New England Journal of Medicine* **329**: 1456–62.

Lewis EJ, Hunsicker LG, Clarke WR, Berl T Pohl MA, Lewis JB *et al.* for the Collaborative Study Group (2001). Renoprotective effect of the angiotensin-receptor antagonist irbesartan in patients with nephropathy due to type 2 diabetes. *New England Journal of Medicine* **345**: 851–60.

Liese AD, Mayer-Davis EJ, Haffner SM (1998). Development of the multiple metabolic syndrome: an epidemiologic perspective. *Epidemiology Reviews* **20**: 157–72.

Lim HS, MacFadyen RJ, Lip GYH (2004). Diabetes mellitus, the renin-angiotensin-aldosterone system, and the heart. *Archives of Internal Medicine* **164**: 1734–8.

Lindholm LH, Ibsen H, Dahlöf B *et al.* for the LIFE Study Group (2002a). Cardiovascular morbidity and mortality in patients with diabetes in the Losartan Intervention For Endpoint reduction in hypertension study (LIFE): a randomised trial against atenolol. *Lancet* **359**: 1004–10.

Lindholm LH, Ibsen H, Borch-Johnsen K *et al.* for the LIFE Study Group (2002b). Risk of new-onset diabetes in the Losartan Intervention For Endpoint reduction in hypertension study. *Journal of Hypertension* **20**: 1879–86.

Lindholm LH, Persson M, Alaupovic P *et al.* (2003). Metabolic outcomes during 1 year in newly detected hypertensives: results of the Antihypertensive Treatment and Lipid Profile in a North of Sweden Efficacy Evaluation (ALPINE study). *Journal of Hypertension* **21**: 1563–74.

Lithell HO (1991). Effect of antihypertensive drugs on insulin, glucose, and lipid metabolism. *Diabetes Care* **14**: 203–9.

Lithell H, Hansson L, Skoog I *et al.* for the SCOPE Study Group (2003). The Study of Cognition and Prognosis in the Elderly (SCOPE): principal results of randomised double-blind intervention trial. *Journal of Hypertension* **21**: 875–86.

Long-Term Intervention with Pravastatin in Ischaemic Disease (LIPID) Study Group (1998). Prevention of cardiovascular events and death with pravastatin in people with coronary heart disease and a broad range of initial cholesterol levels. *New England Journal of Medicine* **339**: 1349–57.

Maki DD, Ma JZ, Louis TA, Kasiske BL (1995). Long-term effects of antihypertensive agents on proteinuria and renal function. *Archives of Internal Medicine* **155**: 1073–80.

Mancia G, Grassi G (2002). Systolic and diastolic blood pressure control in antihypertensive drug trials. *Journal of Hypertension* **29**: 1461–4.

Mancini CBJ, Henry GC, Macaya C *et al.* (1996). Angiotensin-converting enzyme inhibition with quinapril improves endothelial vasomotor dysfuction in patients with coronary artery disease. *Circulation* **94**: 258–65.

Mann JF, Gerstein HC, Pogue J, Bosch J, Yusuf S (2001). Renal insufficiency as a predictor of cardiovascular outcomes and the impact of ramipril: the HOPE randomized trial. *Annals of Internal Medicine* **134**: 629–36.

Marre M, Lievre M, Chatellier G, Mann JFE, Passa P, Menard J on behalf of the DIABHYCAR Study Investigators (2004). Effects of low dose ramipril on cardiovascular and renal outcomes in patients with type 2 diabetes and raised excretion of urinary albumin: randomised, double blind, placebo controlled trial (the DIABHYCAR Study). *British Medical Journal* **328**: 495–9.

Mason JM, Dickinson HO, Nicolson DJ, Campbell F, Ford GA, Williams B (2005). The diabetogenic potential of thiazide-type diuretics and beta-blocker combinations in patients with hypertension. *Journal of Hypertension* **23**: 1777–81.

McInnes GT (2003). Size isn't everything – ALLHAT in perspective. *Journal of Hypertension* **21**: 459–61.

Medalie JH, Papier CM, Goldbourt U *et al.* (1975). Major factors in the development of diabetes mellitus in 10,000 men. *Archives of Internal Medicine* **135**: 811–17.

Miller JA, Floras JS, Zinman B *et al.* (1996). Effect of hyperglycaemia on arterial pressure, plasma renin activity and renal function in early diabetes. *Clinical Science* **90**: 189–95.

Modan M, Halkin H, Almog S *et al.* (1985). Hyperinsulinemia: a link between hypertension, obesity and glucose intolerance. *Journal of Clinical Investigation* **75**: 809–17.

Mogensen C (1984). Microalbuminuria predicts clinical proteinuria and early mortality in maturity-onset diabetes. *New England Journal of Medicine* **310**: 356–60.

Mogensen CE, Keane WF, Bennett PH *et al.* (1995). Prevention of diabetic renal disease with special reference to microalbuminuria. *Lancet* **346**: 1080–4.

Mogensen CE, Neldam S, Tikkanen I, Oran S, Viskoper R, Watts RW *et al.* (2000). Randomised controlled trial of dual blockade of renin-angiotensin system in patients with hypertension, microalbuminuria, and non-insulin dependent diabetes: the candesartan and lisinopril microalbuminuria (CALM) study. *British Medical Journal* **321**: 1440–4.

Morales PA, Mitchell BD, Valdez RA *et al.* (1993). Incidence of NIDDM and impaired glucose tolerance in hypertensive subjects: the San Antonio Heart Study. *Diabetes* **42**: 154–61.

Morris AD, Boyle DI, McMahon AD *et al.* (1997). ACE inhibitor use is associated with hospitalisation for severe hypoglycemia in patients with diabetes. DARTS/MEMO Collaboration. Diabetes Audit and Research in Tayside, Scotland. Medicines Monitoring Unit. *Diabetes Care* **20**: 1363–7.

Mykkanen L, Haffner SM, Kuusisto J *et al.* (1994). Microalbuminuria precedes the development of NIDDM. *Diabetes* **43**: 552–7.

National High Blood Pressure Education Program Working Group (1994). National High Blood Pressure Education Program Working Group Report on Hypertension in the Elderly. *Hypertension* **23**: 275–85.

Neaton JD, Grimm RH, Prineas RJ *et al.* (1993). Treatment of Mild Hypertension Study. Final results. Treatment of Mild Hypertension Study Research Group. *Journal of the American Medical Association* **270**: 713–24.

Nelson RG, Bennett PH, Beck GJ *et al.* (1996). Development and progression of renal disease in Pima Indians with non-insulin-dependent diabetes mellitus. Diabetic Renal Disease Study Group. *New England Journal of Medicine* **335**: 1636–42.

Niskanen L, Hedner T, Hansson L *et al.* (2001). Reduced cardiovascular morbidity and mortality in hypertensive diabetic patients on first-line therapy with an ACE inhibitor compared with a diuretic/beta-blocker-based treatment regimen: A subanalysis of the Captopril Prevention Project. *Diabetes Care* **24**: 2091–6.

Okin PM, Devereux RB, Jern S *et al.* for the Losartan Intervention for Endpoint Reduction in Hypertension Study Investigators (2003). Regression of electrocardiographic left ventricular hypertrophy by losartan versus atenolol: the Losartan Intervention for Endpoint Reduction in Hypertension (LIFE) Study. *Circulation* **108**: 684–90.

Opie LH, Schall R (2004). Old antihypertensives and new diabetes. *Journal of Hypertension* **22**: 1453–8.

Padwal R, Laupacis A (2004). Antihypertensive therapy and evidence of type 2 diabetes. *Diabetes Care* **27**: 247–55.

Pan XR, Li GN, Hu YH *et al.* (1997). Effects of diet and exercise in preventing NIDDM in people with impaired glucose tolerance. The Da Qing IGT and Diabetes Study. *Diabetes Care* **20**: 537–44.

Pahor M, Psaty BM, Alderman MH, Applegate WB, Williamson JD, Furberg CD (2000). Therapeutic benefits of ACE inhibitors and other antihypertensive drugs in patients with type 2 diabetes. *Diabetes Care* **23**: 888–92.

Parving HH (1996). Initiation and progression of diabetic nephropathy. *New England Journal of Medicine* **335**: 1682–3.

Parving HH, Andersen AR, Smidt UM, Hommel E, Mathiesen ER, Svendsen PA (1987). Effect of antihypertensive treatment on kidney function in diabetic nephropathy. *British Medical Journal* **294**: 1443–7.

Parving H-H, Lehnert H, Bröchner-Mortensen J, Gomis R, Andersen S, Arner P for the Irbesartan in Patients with Type 2 Diabetes and Microalbuminuria Study Group (2001a). The effect of irbesartan on the development of diabetic nephropathy in patients with type 2 diabetes. *New England Journal of Medicine* **345**: 870–8.

Parving H, Hommel E, Jensen B *et al.* (2001b). Long-term beneficial effects of ACE inhibition on diabetic nephropathy in normotensive type 1 diabetic patients. *Kidney International* **60**: 228–34.

Pedrini M, Levey A, Lau J *et al.* (1996). The effect of dietary protein restriction on the progression of diabetic and nondiabetic renal disease: A meta-analysis. *Annals of Internal Medicine* **124**: 627–32.

Pell S, D'Alonzo CA (1967). Some aspects of hypertension in diabetes mellitus. *Journal of the American Medical Association* **202**: 104–10.

Pepine CJ, Handberg EM, Cooper-De Hoff RM *et al.* (2003). A calcium antagonist vs a non-calcium antagonist hypertension treatment strategy for patients with coronary artery disease: the International Verapamil-Trandolapril Study (INVEST): a randomised controlled trial. *Journal of the American Medical Association* **290**: 2805–16.

Peto R (1999). Failure of randomisation by "sealed" envelope. *Lancet* **354**: 73.

Petrie JR, Morris AD, Ueda S *et al.* (2000). Trandolapril does not improve insulin sensitivity in patients with hypertension and type 2 diabetes: a double-blind, placebo-controlled cross-over trial. *Journal of Clinical Endocrinology and Metabolism* **85**: 1882–9.

Pfeffer MA, Swedberg K, Granger CB *et al.* (2003). CHARM Investigators and Committees: Effects of candesartan on mortality and morbidity in patients with chronic heart failure: the CHARM-Overall programme. *Lancet* **362**: 759–66.

Pollare T, Lithell H, Berne C (1989). A comparison of the effects of hydrochlorothiazide and captopril on glucose and lipid metabolism in patients with hypertension. *New England Journal of Medicine* **321**: 868–73.

Price DA, Porter LE, Gordon M *et al.* (1999). The paradox of the low-renin state in diabetic nephropathy. *Journal of the American Society of Nephrology* **10**: 2382–9.

Prospective Studies Collaboration (2002). Age-specific relevance of usual blood pressure to vascular mortality: a meta-analysis of individual data for one million adults in 61 prospective studies. *Lancet* **360**: 1903–13.

Pyorala K, Pedersen TR, Kjekshus J, Faergeman O, Olsson AG, Thorgeirsson G (1997). Cholesterol lowering with simvastatin improves prognosis of diabetic people with coronary heart disease. A subgroup analysis of the Scandinavian Simvastatin Survival Study (4S). *Diabetes Care* **20**: 614–20.

Ravid M, Savin H, Jutrin I *et al.* (1993). Long-term stabilising effect of angiotensin-converting enzyme inhibition on plasma creatinine and on proteinuria in normotensive type II diabetic patients. *Annals of Internal Medicine* **118**: 577–81.

Ravid M, Leug R, Rachmanni R, Lisner M (1996). Long-term renoprotective effect of angiotensin converting enzyme inhibitors in non-insulin dependent diabetes: a seven year follow-up. *Archives of Internal Medicine* **156**: 286–9.

Ravid M, Brosh D, Levi Z, Bar-Dayan Y, Ravid D, Rachmani R (1998). Use of enalapril to attenuate decline in renal function in normotensive, normoalbuminuric patients with type 2 diabetes mellitus: a randomized, controlled trial. *Annals of Internal Medicine* **128**: 982–8.

Reaven GM (1988). Banting lecture 1988. Role of insulin resistance in human disease. *Diabetes* **37**: 1595–607.

Reaven GM (1999). Intensive blood pressure/glucose control in type 2 diabetes: why is it so difficult to decrease coronary heart disease? *Journal of Human Hypertension* **13**: S19–23.

Reaven G (2002). Metabolic syndrome: pathophysiology and implications for management of cardiovascular disease. *Circulation* **106**: 286–8.

Reaven GM, Lithell H, Landsberg L (1996). Hypertension and associated metabolic abnormalities – the role of insulin resistance and the sympathoadrenal system. *New England Journal of Medicine* **334**: 378–81.

Rocchini AP (2000). Obesity hypertension, salt sensitivity and insulin resistance. *Nutrition, Metabolism, and Cardiovascular Diseases* **10**: 287–94.

Rubins HB, Robins SJ, Collins D *et al.* (1999). Gemfibrozil for the secondary prevention of coronary heart disease in men with low levels of high-density lipoprotein cholesterol. Veterans Affairs High-Density Lipoprotein Cholesterol Intervention Trial Study Group. *New England Journal of Medicine* **341**: 410–18.

Ruggenenenti P, Fassi A, Ilieva AP *et al.* for the Bergamo Nephrologic Diabetes Complications Trial (BENEDICT) Investigators (2004). Preventing microalbuminuria in type 2 diabetes. *New England Journal of Medicine* **351**: 1941–51.

Ruilope L, Rodicio J (1995). Microalbuminuria in clinical practice: A current survey of world literature. *Kidney International* **4**: 211–16.

Saadine JB, Engelgau MM, Beckles GL *et al.* (2002). A diabetes report card for the United States: quality of care in the 1990s. *Annals of Internal Medicine* **136**: 565–74.

Sacks FM, Svetkey LP, Vollmer WM *et al.* for the DASH–Sodium Collaborative Research Group (2001). Effects on blood pressure of reduced dietary sodium and the Dietary Approaches to Stop Hypertension (DASH) diet. *New England Journal of Medicine* **344**: 3–10.

Sato A, Hayashi K, Naruse M *et al.* (2003). Effectiveness of aldosterone blockade in patients with diabetic nephropathy. *Hypertesnion* **41**: 64–8.

Scheen AJ (2004). Prevention of type 2 diabetes mellitus through inhibition of the renin-angiotensin system. *Drugs* **64**: 2537–65.

Schrier RW, Estacio RO, Esler A, Mehler P (2002). Effects of aggressive blood pressure control in a normotensive type 2 diabetic patients on albuminuria, retinopathy and strokes. *Kidney International* **61**: 1088–97.

Seidell JC, Visscher TL, Hoogeveen RT (1999). Overweight and obesity in the mortality rate data: Current evidence and research issues. *Medicine and Science in Sports and Exercise* **31**: S597–601.

Sever PS, Dahlöf B, Poulter NR *et al.* (2003). Prevention of coronary and stroke events with atorvastatin in hypertensive patients who have average or lower-than-average cholesterol concentration in the Anglo Scandinavian Cardiac Outcomes Trial in Lipid Lowering Arm (ASCOT-LLA): a multicentre randomised controlled trial. *Lancet* **361**: 1149–58.

Shapiro APJ, Benedeck TG, Small JL (1961). Effect of thiazides on carbohydrate metabolism in patients with hypertension. *New England Journal of Medicine* **265**: 1028–33.

Sharma AM (2004). Is there a rationale for angiotensin blockade in the management of obesity hypertension? *Hypertension* **44**: 12–19.

Sharma AM, Janke J, Gorzelniak K, Engeli S, Luft FC (2002). Angiotensin blockade prevents type 2 diabetes by promotion of fat cells. *Hypertension* **40**: 609–11.

Sica DA, Gehr TW (2002). 3-Hydroxy-3-methylglutaryl coenzyme A reductase inhibitors and rhabdomolysis: consideration in the renal failure patient. *Current Opinion in Nephrology and Hypertension* **11**: 123–33.

Simonson DC (1988). Etiology and prevalence of hypertension in diabetic patients. *Diabetes Care* **11**: 821–7.

Skarfors ET, Selinus KI, Lithell HO (1991). Risk factors for developing non-insulin dependent diabetes: a 10 year follow up of men in Uppsala. *British Medical Journal* **303**: 755–60.

Sowers JR, Bakris GL (2000). Antihypertensive therapy and the risk of type 2 diabetes mellitus. *New England Journal of Medicine* **342**: 969–70.

Sowers JR, Haffner S (2002). Treatment of cardiovascular and renal risk factors in the diabetic hypertensive. *Hypertension* **40**: 781–8.

Sowers JR, Epstein M, Frohlich ED (2001). Diabetes, hypertension and cardiovascular disease. *Hypertension* **37**: 1053–9.

Staessen JA, Fagard R, Thijs L *et al.* (1997). Randomised double-blind comparison of placebo and active treatment for older patients with isolated systolic hypertension. The Systolic Hypertension in Europe (Syst-Eur) Trial Investigators. *Lancet* **350**: 757–64.

Stamler J, Vaccaro O, Neaton J *et al.* (1993). Diabetes, other risk factors, and 12-year cardiovascular mortality for men screened for the Multiple Risk Factor Intervention Trial. *Diabetes Care* **16**: 434–9.

Stevens J, Cai J, Pamuk ER *et al.* (1998). The effect of age on the association between body-mass index and mortality. *New England Journal of Medicine* **338**: 1–7.

Strippoli GFM, Craig M, Deeks JJ, Schena FP, Craig JC (2004). Effects of angiotensin converting enzyme inhibitors and angiotensin II receptor antagonists on mortality and renal outcomes in diabetic nephropathy: systemic review. *British Medical Journal* **329**: 823–38.

Swislocki ALM, Hoffman BB, Reaven GM (1989). Insulin resistance, glucose intolerance and hyperinsulinemia in patients with hypertension. *American Journal of Hypertension* **2**: 419–23.

Tarnow L, Rossing P, Gall MA, Nielson FS, Parving HH (1994). Prevalence of arterial hypertension in diabetic patients before and after JNC-V. *Diabetes Care* **17**: 1247–51.

Tatti P, Pahor M, Byington RP, Di Mauro P, Guarisco R, Strollo G, Strollo F (1998). Outcome results of the Fosinopril versus Amlodipine Cardiovascular Events randomized Trial in patients with hypertension and NIDDM. *Diabetes Care* **21**: 597–605.

Thamer M, Ray NF, Taylor T *et al.* (1999). Association between antihypertensive drug use and hypoglycemia: a case-control study of diabetic users of insulin or sulfonylureas. *Clinical Therapeutics* **21**: 1387–400.

Torlone E, Rambotti AM, Perriello G *et al.* (1991). ACE-inhibition increases hepatic and extrahepatic sensitivity to insulin in patients with type 2 (non-insulin-dependent) diabetes mellitus and arterial hypertension. *Diabetologia* **34**: 119–25.

Torlone E, Britta M, Rambotti AM *et al.* (1993). Improved insulin action and glycaemic control after long-term angiotensin-converting enzyme inhibition in subjects with arterial hypertension and type 2 diabetes. *Diabetes Care* **16**: 1347–55.

Tuomilehto J, Rastenyte D, Birkenhager WH, Thijs L, Antikainen R, Bulpitt CJ, Fletcher AE, Forette F, Goldhaber A, Palatini P, Sarti C, Fagard R, Staessen JA for the Systolic Hypertension in Europe Trial Investigators (1999). Effects of calcium channel blockers in older patients with diabetes and systolic hypertension. *New England Journal of Medicine* **340**: 677–84.

Tuomilehto J, Lindstrom J, Eriksson JG *et al.* (2001). Prevention of type 2 diabetes mellitus by changes in lifestyle among subjects with impaired glucose tolerance. *New England Journal of Medicine* **344**: 1343–50.

UK Prospective Diabetes Study Group (1998a). Tight blood pressure control and risk of macrovascular and microvascular complications in type 2 diabetes: UKPDS 38. *British Medical Journal* **317**: 703–13.

UK Prospective Diabetes Study Group (1998b). Efficacy of atenolol and captopril in reducing risk of macrovascular and microvascular complications in type 2 diabetes: UKPDS 39. *British Medical Journal* **317**: 713–20.

UK Prospective Diabetes Study (UKPDS) Group (1998). Intensive blood-glucose control with sulphonylureas or insulin compared with conventional treatment and risk of complications in patients with type 2 diabetes (UKPDS 33). *Lancet* **352**: 837–53.

Vasan RS, Larson MG, Leip EP *et al.* (2001). Impact of high-normal pressure on the risk of cardiovascular disease. *New England Journal of Medicine* **345**: 1291–7.

Verdecchia P, Reboldi G, Angeli F *et al.* (2004). Adverse prognostic significance of new diabetes in treated hypertensive subjects. *Hypertension* **43**: 963–9.

Verma S, Strauss M (2004). Angiotensin receptor blockers and myocardial infarction. *British Medical Journal* **329**: 1248–9.

Viberti G, Mogensen C, Groop L *et al.* for the European Microalbuminuria Captropril Study Group (1994). Effect of captopril on progression to clinical proteinuria in patients with insulin-dependent diabetes mellitus and microalbuminuria. *Journal of the American Medical Association* **271**: 275–9.

Viberti G, Wheeldon NM for the MicroAlbuminuria Reduction with VALsartan (MARVAL) Study Investigators (2002). Microalbuminuria reduction with valsartan in patients with type 2 diabetes mellitus. A blood pressure-independent effect. *Circulation* **106**: 672–8.

Von Eckardstein A, Schulte H, Assmann G (2000). Risk for diabetes mellitus in middle-aged Caucasian male participants of the PROCAM study: implications for the definition of impaired fasting glucose by the American Diabetes Association. *Journal of Clinical Endocrinology and Metabolism* **85**: 3101–8.

Walker WG (1993). Hypertension-related renal injury: a major contributor to end-stage renal disease. *American Journal of Kidney Diseases* **22**: 164–73.

Wasserman DH, Zinman B (1994). Exercise in individuals with IDDM. *Diabetes Care* **17**: 924–37.

Whelton PK, Appel LJ, Espeland MA *et al.* (1998). Sodium reduction and weight loss in the treatment of hypertension in older persons: a randomized controlled trial of non-pharmacological intervention in the elderly (TONE). TONE Collaborative Research Group. *Journal of the American Medical Association* **279**: 839–46.

Whelton PK, He J, Appel LJ *et al.* (2002). Primary prevention of hypertension. Clinical and public health advisory from the National High Blood Pressure Education Program. *Journal of the American Medical Association* **288**: 1882–8.

Williams B (1999). The unique vulnerability of diabetic patients to hypertensive injury. *Journal of Human Hypertension* **13**: S3–8.

Williams B, Poulter NR, Brown MJ *et al.* (2004). Guidelines for management of hypertension: report of the fourth working party of the British Hypertension Society, 2004 – BHS IV. *Journal of Human Hypertension* **18**: 139–85.

World Health Organization International Society of Hypertension Writing Group (2003). 2003 World Health Organization (WHO)/International Society of Hypertension (ISH) statement on management of hypertension. *Journal of Hypertension* **21**: 1983–92.

Xin X, He J, Frontini MG , Ogden LG, Motsamai OK, Whelton PK (2001). Effects of alcohol reduction on blood pressure: A meta-analysis of randomised controlled trials. *Hypertension* **38**: 1112–17.

Yosefy C, Magen E, Kiselevich A *et al.* (2004). Rosiglitazone improves, while glibenclamide worsens blood pressure control in treated hypertensive diabetic and dyslipidemic subjects via modulation of insulin resistance and sympathetic activity. *Journal of Cardiovascular Pharmacology* **44**: 215–22.

Zanchetti A, Ruilope LM (2002). Antihypertensive treatment in patients with type 2 diabetes mellitus: what guidance from recent randomized controlled trials? *Journal of Hypertension* **20**: 2099–110.

Zimmermann M, Unger T (2004). Challenges in improving prognosis and therapy: the Ongoing Telmisartan Alone and in Combination with Ramipril Global End point Trial Programe. *Expert Opinion on Pharmacotherapy* **5**: 1201–8.

7 Diabetes and Stroke / Transient Ischaemic Attacks

Christopher S. Gray and *Janice E. O'Connell*

7.1 Introduction

It is generally accepted that both type 1 and type 2 diabetes are important risk factors for stroke (Kannel and McGee, 1979; Fuller *et al.*, 1983) (see also Chapter 1). Although it is often quoted that diabetes confers a two- to threefold increased risk of first ever and recurrent stroke it is important to recognise that this risk is primarily for ischaemic stroke, there being no proven association with primary intracerebral haemorrhage (Alex *et al.*, 1962; Peress *et al.*, 1972; Laing *et al.*, 2003).

Definition of stroke and transient ischaemic attacks

Stroke is an imprecise diagnostic label that contributes little to disease prevention or management. Historically a simple and arbitrary time distinction has been made between transient ischaemic attacks (TIAs, where transient neurological dysfunction lasts less than 24 h) and the completed stroke (where neurological dysfunction persists beyond 24 h). Most recent evidence suggests that not only do most TIAs resolve within 60 min but, in addition, nearly all TIA patients have neuroradiological evidence of ischaemic damage when symptoms persist beyond 6 h. Thus a new definition for TIA has been proposed: 'a brief episode of neurological dysfunction with symptoms lasting less than one hour and without evidence of acute infarction' (Albers *et al.*, 2002).

Within the definition of ischaemic stroke there is a spectrum ranging from large- to small-vessel occlusive disease, which may be symptomatic (disabling or non-disabling) or asymptomatic (so-called silent-strokes). Furthermore, ischaemic stroke

Diabetic Cardiology Editors Miles Fisher and John J. McMurray
© 2007 John Wiley & Sons, Ltd.

is an important cause of vascular dementia and, as we discuss in this chapter, also contributes to the underlying pathology of Alzheimer's dementia.

Burden of stroke

The burden of stroke has been well described but is often under-emphasised. Accounting for 6% of the total clinical budget, stroke is the third major cause of death and the major cause of severe disability in the community in the United Kingdom. (Isarol and Forbes, 1992; MacDonald *et al.*, 2000) Although primarily a disorder of older people, with the peak age incidence occurring in those over 75 years of age, a significant proportion of patients are younger with readily identifiable and potentially reversible risk factors, including diabetes. In the United Kingdom alone, stroke is estimated to occur in over 150 000 people per annum (MacDonald *et al.*, 2000).

The last 70 years have witnessed a major and progressive demographic shift in populations toward the extremes of old age with maximal population expansion in those aged over 75 years. Older people have a higher prevalence of established cardiovascular risk factors and, despite the earlier recognition and management of these factors, demographic trends mean that the incidence of stroke is likely to continue to rise in the future (Brown *et al.*, 1996). Although major vascular risk factors may be readily identified and appropriately treated, some often go under-recognised, especially in the older population. The prevalence of recognised type 2 diabetes in older people has been estimated to be approximately 7%. In addition, a further 7.7–14.8% of persons over 65 years of age may have previously unrecognised type 2 diabetes according to American Diabetes Association and World Health Organization criteria, respectively (Wahl *et al.*, 1998) (see Chapter 11).

In the last few years the management of acute stroke has changed considerably in response to evidence demonstrating the benefits of stroke units and specialist stroke teams (Stroke Unit Trialists' Collaboration, 1997). Furthermore, the emerging evidence for thrombolysis as a treatment in acute stroke has at last offered a potential treatment for some stroke patients (Wardlaw *et al.*, 2002). It has been estimated that up to one-third of acute stroke patients may have diabetes (Gray *et al.*, 2004a). Beyond the evidence demonstrating a causal relationship between diabetes and stroke there is now accumulating evidence to direct the early management and prevention of stroke in diabetic patients.

7.2   Diabetes as a Risk Factor for Stroke

The majority of diabetic patients have multiple risk factors for vascular disease, however diabetes remains an independent risk factor for stroke across all age groups (Wolf *et al.*, 1983). This increased risk is not confined to patients with diabetes but also includes patients with impaired glucose tolerance (IGT), asymptomatic non-fasting hyperglycaemia and hyperinsulinaemia (Coutinho *et al.*, 1999). The increase in risk conferred by diabetes also extends to patients with hypertension who already have a high absolute risk of cardiovascular disease (Kannel and McGee, 1979; Stamler *et al.*, 1993).

It has long been recognised that usual blood pressure levels are directly and continuously associated with risk of stroke in patients with or without a previous history of hypertension (Prospective Studies Collaboration, 1995; Eastern Stroke and Coronary Heart Disease Collaborative Research Group, 1998). A meta-analysis of studies examining the relationship between fasting, postprandial and casual glucose levels has demonstrated a similar relationship between glucose levels and cardiovascular risk. Furthermore, like blood pressure, this increased risk extends below diabetic and IGT thresholds and into the 'normal' range (Coutinho et al., 1999).

Accepting that type 2 diabetes is the predominant form of diabetes in stroke patients, the United Kingdom Prospective Diabetes Study (UKPDS) has demonstrated that over a 9-year period 20% of type 2 diabetic patients are likely to experience macrovascular complications (UK Prospective Diabetes Study Group, 1996). This is in contrast to an estimated 9% experiencing microvascular complications over a similar period. Overall, macrovascular complications account for 50% of deaths in such patients (Reichard et al., 1991; Ohkubo et al., 1995; UK Prospective Diabetes Study Group, 1996). Diabetes confers an increased risk of stroke through a number of different mechanisms, both direct and indirect. Against this background of increased risk, the diagnosis of ischaemic stroke potentially encompasses five pathophysiological categories: those due to thrombosis in situ (29–44%); cardio-embolism (20–25%); small artery disease or lacunar strokes (13–21%); and those due to mixed or undetermined aetiologies (15–17%) (Adams et al., 1993).

Carotid disease

Within the large extracranial carotid arteries it is well established that atherosclerotic changes (especially with advanced stenosis) increase the risk of atherothrombotic stroke. Carotid stenosis is a prevalent finding in the general elderly population with estimates ranging from 1% below 60 years of age to 10% over 80 years (Carolei and Marini, 2000). In both diabetic patients and those with IGT atherosclerotic changes in the vascular intima and media are accelerated, leading to significantly increased risk. It has been estimated that type 2 diabetes confers a threefold increased risk for the development of asymptomatic carotid artery stenosis when compared with non-diabetic subjects (De Angelis, 2003). The finding of a stenosed extracranial carotid artery (> 70%) in an individual with no previous history of stroke or TIA increases the estimated annual risk of stroke from 1% to 2–3%. For a patient with a previous history of stroke or TIA in the distribution of a stenosed carotid artery (> 70%) the risk of a further ischaemic stroke in the same carotid distribution is increased to 11% over a 3-year period (European Carotid Surgery Trialists' Collaborative Group, 1991, 1998; Norris et al., 1991). Thus for carotid stenosis, the most important marker of increased risk is a previous symptomatic TIA or stroke in the distribution of the affected artery.

The relevance of diabetes as a risk factor for early recurrence of stroke was recently highlighted in a study of patients presenting to an emergency department in North America with TIA. The risk of early (2 days) stroke or TIA recurrence was 5% compared with previous estimates of 1–2% at 7 days. At 90 days, 23.2% had re-presented with either stroke or TIA compared with previous estimates of risk of 2–4% at 30 days. Importantly, a previous history of diabetes increased the risk of recurrence twofold (Hankey 1996; Gubitz *et al.*, 1999; Johnston *et al.*, 2000a; Warlow *et al.*, 2001). Such data provide important guidance for clinicians involved in the care of patients with TIA: the risk of early recurrence is approximately five times that previously reported, and diabetic patients are at greatest risk.

Other vessels

Beyond the large extracranial vessels, diabetes increases the risk of atheroma formation throughout the large, medium and smaller arteries and arterioles of the cerebral circulation. In the small intraparenchymal vessels there is increased microatheroma, basement membrane thickening, lipid transformation of the vessel wall and endothelial proliferation. These changes lead to vessel occlusion within the microcirculation, increasing the risk of lacunar infarction in the territory of single deep perforating arteries (Alex *et al.*, 1962; Peress *et al.*, 1972). Such pathophysiological changes explain why lacunar infarction is more prevalent in diabetics than is widely recognised (Alex *et al.*, 1962; Megherbi *et al.*, 2003).

When managing diabetic patients with stroke, the distinction between haemorrhagic or ischaemic pathology is clearly important if considering patients for acute treatment with thrombolysis or secondary prevention with antiplatelet or antithrombotic therapy. Furthermore, some understanding of the pathophysiological process leading to the acute event further informs acute treatment strategies and prevention.

Beyond classifying strokes according to their likely pathology it is possible to further describe them according to the vascular territory affected within the brain, or according to the clinical syndrome with which they present. Describing stroke patients by their clinical syndrome is of practical value in that it enables non-stroke specialists to predict the likely underlying pathogenesis and make some estimation of early prognosis. One such classification as described by Bamford *et al.* (1991) utilises a description of the patient's neurological deficits as demonstrated on clinical examination to create one of four stroke syndromes, each with its own likely prognosis for survival, recurrence and recovery of functional independence (Table 7.1). For the cardiologist or diabetologist, the clinical relevance of such a distinction is that the prevalent lacunar strokes have a good prognosis in terms of survival, although almost half will have persisting disability up to 1 year after the incident event, with a risk of symptomatic recurrence in the first year of approximately 9% (Bamford *et al.*, 1991).

7.3   Diabetes, Post-stroke Hyperglycaemia and Outcome from Stroke

Prognosis of stroke

Diabetes not only increases the risk of stroke two- to threefold but also confers a poor prognosis following the acute event with increased mortality, reduced neurological recovery and poor functional outcomes (Kannel and McGee, 1979; Pulsinelli *et al.*, 1983; Oppenheimer *et al.*, 1985; Olsson *et al.*, 1990). Such an association also extends

Table 7.1 Clinical stroke syndromes and their prognosis. Adapted from Bamford *et al.*, 1991.

Clinical syndrome	Symptoms and signs at the time of maximum deficit	Mortality (12 months)	Independent function (12 months)	Recurrence (12 months)
Total Anterior Circulation Infarcts (TACI)	Combination of: • New higher cerebral dysfunction • Homonymous visual field defect • Ipsilateral motor and/or sensory deficit of at least two areas of the face, arm or leg	60%	4%	6%
Partial Anterior Circulation Infarcts (PACI)	• Only two of three components of TACI • Higher cerebral dysfunction alone, or with motor/sensory deficit more restricted than those classified as LACI	10%	55%	17%
Lacunar Infarcts (LACI)	• Pure motor stroke • Pure sensory stroke • Sensory-motor stroke • Ataxic hemiparesis (including dysarthria, clumsy hand syndrome, homolateral ataxia and crural paresis)	11%	60%	9%
Posterior Circulation Infarcts (POCI)	• Ipsilateral cranial nerve palsy with contralateral motor and/or sensory deficit • Bilateral motor and/or sensory deficit • Disorder of conjugate eye movement • Cerebellar dysfunction without ipsilateral long tract deficit • Isolated hemianopia or cortical blindness	19%	62%	20%

to the finding of hyperglycaemia in the immediate aftermath of stroke. Several large clinical studies have now demonstrated a positive association between a raised blood glucose concentration and poor outcome from stroke: greater mortality and reduced functional recovery (Gray et al., 1987, 1992; Power et al., 1988; Weir et al., 1997). In a meta-analysis of clinical studies of hyperglycaemia and stroke outcome, Capes found that the relative risk of death in hyperglycaemic non-diabetic stroke patients was increased by 3.3 (95% CI 2.3–4.6) (Capes et al., 2001). Thus there is evidence for an association between post-stroke hyperglycaemia and stroke outcome both in the presence and absence of underlying IGT or diabetes. There is also some evidence to suggest that the finding of both stress hyperglycaemia and impaired glucose metabolism is associated with the worst prognosis (Gray et al., 1987).

Post-stroke hyperglycaemia (PSH)

In any given population of acute stroke patients it has been estimated that 8–20% will have a past history of diabetes, with a further 6–42% having previously unrecognised diabetes prior to the acute event (Riddle and Hart, 1982; Oppenheimer et al., 1985; Gray et al., 1987; Kiers et al., 1992). Variations in the populations studied, the criteria applied for the diagnosis of diabetes and the use of blood fructosamine and glycosylated haemoglobin as indirect diagnoses of diabetes have contributed to such wide estimates. The frequent finding of hyperglycaemia in the immediate aftermath of stroke, so-called post-stroke hyperglycaemia (PSH), further complicates estimates of the prevalence of diabetes or impaired glucose tolerance. In one series of acute stroke patients it was estimated that up to 68% had PSH, defined by a plasma glucose concentration > 6.0 mmol/l (Scott et al., 1999). Like diabetes, the finding of PSH has been reported to be associated with a poor prognosis: increased mortality and poor functional outcomes (Capes et al., 2001).

It has previously been suggested that PSH is a stress response occurring in those stroke patients most severely affected and for whom a poor prognosis is predetermined (Woo et al., 1988; O'Neill et al., 1991). Most recent evidence, however, has demonstrated that hyperglycaemia is prevalent across all clinical subtypes and severities of stroke and is not restricted to those most severely affected (Scott et al., 1999). It is also probable that in a small number of patients stress hyperglycaemia occurs as the result of neuroendocrine dysregulation in response to specific cortical lesions (Allport et al., 2004).

Following acute stroke, a diagnosis of diabetes mellitus or IGT should ideally be made when the stress of the acute event has dissipated and the patient is clinically stable. In one cohort study, oral glucose tolerance testing when performed 3 months after stroke onset in patients presenting with PSH (admission plasma glucose > 6.0 mmol/l) found IGT or diabetes in 58% of subjects, with the estimated prevalence of previously unrecognised diabetes being 16–24%. The finding of admission plasma glucose > 6.0 mmol/l plus HbA1c > 6.2% was highly predictive of diabetes at 3 months (positive predictive value 80%, negative predictive value 96%) (Gray et al., 2004a).

In summary, PSH is a frequent finding and occurs in up to two-thirds of acute stroke patients. Although in some patients this may reflect the stress of the acute event, it is not a phenomenon confined to those most severely affected and in the majority (two-thirds) it reflects underlying dysglycaemia (diabetes mellitus or IGT).

7.4 Hyperglycaemia and Ischaemic Cerebral Damage

Patholophysiology

Following ischaemic stroke, cerebral blood flow to the affected area rapidly falls leading to cell death within the core of the ischaemic area. The sequence of events leading to cell death has been termed the ischaemic cascade (Pulsinelli *et al.*, 1985; Pulsinelli 1992). Around the infarct core is a zone in which cerebral blood flow is reduced but not sufficient to cause irreversible cell damage. This zone, within which some spontaneous recovery of cellular activity may occur, has been described as the ischaemic penumbra (Astrup *et al.*, 1977, 1981). Within the infarct core there is an increase in glycolysis with the result that tissue glucose levels rapidly fall and metabolism decreases (Ginsberg *et al.*, 1977; Vázquez-Cruz *et al.*, 1990). As a consequence of prolonged hypoxia, cellular metabolism fails and there is an accumulation of cerebral lactate. These changes lead to failure of the membrane ion pump, an efflux of potassium and an influx of sodium and calcium ions along with water and the formation of cytotoxic oedema. Enzymatic lipolysis of the cell membrane is enhanced by calcium ions and there is a release of free fatty acids, which in turn facilitate production of toxic free radicals, inflammatory responses and prostaglandins. This sequence of events leads to membrane depolarisation and cell death. The ischaemic cascade is further enhanced by the toxic effects of high concentrations of excitatory neurotransmitters (aspartate, glutamate), which are released from damaged cells. Finally, within the penumbra, secondary vasogenic oedema forms as a consequence of the disrupted blood–brain barrier. This further contributes to ischaemic damage through a direct effect upon small vessels whilst also increasing the oxygen diffusion distance. There is accumulating evidence that this sequence of events leading to cell death may be influenced by hyperglycaemia.

Effects of hyperglycaemia

Hyperglycaemia occurring at the onset of cerebral ischaemia is thought to increase infarction by enhancing intracellular and extracellular acidosis. Following focal cerebral ischaemia there is a local increase in glycolysis and a rapid decline in tissue glucose levels. Consequently, glucose metabolism at the centre of the ischaemic area decreases whereas at the periphery glucose metabolism is enhanced. With prolonged hypoxia, cellular metabolism fails and cerebral lactate levels increase rapidly. Although clinical studies have shown that hyperglycaemia is associated with poor outcome across a range of plasma glucose concentrations, it seems probable that extent of the metabolic changes and thereby the ensuing cerebral damage is dependent upon the degree of hyperglycaemia (Capes *et al.*, 2001).

The deleterious effect of hyperglycaemia upon stroke outcome is not confined to stroke due to cerebral infarction. Animal studies have also shown enhanced cell death and increased brain oedema in the presence of hyperglycaemia following experimental intracranial haemorrhage (Song *et al.*, 2003).

Beyond a direct effect upon cellular metabolism, hyperglycaemia may also increase the permeability of ischaemic capillary endothelium thus contributing to haemorrhagic transformation of an infarct. These changes further enhance ischaemic damage through energy depletion and lactate accumulation (Siemkowicz and Hanson, 1978; Beghi *et al.*, 1989).

In addition to the experimental evidence for an association between hyperglycaemia and poor stroke outcome, recent advances in neuroradiogical imaging have permitted detailed estimates of cerebral infarct volumes in clinical studies. Using serial estimates of infarct volume there is some evidence to suggest that persistent PSH is independently associated with infarct expansion and worse clinical outcome (Baird *et al.*, 2003).

Beyond a direct negative influence upon outcome from stroke there is accumulating evidence that hyperglycaemia may also influence the safety and effectiveness of acute stroke therapies. In the first major clinical trial demonstrating a significant clinical benefit from thrombolysis with recombinant tissue plasminogen activator (rt-PA) in ischaemic stroke, admission hyperglycaemia was associated with reduced odds for good clinical outcomes and a higher risk of intracranial haemorrhage (Bruno *et al.*, 2002). Similarly, in a North American clinical series, hyperglycaemia (plasma glucose > 11.2 mmol/l) at the time of rt-PA treatment was associated with a fivefold increased risk of intracranial haemorrhage (Demchuk *et al.*, 1999).

In summary, although the totality of the clinical and experimental evidence tends to support a direct relationship between hyperglycaemia and stroke outcome, cause and effect have not as yet been proven through appropriate clinical trials.

7.5 Management of Diabetes and Hyperglycaemia following Stroke

There is still no safe, simple and effective medical therapy for the majority of acute stroke patients. Although thrombolysis with rt-PA when given within 3 h of symptom onset following ischaemic stroke has been shown to improve functional recovery, there remains concern regarding the risk/benefit of such treatment. Routine use of thrombolysis for stroke in the UK is minimal and even in experienced North American centres less than 20% of potentially eligible patients receive such therapy (Johnston *et al.*, 2000b).

Apart from thrombolysis, recent advances in acute stroke treatments have been consistently disappointing (neuroprotective therapy) and attention is once again being directed towards monitoring and modifying physiological variables that may influence stroke outcome. In the absence of a simple and effective medical therapy there is increasing evidence that the provision of specialist stroke care within acute and rehabilitation stroke units is associated with improved outcome (Stroke Unit Trialists' Collaboration, 1997). Such evidence has led to the widespread introduction of stroke units. An essential component of acute stroke unit care is the intensive monitoring of physiological variables (hydration, glucose, temperature, blood pressure, oxygen saturation) and their early correction. It remains to be determined, however, whether such intervention does actually improve patient outcomes.

The Royal College of Physicians (UK) National Clinical Guidelines for Stroke highlight the importance of organised stroke care and the need to consider the early management of hyperglycaemia, blood pressure, hydration and pyrexia (Intercollegiate Working Party for Stroke, 2000). Whilst there is accumulating evidence for a link between hyperglycaemia, diabetes and enhanced ischaemic cerebral damage, such an association has never been confirmed by any clinical trial. Similarly, any potential insulin treatment effect has not been examined in appropriate clinical trials.

Management of hyperglycaemia

In contrast, evidence from clinical trials in acute myocardial infarction and critically ill patients in intensive care support the concept of treating hyperglycaemia and maintaining euglycaemia with insulin. An overview of trials in acute myocardial infarction has shown that treatment of acute myocardial infarction with a glucose–potassium–insulin (GKI)-based regimen reduces in-hospital mortality by 28% (Fath-Ordoubadi and Beatt, 1997). Furthermore, insulin treatment in acute myocardial infarction may also confer survival benefits in the absence of initial hyperglycaemia (Diaz *et al.*, 1998). Consistent with these findings is the evidence supporting intensive insulin therapy and euglycaemic control in patients admitted to intensive care (Van den Berghe *et al.*, 2001). In the first DIGAMI study, patients presenting with acute myocardial infarction and admission plasma glucose > 11 mmol/l (with or without a past history of diabetes) were randomised to an insulin infusion for > 24 h and then subcutaneous insulin four times daily for > 3 months (Malmberg *et al.*, 1995). Treatment conferred a significant 52% relative reduction in mortality up to 12 months after the acute event, although a more recent study did not show any benefit (see also Chapter 4).

Such a prolonged insulin treatment regimen in acute stroke patients is not feasible in routine practice where the complexity of clinical stroke care combined with the practical difficulties in maintaining hydration and nutrition potentially makes routine treatment with insulin beyond 24 h both illogical and unsafe. Furthermore, whilst the majority of acute stroke patients may present with hyperglycaemia, this is usually mild with mean plasma glucose concentrations of 8–9 mmol/l (Gray *et al.*, 2004b). The management of diabetes and hyperglycaemia following stroke is further complicated by the fact that up to one-third of all stroke patients have swallowing difficulties in the immediate aftermath of the acute event. Although these usually resolve in two-thirds of cases during the first week, nutritional support and supplementation in acute stroke patients are often fraught with practical and ethical difficulties, thus creating a challenge for tight euglycaemic control in the first few days. There is accumulating evidence to suggest that PSH is maximal in the first 12–18 h following stroke and that glucose levels will decline spontaneously without specific intervention. Treatment with a variable-dose GKI regimen can safely induce and maintain stable euglycaemia during the first 24 h of hospitalisation although the clinical benefit of such intervention is currently being examined in the ongoing Glucose Insulin in Stroke Trial (GIST-UK) (Gray *et al.*, 2004b).

For clinicians caring for stroke patients it is important to recognise that up to 40% will deteriorate neurologically following admission to hospital (Toni *et al.*, 1995). This neurological deterioration may reflect natural progression of the initial stroke, but may also be due to enhanced ischaemic damage through changes in physiological variables such as glucose, temperature and blood pressure. Although there is similar evidence to that for glucose for associating these additional variables with stroke outcome, it is probable that they are inexorably linked and treatment of one will have effects upon the other.

In summary, on the basis of current evidence should clinicians actively manage hyperglycaemia following stroke and how? The National Service Framework for Older People (UK) Standard 5 (Stroke) specifically states that 'immediate management to improve chances of survival and minimise risk of complications should include: appropriate control of blood pressure, maintenance of hydration and oxygen saturation and *management of hyperglycaemi*a and fever'. Unfortunately these are areas in which our evidence base derives purely from clinical and experimental associations and there is a pressing need for clinical trials to clarify the risks/benefits of routine interventions. Thresholds for the routine management of hyperglycaemia vary across centres and between clinicians, although the evidence does suggest that no true threshold exists above which risk is suddenly conferred. Local policies for the management of PSH also vary considerably and the safety and efficacy of these local regimens have not been examined in safety or outcome studies. Treatment with a variable-insulin-dose GKI infusion regimen has been shown to be associated with a physiological lowering of plasma glucose mimicking the 'normal' hyperglycaemic response to stroke with no adverse effect upon patient outcome (Figure 7.1). Although it is feasible to routinely deliver euglycaemic treatment to acute stroke patients in the first 24 h, the clinical efficacy of such an intervention remains unproven and results of the ongoing randomised controlled clinical trial to evaluate GKI-maintained euglycaemia are awaited (Gray *et al.*, 2001). In the absence of specific euglycaemic intervention, mild to moderate PSH should still be actively managed with intravenous saline hydration, with which mean plasma glucose levels have been shown to decline although not achieving truly 'normal' levels (Figure 7.1). Significant hyperglycaemia that may contribute to dehydration should be actively corrected with insulin and adequate intravenous fluid replacement.

In patients for whom thrombolysis is contemplated it would seem prudent to attempt to correct hyperglycaemia and maintain euglycaemia, although the therapeutic time window for thrombolytic therapy is so short (<3 h from symptom onset) that effective glycaemic control may actually follow rather than precede such treatment.

Advances in the management of stroke have been extremely limited when compared with acute myocardial infarction. It is only following the widespread introduction of specialist stroke services that comparable clinical trials can now be undertaken. Diabetes and hyperglycaemia are not only major risk factors for stroke but also important prognostic factors for stroke outcome. Beyond the acute phase of the disease it is clear that intensive management of vascular risk factors confers major benefits for stroke patients. Until a safe, simple and effective therapy is developed for the majority of stroke patients our priority is to reduce mortality, disability and dependency through the implementation of proven strategies to prevent first ever and recurrent stroke.

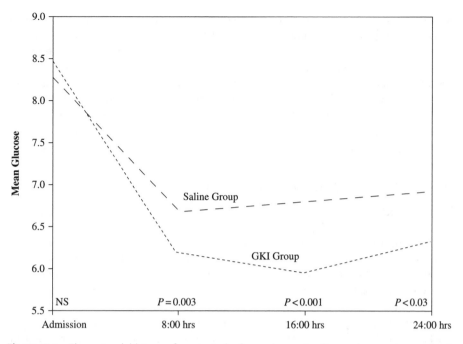

Figure 7.1 The natural history of post stroke hyperglycaemia. Mean plasma glucose levels in the GKI and Saline treatment groups. Reprinted with permission from Lippincott Williams and Wilkins from Gray CS, Hildreth AJ, Alberti KGMM, O'Connell JE, on behalf of the GIST Collaboration (2004b). Post stroke hyperglycemia; natural history and immediate management. *Stroke* **35:**122–6.

7.6 Prevention of Stroke in Diabetic Patients

Hypertension

Hypertension is the single most important and potentially reversible risk factor for cerebrovascular disease in both diabetic and non-diabetic individuals (see also Chapter 6). Epidemiological studies confirm that usual systolic and diastolic blood pressure levels are directly and continuously associated with risk of stroke (both cerebral infarction and primary intracerebral haemorrhage) in patients with and without a previous history of hypertension (Prospective Studies Collaboration, 1995; Eastern Stroke and Coronary Heart Disease Collaborative Research Group, 1998). In addition, a similar linear relationship exists between systolic and diastolic blood pressure and risk of recurrent cerebrovascular events in survivors of stroke and TIA (Rodgers *et al.*, 1996). Reducing diastolic blood pressure by 5–6 mmHg in people with hypertension and no history of cerebrovascular disease reduces their risk of stroke by approximately one-third, with all major classes of antihypertensive agents appearing equally effective (Blood Pressure Lowering Treatment Trialists' Collaboration, 2000). Furthermore, drug interventions to lower blood pressure have been shown to reduce the risk of stroke recurrence in hypertensive stroke survivors (INDANA Project Collaborators, 1997). Whilst it is accepted that hypertension is a major determinant of stroke risk in diabetics, the majority of patients have multiple risk factors such as dyslipidaemia, ischaemic heart disease and peripheral vascular disease that may influence the choice of antihypertensive therapy. Trial evidence suggests that tight diabetic control may not directly reduce the risk of stroke and TIA (UK Prospective Diabetes Study (UKPDS) Group, 1998) and clinicians therefore also need to direct attention towards the management of other modifiable vascular risk factors such as hypertension.

The United Kingdom Prospective Diabetes Study

The United Kingdom Prospective Diabetes Study incorporated a randomised controlled trial (also called the 'Hypertension in Diabetes Study', or HDS) to establish if tight control of blood pressure ($< 150/85$ mmHg) reduced morbidity and mortality in patients with type 2 diabetes (UK Prospective Diabetes Study Group, 1998). Treated hypertensive diabetics whose blood pressure was above this target level and those who were previously untreated ($\geq 160/ \geq 90$ mmHg) were randomised to receive either intensive or less intensive blood pressure lowering therapy. The intensive treatment comprised an angiotensin-converting enzyme (ACE) inhibitor (captopril) or a beta-blocker (atenolol), with a target blood pressure of $< 150/85$. The other treatment limb aimed for less tight control of blood pressure ($< 180/105$), avoiding ACE inhibitors and beta-blockers. Almost one-third (29%) of patients randomised to the tight control group needed three or more agents to control their blood pressure, compared with 11% in the less intensive treatment group. Tight control resulted in significantly lower blood pressure; the mean blood pressure over 9 years of follow-up was 144/82 in the intensive treatment group compared with 154/87 in the other limb. After a median follow-up period of 8.4 years, intensive management of hypertension in these UKPDS patients resulted in a 24% relative risk reduction for the development of any endpoint related to diabetes. There was no significant difference in diabetic control between the intensive and less-intensive treatment groups (mean HbA1c 7.2% for both). Intensive treatment led to a highly significant 44% relative reduction in fatal or non-fatal stroke, but no significant decrease in rates of myocardial infarction.

These results are comparable with those seen in other trials of blood-pressure-lowering treatment in older people (Dahlof *et al.*, 1991; SHEP Co-operative Research Group, 1991). Thus, intensive glycaemic control in patients with type 2 diabetes is not sufficient to reduce their risk of stroke; simultaneous management of hypertension is also necessary. The UK Prospective Diabetes Study Group (1998) also showed that intensive blood pressure treatment would probably require combination therapy, including beta-blockers or ACE inhibitors. It should be noted that even in the their tight control group, the mean level of blood pressure achieved was still higher than the current UK recommended target of $< 130/80$ mmHg for clinic readings (Williams *et al.*, 2004). However, this trial did demonstrate that the lowest risk of complications due to diabetes was seen in patients with systolic blood pressure < 120 mmHg, in line with current recommendations (Adler *et al.*, 2000).

Renin–angiotensin system blockade

Heart Outcomes Prevention Evaluation (HOPE) study

We know that adequate management of hypertension in diabetic patients is essential in order to reduce their risk of TIA and stroke. There is also accumulating evidence that for patients at high risk of vascular disease, including diabetics, the benefits of antihypertensive therapy probably extend beyond the blood-pressure-lowering effect. In the HOPE study, 9297 high-risk vascular patients aged 55 years or older, including 3577 (38%) with diabetes plus one additional risk factor (including stroke or TIA), were randomised to treatment with the ACE inhibitor ramipril or placebo (Heart Outcomes Prevention Evaluation Study Investigators, 2000). Ramipril resulted in modest reductions in office blood pressure compared with placebo (3.8/2.8 mmHg). Nevertheless, overall results confirmed that the relative risk of any stroke or fatal stroke was decreased by 32% and 61%, respectively. Ramipril was beneficial even in those who were normotensive at baseline. Further analysis of the results for the diabetic subgroup ($n = 3577$) confirmed a significant 33% reduction in stroke risk, again irrespective of baseline blood pressure (Heart Outcomes Prevention Evaluation (HOPE) Study Investigators, 2000).

Thus, as in the UKPDS, the benefits observed in the HOPE study with fairly modest reductions in office blood pressure were greater than might be predicted from epidemiological data (Bosch *et al.*, 2002). Explanations for this observation include a protective effect on the vasculature by drugs like ACE inhibitors or beta-blockers or enhanced control of ambulatory blood pressure levels compared with clinic readings (Svensson *et al.*, 2001).

PROGRESS

Further evidence for the beneficial effect of ACE inhibitors in reducing risk of recurrent stroke comes from the PROGRESS trial (PROGRESS Collaborative Group, 2001). This study recruited 6105 hypertensive and normotensive patients with a history of stroke or TIA, of whom 13% were diabetic. The maximum beneficial effect was seen in patients on combined therapy with the ACE inhibitor perindopril plus the diuretic indapamide. Mean blood pressure lowering on combined therapy was 12/5 mmHg compared with perindopril monotherapy (mean 5/3 mmHg). Treatment with perindopril plus indapamide resulted in a relative risk reduction for recurrent stroke of 43%, compared with a non-significant 5% decrease with perindopril alone. A *post hoc* diabetes subgroup analysis was done for the diabetic patients enrolled in this study, and the results were very similar (Berthet *et al.*, 2004).

Intensive blood pressure lowering

HOT trial

It appears therefore that in hypertensive diabetic patients, the intensity of blood pressure therapy is important in order to maximally decrease their risk of stroke and other vascular events. In order to further investigate the intensity of blood pressure lowering, the HOT study aimed to determine the optimum treatment level for diastolic blood pressure. The HOT investigators found that there was a twofold increase in the incidence of cardiovascular events in hypertensive diabetic patients and that in these individuals intensive treatment to reduce diastolic blood pressure to <80 mmHg resulted in a 30% reduction in the risk of stroke compared with more modest reductions in blood pressure to <90 mmHg (Hansson *et al.*, 1998). Treatment in the HOT study was with a calcium channel blocker-based regime, but for many patients this was combined with a beta-blocker or ACE inhibitor.

Some international management guidelines recommend a target systolic blood pressure of <130 mmHg for diabetic patients (see Chapter 6). However, accumulating evidence, including the clinical trials quoted above, suggests that high-risk vascular patients such as diabetics should be treated even more aggressively irrespective of their baseline blood pressure in order to reduce the risk of cerebrovascular events. The management of hypertension immediately following acute stroke is more contentious (O'Connell and Gray, 1994). The majority of acute stroke patients are hypertensive on admission to hospital and, for many, blood pressure falls spontaneously over the first 7–10 days. Cerebral vasoreactivity and autoregulation of blood flow are impaired immediately after stroke so that cerebral perfusion may become dependent upon systemic blood pressure levels. Thus lowering the blood pressure in the acute phase after stroke may be potentially harmful and ongoing clinical trials are addressing this issue. In the PROGRESS and HOPE trials, ACE inhibitor therapy was delayed for 2–4 weeks after stroke. Based on current evidence, it would seem prudent to withhold antihypertensive therapy until stroke patients are clinically and neurologically stable, except for specific clinical circumstances such as accelerated hypertension where immediate blood pressure lowering is mandatory (Robinson and Potter, 2004).

Dyslipidaemia, diabetes and stroke

The relationship between dyslipidaemia and cardiovascular disease is qualitatively similar in diabetic and non-diabetic patients, but for any given level of cholesterol the absolute risk is higher for diabetics. The evidence that dyslipidaemia is a risk factor for stroke is conflicting, with a recent meta-analysis showing no apparent association (Prospective Studies Collaboration, 1995). Many studies, however, fail to distinguish between strokes caused by cerebral infarction or primary intracerebral haemorrhage. Evidence from Caucasian and Asian population studies confirms a positive association between total cholesterol levels and risk of cerebral infarction, which may be offset by a negative correlation between cholesterol and risk of intracerebral haemorrhage (Iso *et al.*, 1989; Yano *et al.*, 1989). Epidemiological evidence of such associations does not prove cause and effect, but leads to concern that extrapolation from such data to clinical practice may put patients at risk. Indeed, the early trials of cholesterol-lowering therapies such as diet, fibrates, niacin, colestipol and surgery showed no effect on risk of stroke. These early studies did demonstrate a reduction in ischaemic heart disease, although not to the extent that might have been predicted by the epidemiological evidence. More recent trials with the HMG-CoA reductase inhibitors (statins) have demonstrated much greater lowering of cholesterol (total and low-density lipoprotein,

LDL) and triglyceride concentrations, together with small increases in high-density lipoprotein (HDL)-cholesterol, accompanied by much larger reductions in ischaemic heart disease. Analysis of data from the large secondary prevention statin trials confirms that the beneficial effects of lowering cholesterol were similar in diabetic and non-diabetic patients.

It should be remembered that the majority of diabetic patients at risk of stroke are older and have type 2 diabetes. In these individuals, the predominant lipid abnormalities are raised triglycerides and reduced HDL-cholesterol. In contrast to the evidence linking dyslipidaemia to ischaemic heart disease, it is only recently that statin therapy has also been shown to be effective in reducing cerebrovascular disease. A meta-analysis of the statin trials confirmed that, in patients with known ischaemic heart disease, cholesterol-lowering therapy was associated with a 30% reduction in the risk of stroke (Bucher *et al.*, 1998). Furthermore, statins did not seem to increase the risk of haemorrhagic stroke, despite the epidemiological evidence for an association between low cholesterol and intracerebral haemorrhage. Although statins are also very effective in primary prevention of ischaemic heart disease, the results for primary stroke prevention are less impressive, with a much smaller reduction in stroke risk observed in clinical trials (Hess *et al.*, 2000). This may simply reflect the lower overall rate of stroke in the study populations.

More recently, cholesterol-lowering therapy in diabetics and other patients at high risk of vascular disease was studied in the United Kingdom Medical Research Council / British Heart Foundation-coordinated Heart Protection Study (Heart Protection Study Collaborative Group, 2002) This large clinical trial included 20 536 patients aged 40–80 years in whom there was uncertainty regarding the benefits of lipid lowering: diabetics, people > 70 years old, those with non-coronary vascular disease and those with average to below average cholesterol levels. The participants were randomised to receive high-dose simvastatin (40 mg daily) or placebo, with a mean follow-up of 5 years (Figure 7.2). This important study confirmed that benefit was conferred irrespective of baseline cholesterol concentration, with significant reductions in vascular events (major coronary events, stroke or revascularisations) seen in all patient groups. The beneficial effects of statins appeared to be additional to those of other vasculoprotective therapies such as aspirin, ACE inhibitors and beta-blockers. There was a 25% reduction in incidence of first ever stroke (4.3% vs. 5.7%), which was seen in all patient groups, including diabetic patients. This was mainly due to a reduction in cerebral infarction, with no observed increase in intracerebral haemorrhage. The risk of TIA was also substantially decreased by simvastatin therapy (2.0% vs. 2.4%). For all patient groups, including diabetics, these benefits were seen in patients with and without a previous history of ischaemic heart disease.

Further analysis of results for the 5963 diabetics enrolled in the Heart Protection Study confirmed a 22% reduction in risk of vascular events with simvastatin, similar to the other high-risk individuals in the study (Heart Protection Study Collaborative Group, 2003). Furthermore, there were highly significant reductions in vascular events of 33% amongst the 2912 diabetic participants with no occlusive arterial disease at study entry and of 27% amongst the 2426 diabetics with pretreatment LDL-cholesterol less than 3 mmol/l. The results of the Heart Protection Study suggest that statin therapy should be part of the vascular risk reduction strategy for all diabetic patients, even if

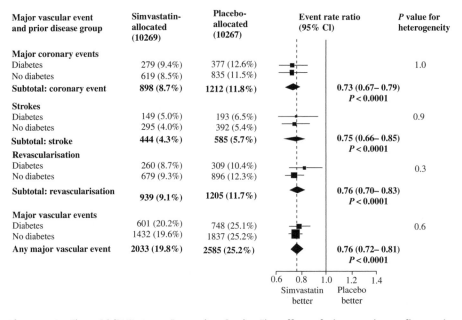

Major vascular event and prior disease group	Simvastatin-allocated (10269)	Placebo-allocated (10267)	Event rate ratio (95% CI)	P value for heterogeneity
Major coronary events				
Diabetes	279 (9.4%)	377 (12.6%)		1.0
No diabetes	619 (8.5%)	835 (11.5%)		
Subtotal: coronary event	**898 (8.7%)**	**1212 (11.8%)**	0.73 (0.67– 0.79) P < 0.0001	
Strokes				
Diabetes	149 (5.0%)	193 (6.5%)		0.9
No diabetes	295 (4.0%)	392 (5.4%)		
Subtotal: stroke	**444 (4.3%)**	**585 (5.7%)**	0.75 (0.66– 0.85) P < 0.0001	
Revascularisation				
Diabetes	260 (8.7%)	309 (10.4%)		0.3
No diabetes	679 (9.3%)	896 (12.3%)		
Subtotal: revascularisation	**939 (9.1%)**	**1205 (11.7%)**	0.76 (0.70– 0.83) P < 0.0001	
Major vascular events				
Diabetes	601 (20.2%)	748 (25.1%)		0.6
No diabetes	1432 (19.6%)	1837 (25.2%)		
Any major vascular event	**2033 (19.8%)**	**2585 (25.2%)**	0.76 (0.72– 0.81) P < 0.0001	

0.6   0.8   1.0   1.2   1.4
Simvastatin   Placebo
better   better

Figure 7.2 The MRC/BHF Heart Protection Study. The effect of simvastatin on first major coronary event, stroke or revascularisation in participants with or without diabetes. Reprinted with permission from Elsevier Science from Heart Protection Study Collaborative Group (2003). MRC/BHF Heart Protection Study of cholesterol-lowering with simvastatin in 5963 people with diabetes: a randomised placebo-controlled trial. *Lancet* **361**: 2005–16.

they do not have manifest coronary or cerebrovascular disease and irrespective of their cholesterol level. This is particularly important for older patients with type 2 diabetes who have the greatest absolute risk of first ever and recurrent stroke.

Antiplatelet agents

Antiplatelet therapy is a proven component of secondary prevention in patients with TIA or stroke. The Antiplatelet Trialists' Collaboration meta-analysis in 1994 demonstrated a significant reduction in vascular events (non-fatal myocardial infarction, non-fatal stroke or vascular death) in diabetic patients with vascular disease treated with antiplatelet therapy (Antiplatelet Trialists' Collaboration, 1994). Recently, the Management of Atherothrombosis with Clopidogrel in High-risk Patients (MATCH) trial assessed the role of combined antiplatelet therapy in patients with ischaemic cerebrovascular disease, with a combined vascular endpoint including ischaemic stroke and rehospitalisation for transient ischaemic attack (Diener *et al.*, 2004). Combined therapy in ischaemic stroke produced a relative risk reduction that was not statistically significant and was countered by a higher bleeding event rate in this population. Combined therapy in the 68% of the MATCH population that had diabetes produced a slightly higher relative risk reduction than in the rest of the study population, but again this did not achieve statistical significance and was associated with increased bleeding.

7.7 Diabetes, Cognitive Impairment and Dementia

As with type 2 diabetes, the prevalence of cognitive impairment leading to dementia increases with advancing age (Park et al., 2003). Identification of any aetiological factors predisposing to cognitive decline is important in order to reduce the burden on patients, their carers and health and social services. Epidemiological evidence from both cross-sectional and longitudinal studies suggests that individuals with diabetes have a twofold increased risk of cognitive impairment and dementia compared with the general population (Areosa Sastre and Grimley Evans, 2003). This association between impaired cognition and diabetes appears to be strengthened by duration of the disease and the use of insulin therapy, likely reflecting illness severity in the case of type 2 diabetes.

Longitudinal population-based studies confirm that diabetes is a risk factor for both vascular dementia and Alzheimer's disease (Peila et al., 2002; Areosa Sastre and Grimley Evans, 2003) Vascular dementia is a general diagnostic label for loss of cognitive function caused by ischaemic or haemorrhagic cerebral lesions due to cerebrovascular disease or other cardiovascular pathology (Roman, 2003). There are a number of different diagnostic criteria and scoring systems for vascular dementia but this label should only be applied when there is evidence of cerebrovascular disease, dementia and a temporal relationship between these two disorders. Vascular dementia is the second most common cause of dementia in the elderly, accounting for 10–30% of all cases. The ischaemic types of vascular dementia are divided into two broad groups: large vessel and small vessel. In the large-vessel subtype, post-stroke dementia is the commonest form of acute-onset vascular dementia and has an estimated prevalence of 10–16% (Barba et al., 2000). Dementia after stroke may be caused by a single strategically located cortical or subcortical stroke, or by multiple strokes, so-called multi-infarct dementia. Small-vessel vascular dementia may be of abrupt onset (e.g. due to lacunar infarction) but more commonly develops more slowly due to diffuse subcortical disease. These patients may have characteristic computed tomography (CT) features of symmetrically decreased density of periventricular and subcortical white matter, and correlation has been shown between the extent of these lesions and the degree of cognitive impairment.

The risk of dementia is substantially increased in people with both diabetes and stroke. A longitudinal study in Hispanic Americans aged over 60 years confirmed that 43% of all incident dementia cases were attributable to type 2 diabetes, stroke or a combination of these two risk factors (Haan et al., 2003). Longitudinal population studies suggest that diabetes is also associated with an increased risk of developing Alzheimer-type dementia (Peila et al., 2002; Honig et al., 2003). The association between diabetes and Alzheimer's disease is more difficult to explain. For some diabetic patients, cerebral infarction may play an additive role in the development of Alzheimer's disease, for example by a critical silent-stroke uncovering early and previously asymptomatic dementia. A study of 1766 Medicare recipients without dementia at baseline confirmed that the annual incidence of Alzheimer's disease was 5.2% in people with a history of stroke compared with 4% in those without clinically apparent cerebrovascular disease (Honig et al., 2003). In these patients, the presence of both stroke and diabetes led to a significant increase in the risk of Alzheimer's disease (relative risk 4.6). More importantly, amongst vascular risk factors, only diabetes was related to the risk of Alzheimer's disease in the absence of stroke. This and evidence from other studies suggest that cerebrovascular disease alone cannot solely account for the increased likelihood of Alzheimer's disease in diabetic individuals (den Heiger *et al.*, 2003; Honig *et al.*, 2003).

There are a number of other potential mechanisms to explain the observed association between diabetes and Alzheimer's disease. These include impairment of insulin transport into the brain or dysfunction of insulin signal transduction. Any disturbance of cerebral insulin pathways could result in impaired amyloid metabolism and less prevention of tau phosphorylation, leading to accumulation of plaques and neurofibrillary tangles, the pathological hallmarks of Alzheimer's dementia. Of note, non-enzymatic advanced glycosylation end-products (so-called AGEs) can cause cross-linking of amyloid proteins, and AGEs have been detected within the plaques and tangles in the brains of those with Alzheimer's disease (Thomas *et al.*, 1996; Munch *et al.*, 1998). In addition, there may be a genetic explanation for the relationship between diabetes and Alzheimer's disease. The major gene associated with increased risk of Alzheimer's is apolipoprotein E (ApoE), with the ApoE4 variant in particular conferring a substantial risk. The association between diabetes and Alzheimer's dementia is particularly strong for type 2 diabetics with this allele, with a relative risk of 5.5 compared with individuals without these two risk factors (Peila *et al.*, 2002). These data are supported by autopsy evidence, which demonstrated increased numbers of plaques and neurofibrillary tangles in diabetic carriers of the ApoE4 genotype. Further support for an aetiological role for diabetes in Alzheimer's disease comes from the Rotterdam study, a large population-based cohort study of chronic disease in older people (den Heiger *et al.*, 2003). *In vivo* assessment of the volume of the hippocampus and amygdala by volumetric magnetic resonance imaging (MRI) provides a good estimate of the degree of Alzheimer's pathology, even in older people with no clinical features of dementia. Type 2 diabetes was associated with atrophy of the hippocampus and amygdala on MRI, and this was not related to any coexistent vascular disease.

Vascular dementia and Alzheimer's disease share certain vascular risk factors such as diabetes, hypertension and smoking. Nevertheless, current research suggests that cognitive decline and dementias are linked to diabetes by mechanisms over and above cerebrovascular disease. There is evolving evidence for an overlap between pathophysiological changes such as AGEs, which lead to complications of diabetes and also degenerative brain disease due to Alzheimer's pathology. However, there is as yet no convincing evidence relating the type or intensity of diabetic therapy to the prevention or treatment of cognitive impairment in type 2 diabetes (Areosa Sastre and Grimley Evans, 2003).

7.8 Conclusions

Older patients with type 2 diabetes are at high risk of macrovascular complications, including stroke and TIA. A reduction in cerebrovascular disease can be achieved by a comprehensive strategy of vascular risk reduction aimed at multiple risk factors (Gaede *et al.*, 2003). Treatment should encompass lifestyle changes, tight control of glycaemia and hypertension and specific drug therapies such as ACE inhibitors, statins and antiplatelet agents. In our ageing populations the financial and social burden of stroke is likely to increase for the foreseeable future. The introduction of any new acute stroke treatment is unlikely to significantly reduce this burden and our priority remains the prevention of first ever and recurrent stroke. The importance of diabetes as both a risk and prognostic factor for cerebrovascular disease is now well established. Large randomised controlled clinical trials have consistently demonstrated benefit following intensive management of vascular risk factors in diabetes. The challenge for the future is in identifying those at maximal risk of stroke and delivering optimal prevention within managed healthcare economies.

References

Adams HP, Bendixen B, Kapelle J *et al.* (1993). Classification of subtypes of acute ischaemic stroke. *Stroke* **24**: 35–41.

Adler A, Stratton IM, Neil HAW, Yudkin JS, Matthews DR, Cull CA *et al.* (2000). Association of systolic blood pressure with macrovascular and microvascular complications of type-2 diabetes (UKPDS 36): prospective observational study. *British Medical Journal* **321**: 412–9.

Albers GW, Caplan LR, Easton JD, Fayad PB, Mohr JP, Saver JL, Sherman DG for the TIA Working Group (2002). Transient ischaemic attack – proposal for a new definition. *New England Journal of Medicine* **347**: 1713–6.

Alex M, Baron EK, Goldenberg S, Blumenthal HT (1962). An autopsy study of cerebrovascular accident in diabetes mellitus. *Circulation* **25**: 663–73.

Allport L, Butcher K, Baird T *et al.* (2004). Insular cortical ischemia is independently associated with acute stress hyperglycemia. *Stroke* **35**: 1886–91.

Antiplatelet Trialists' Collaboration (1994). Collaborative overview of randomised trials of antiplatelet therapy – I: Prevention of death, myocardial infarction, and stroke by prolonged antiplatelet therapy in various categories of patients. *British Medical Journal* **308**: 81–106.

Areosa Sastre A, Grimley Evans J (2003). Effect of the treatment of type II diabetes mellitus on the development of cognitive impairment and dementia (Cochrane Review). *The Cochrane Library*, Issue 4. Oxford: Oxford Update Software.

Astrup J, Symon L, Branston NM *et al.* (1977). Cortical evoked potential and extracellular K+ and H+ at critical levels of brain ischemia. *Stroke* **8**: 51–7.

Astrup J, Siesjo BK, Symon L (1981). Thresholds in cerebral ischemia – the ischemic penumbra. *Stroke* **12**: 723–5.

Baird TA, Parsons MW, Phanh T *et al.* (2003). Persistent poststroke hyperglycemia is independently associated with infarct expansion and worse clinical outcome. *Stroke* **34**: 2208–14.

Bamford J, Sandercock P, Dennis M, Burn J, Warlow C (1991). Classification and natural history of clinically identifiable subtypes of cerebral infarction. *Lancet* **337**: 1521–6.

Barba R, Martinez-Espinosa S, Rodriguez-Garcia E, Podal M, Vivancos J, Del Ser T (2000). Poststroke dementia: clinical features and risk factors. *Stroke* **31**: 1494–501.

Beghi E, Boglium G, Cavaleth G, Sanguinetti I, Agliabue M, Agostoni F, Macchi I (1989). Haemorrhagic infarction, risk factors, clinical and tomographic features and outcome. A case control study. *Acta Neurologica Scandinavica* **80**: 226–31.

Berthet K, Neal BC, Chalmers JP, *et al.* (2004). Reductions in the risks of recurrent stroke in patients with and without diabetes: the PROGRESS Trial. *Blood Pressure* **13**: 1–7.

Blood Pressure Lowering Treatment Trialists' Collaboration (2000). Effects of ACE inhibitors, calcium antagonists and other blood pressure lowering drugs: results of prospectively designed overviews of randomised trials. *Lancet* **356**: 1955–64.

Bosch J, Yusuf S, Pogue J *et al.* (2002). Use of Ramipril in preventing stroke: double blind randomised trial. *British Medical Journal* **324**: 799–802.

Brown RD, Whisnant JP, Sicks JD, O'Fallon WM, Weibers DO (1996). Stroke incidence, prevalence and survival: secular trends in Rochester, Minnesota, through 1989. *Stroke* **27**: 373–80.

Bruno A, Levine SR, Frankel MR, Brott TG, In Y, Tilley BC, Lyden PD, Broderick JP, Kwaitowski TG, Fineberg SE for the NINDS rt-PA Stroke Study Group (2002). Admission glucose levels and clinical outcomes in the NINDS rt-PA Stroke Trial. *Neurology* **59**: 669–74.

Bucher HC, Griffith LE, Guyatt GH (1998). Effect of HMGcoA reductase inhibitors on stroke. A meta-analysis of randomised controlled trials. *Annals of Internal Medicine* **128**: 89–95.

Capes SE, Hunt D, Malmberg K, Pathak P, Gerstein GH (2001). Stress hyperglycaemia and prognosis of stroke in nondiabetic and diabetic patients. *Stroke* **32**: 2426–32.

Carolei A and Marini C (2000). Surgical and medical therapy in asymptomatic carotid lesions. In: Fieschi C, Fisher M (eds) *Prevention of Ischaemic Stroke.* London: Martin Dunitz, pp. 217–230.

Coutinho M, Wang Y, Gerstein HC, Yusuf S (1999). The relationship between glucose and incident cardiovascular events. *Diabetes Care* **22**: 233–40.

Dahlof B, Lindholm LH, Hansson L *et al.* (1991). Morbidity and mortality in the Swedish trial in old Patients with Hypertension (STOP-Hypertension). *Lancet* **338**: 1281–5.

De Angelis M (2003). Prevalence of carotid stenosis in type 2 diabetic patients asymptomatic for cerebrovascular disease. *Diabetes Nutrition and Metabolism* **16**: 48–55.

Demchuk AM, Morgenstern LB, Krieger DW, Chi TL, Hu W, Wein TH, Hardy RJ, Grotta JC, Buchan AM (1999). Serum glucose level and diabetes predict tissue plasminogen activator related intracerebral haemorrhage in acute ischemic stroke. *Stroke* **30**: 34–9.

Diaz R, Ernesto A, Paolasso A, *et al.* (1998). Metabolic modulation of acute myocardial infarction. The ECLA Glucose Insulin-Potassium Pilot Trial. *Circulation* **98**: 2227–34.

Diener H-C, Bogousslavsky J, Brass LM, Cimminiello C, Csiba L, Kaste M, Leys D, Matias-Guiu J, Rupprecht H-J on behalf of the MATCH Investigators (2004). Aspirin and clopidogrel compared with clopidogrel alone after recent ischaemic stroke or transient ischaemic attack in high-risk patients (MATCH): randomised, double-blind, placebo controlled trial. *Lancet* **364**: 331–7.

Eastern Stroke and Coronary Heart Disease Collaborative Research Group (1998). Blood pressure, cholesterol and stroke in eastern Asia. *Lancet* **352**: 1801–7.

European Carotid Surgery Trialists' Collaborative Group (1991). MRC European Carotid Surgery Trial: interim results for symptomatic patients with severe (70–99%) or with mild (0–29%) carotid stenosis. *Lancet* **337**: 1235–43.

European Carotid Surgery Trialists' Collaborative Group (1998). Randomised trial of endarterectomy for recently symptomatic carotid stenosis: final results of the MRC European Carotid Surgery Trial (ECST). *Lancet* **351**: 1379–87.

Fath-Ordoubadi F, Beatt KJ (1997). Glucose–insulin–potassium therapy for treatment of acute myocardial infarction: an overview of randomised placebo controlled trials. *Circulation* **96**: 1152–6.

Fuller JH, Shipley MJ, Rose G, Jarret RJ, Keen M (1983). Mortality from coronary heart disease and stroke in relation to degree of glycaemia: The Whitehall Study. *British Medical Journal* **287**: 867–70.

Gaede P, Vedel P, Larson N, Jenson GVH, Parving H-H, Pedersen O (2003). Multifactorial intervention and cardiovascular disease in patients with type 2 diabetes. *New England Journal of Medicine* **348**: 383–93.

Ginsberg MP, Reivich M, Giandomenico A, Greenberg JH (1977). Local glucose utilization in acute local cerebral ischemia: local dysmetabolism and diaschisis. *Neurology* **27**: 1042–8.

Gray CS, Taylor R, French JM *et al.* (1987). The prognostic value of stress hyperglycaemia and previously unrecognised diabetes following acute stroke. *Diabetic Medicine* **4**: 237–40.

Gray CS, Taylor R, French JM *et al.* (1992). The prognostic value of stress hyperglycaemia and previously unrecognised diabetes mellitus in acute stroke. *Journal of Neurology, Neurosurgery, and Psychiatry* **55**: 263–70.

Gray CS, O'Connell JE, Lloyd H (2001). Diabetes, hyperglycaemia and recovery from stroke. *Geriatrics and Gerontology International* **1**: 2–7.

Gray CS, Scott JF, French JM, Alberti KGMM, O'Connell JE (2004a). Prevalence and prediction of unrecognised diabetes mellitus and impaired glucose tolerance following acute stroke. *Age and Ageing* **33**: 71–7.

Gray CS, Hildreth AJ, Alberti KGMM, O'Connell JE on behalf of the GIST Collaboration (2004b). Post stroke hyperglycemia; natural history and immediate management. *Stroke* **35**: 122–6.

Gubitz G, Phillips S, Dwyer V (1999). What is the cost of admitting patients with transient ischaemic attack to hospital? *Cerebrovascular Diseases* **9**: 210–4.

Haan MN, Mungas DM, Gonzalez HM, Ortiz TA, Acharya A, Jagust WJ (2003). Prevalence of dementia in older Latinos: the influence of type 2 diabetes mellitus, stroke and genetic factors. *Journal of the American Geriatrics Society* **51**: 169–77.

Hankey GJ (1996). Impact of treatment of people with transient ischaemic attacks on stroke incidence and public health. *Cerebrovascular Diseases* **6** (Suppl 1): 26–33.

Hansson L, Zanchetti A, Carruthers SG *et al.* (1998). Effects of intensive blood pressure lowering and low dose aspirin in patients with hypertension: principal results of the Hypertension Optimal treatment (HOT) randomised trial. *Lancet* **351**: 1755–62.

Heart Outcomes Prevention Evaluation (HOPE) Study Investigators (2000). Effects of ramipril on cardiovascular and microvascular outcomes in people with diabetes mellitus: results of the HOPE study and MICRO-HOPE substudy. *Lancet* **355**: 253–9.

Heart Outcomes Prevention Evaluation Study Investigators (2000) Effects of an angiotensin-converting enzyme inhibitor, ramipril, on cardiovascular events in high-risk patients. *New England Journal of Medicine* **342**: 145–53.

Heart Protection Study Collaborative Group (2002). MRC/BHF Heart Protection Study of cholesterol lowering with simvastatin in 20 536 high-risk individuals: a randomised placebo controlled trial. *Lancet* **360**: 7–22.

Heart Protection Study Collaborative Group (2003). MRC/BHF Heart Protection Study of cholesterol-lowering with simvastatin in 5963 people with diabetes: a randomised placebo-controlled trial. *Lancet* **361**: 2005–16.

den Heiger T, Vermeer SE, Van Dijk EJ *et al.* (2003). Type 2 diabetes mellitus and atrophy of medial temporal lobe structures on brain MRI. *Diabetologia* **46**: 1604–10.

Hess DC, Demchuk AM, Brass LM, Yatsu FM (2000). HMG-CoA reductase inhibitors (statins). A promising approach to stroke prevention. *Neurology* **54**: 790–6.

Honig LS, Tang M-X, Albert S *et al.* (2003). Stroke and the risk of Alzheimer disease. *Archives of Neurology* **60**: 1707–12.

INDANA Project Collaborators (1997). Effect of antihypertensive treatment in patients already having suffered from stroke. Gathering the evidence. *Stroke* **28**: 2557–62.

Intercollegiate Working Party for Stroke (2000). *National Clinical Guidelines for Stroke*. London: Royal College of Physicians.

Isarol PA, Forbes JF (1992). The cost of stroke to the National Health Service in Scotland. *Cerebrovascular Diseases* **1**: 47–50.

Iso H, Jacobs DR Jr, Wentworth D, Neaton JD, Cohen JD for the MRFIT Research Group (1989). Serum cholesterol levels and six year mortality from stroke in 350,977 men screened for the Multiple Risk Factor Intervention Trial. *New England Journal of Medicine* **320**: 904–10.

Johnston SC, Gress DR, Browner WS, Sidney S (2000a). Short tem prognosis after emergency department diagnosis of TIA. *Journal of the American Medical Association* **284**: 2901–6.

Johnston SC, Fung LH, Gillum LA *et al.* (2000b). Utilisation of intravenous tissue-type plasminogen activator for ischaemic stroke: the Cleveland Area Experience. *Journal of the American Medical Association* **283**: 1151–8.

Kannel WB, McGee DL (1979). Diabetes and cerebrovascular disease. The Framingham Study. *Journal of the American Medical Association* **241**: 2035–8.

Kiers L, Davis SM, Larkins R *et al.* (1992). Stroke topography and outcome in relation to hyperglycaemia and diabetes. *Journal of Neurology, Neurosurgery, and Psychiatry* **55**: 263–70.

Laing SP, Swerdlow AJ, Carpenter LM, Slater SD, Burden AC, Botha JL, Morris AD, Waugh NR, Gatling W, Gale EAM, Patterson CC, Zongkai Q, Keen H (2003). Mortality from cerebrovascular disease in a cohort of 23000 patients with insulin-treated diabetes. *Stroke* **34**: 418–21.

MacDonald BK, Cockerell OC, Sander JWAS, Shorvon SD (2000). The incidence and lifetime prevalence of neurological disorders in a prospective community based study in the UK. *Brain* **123**: 665–75.

Malmberg K, Ryden L, Efendic S *et al.* (1995). Randomised trial of insulin glucose infusion followed by subcutaneous insulin treatment in diabetic patients with acute myocardial infarction (DIGAMI study): Effects on mortality at one year. *Journal of the American College of Cardiology* **26**: 57–65.

Megherbi SE, Milan C, Couvreur G, Osseby GV, Tilling K, di Carlo A, Inzitari D, Wolf CD, Moreau T, Giroud M; European BIOMED Study of Stroke Care Group (2003). Association between diabetes and stroke subtype on survival and functional outcome 3 months after stroke: data form the European BIOMED Stroke Project *Stroke* **34**: 688–94.

Munch G, Schinzel R, Loske C *et al.* (1998). Alzheimer's disease – synergistic effects of glucose deficits, oxidative stress and advanced glycosylation end products. *Journal of Neural Transmission* **105**: 439–61.

Norris JW, Zhu CZ, Bornstein NM, Chambers BR (1991). Vascular risks of asymptomatic carotid stenosis. *Stroke* **22**: 1485–90.

O'Connell JE, Gray CS (1994). Treating hypertension after stroke *British Medical Journal* **308**: 1523–4.

Ohkubo Y, Kishikawa H, Araki E *et al.* (1995). Intensive insulin therapy prevents the progression of diabetic microvascular complications in Japanese patients with non-insulin dependant diabetes mellitus: a randomised prospective study. *Diabetes Research and Clinical Practice* **28**: 103–17.

Olsson T, Viitanen M, Asplund K, Eriksson S, Hagg E (1990). Prognosis after stroke in diabetic patients. A controlled prospective study. *Diabetologia* **33**: 244–9.

O'Neill PA, Davis I, Fullerton KJ, Bennett D (1991). Stress hormone and blood glucose response following acute stroke in the elderly. *Stroke* **22**: 842–7.

Oppenheimer SM, Hoffbrand B, Oswald GA, Yudkin JS (1985). Diabetes mellitus and early mortality from stroke. *British Medical Journal* **291**: 1014–5.

Park HL, O'Connell JE, Thomson RG (2003). A systematic review of cognitive decline in the general elderly population. *International Journal of Geriatric Psychiatry* **18**: 1121–34.

Peila R, Rodriguez BL, Launer LJ (2002). Type 2 diabetes, APOE gene, and the risk for dementia and related pathologies: the Honolulu-Asia Aging study. *Diabetes* **51**: 1256–62.

Peress NS, Kane WC, Aronson SM (1972). Central nervous system findings in a tenth decade autopsy population. *Progress in Brain Research* **40**: 473–83.

Power MJ, Fullerton KJ, Stout RW (1988). Blood glucose and prognosis of acute stroke. *Age and Ageing* **17**: 164–70.

PROGRESS Collaborative Group (2001). Randomised trial of a perindopril-based blood pressure-lowering regimen among 6105 individuals with previous stroke or transient ischaemic attack. *Lancet* **358**: 1033–41.

Prospective Studies Collaboration (1995). Cholesterol, diastolic blood pressure and stroke. 13000 strokes in 450,000 people in 45 prospective cohorts. *Lancet* **346**: 1647–53.

Pulsinelli WA (1992). Pathophysiology of acute stroke. *Lancet* **339**: 533–6.

Pulsinelli WA, Levy DE, Sigsbee B, Scherer P, Plum F (1983). Increased damage after ischaemic stroke in patients with hyperglycaemia with or without established diabetes mellitus. *American Journal of Medicine* **74**: 540–3.

Pulsinelli WA, Kraig RP, Plum F (1985). Hyperglycaemia, cerebral acidosis and ischaemic brain damage. In: Plum F, Pulsinelli WA (eds) *Cerebrovascular Diseases 14th Princeton Conference*. New York: Raven Press, pp. 201–10.

Reichard P, Berglund B, Britz A, Cars I, Nilsson BY, Rosenqvist U (1991). Intensified conventional insulin treatment retards the microvascular complications of insulin dependant diabetes mellitus (IDDM): the Stockholm Diabetes International Study (SDIS) after 5 years. *Journal of Internal Medicine* **230**: 101–8.

Riddle MC, Hart J (1982). Hyperglycemia, recognised and unrecognised, as a risk factor for stroke and transient ischemic attacks. *Stroke* **13**: 356–9.

Robinson TG, Potter JF (2004). Blood pressure in acute stroke. *Age and Ageing* **33**: 6–12.

Rodgers A, McMahon S, Gamble G *et al.* on behalf of the United Kingdom Transient Ischaemic Attack Collaborative Group (1996). Blood pressure and risk of stroke in patients with cerebrovascular disease. *British Medical Journal* **313**: 147.

Roman GC (2003). Vascular dementia: distinguishing characteristics, treatment and prevention. *Journal of the American Geriatrics Society* **51**: S296–304.

Scott JF, Robinson G, O'Connell JE, Alberti KGMM, Gray CS (1999). Prevalence of admission hyperglycaemia across clinical sub types of acute stroke. *Lancet* **353**: 376–7.

SHEP Co-operative Research Group (1991). Prevention of stroke by hypertensive drug therapy in older persons with isolated systolic hypertension: final results of the systolic hypertension in the elderly programme. *Journal of the American Medical Association* **265**: 3255–64.

Siemkowicz E, Hanson AJ (1978). Clinical restitution following cerebral ischaemia in hypo-, normo- and hyperglycaemic rats. *Acta Neurologica Scandinavica* **58**: 1–8.

Song EC, Chu K, Jeong SW *et al.* (2003). Hyperglycemia exacerbates brain edema and perihematomal cell death after intracerebral hemorrhage. *Stroke* **34**: 2215–20.

Stamler J, Vaccaro O, Neaton JD, Wentworth D (1993). Diabetes, other risk factors and 12 year cardiovascular mortality for men screened in Multiple Risk Factor Intervention Trial. *Diabetes Care* **16**: 434–44.

Stroke Unit Trialists' Collaboration (1997). Collaborative systematic review of the randomised trials of organised in patient (stroke unit) care after stroke. *British Medical Journal* **314**: 1151–9.

Svensson P, de Faire U, Sleight P, Ostergren J (2001). Comparative effects of ramipril on ambulatory and office blood pressures: a HOPE substudy. *Hypertension* **38**: e28–32.

Thomas T, Thomas G, McLendon C, Sutton T, Mullan M (1996). β Amyloid mediated vasoactivity and vascular endothelial damage. *Nature* **380**: 168–71.

Toni D, Fiorelli M, Gentile M *et al.* (1995). Deteriorating neurological deficit secondary to acute ischaemic stroke: a study on predictability, pathogenesis and prognosis. *Archives of Neurology* **52**: 670–5.

UK Prospective Diabetes Study Group (1996). UK Prospective Diabetes Study 17: a nine year update of a randomised controlled trial on the effect of improved metabolic control on complications in non insulin dependant diabetes mellitus. *Annals of Internal Medicine* **124**: 136–45.

UK Prospective Diabetes Study Group (1998). Tight blood pressure control and risk of macrovascular and microvascular complications in type 2 diabetes (UKPDS 38). *British Medical Journal* **317**: 703–13.

UK Prospective Diabetes Study (UKPDS) Group (1998). Intensive blood-glucose control with sulphonylureas or insulin compared with conventional treatment and risk of complications in patients with type 2 diabetes (UKPDS 33). *Lancet* **352**: 837–53.

Van den Berghe G, Wouters P, Weekers F, Verwaest C, Bruyninckx, Schetz M, Vlasselaers D, Ferdinande P, Lauwers P, Bouillon R (2001). Intensive insulin therapy in critically ill patients. *New England Journal of Medicine* **345**: 1359–67.

Vázquez-Cruz J, Martí-Vilalta JL, Ferrer I, Pérez-Gallofré A, Folch J (1990). Progressing cerebral infarction in relation to plasma glucose in gerbils. *Stroke* **21**: 1621–4.

Wahl PW, Savage PJ, Psaty BM, Orchard TJ, Robbins JA, Tracy RP (1998). Diabetes in older adults: comparison of 1997 American diabetes Association classification of diabetes mellitus with 1985 WHO classification. *Lancet* **352**: 1012–5.

Wardlaw J, Yamaguchi T, Del Zoppo G (2002). Thrombolysis for acute ischaemic stroke (Cochrane Review). *The Cochrane Library*, Issue 2. Oxford: Oxford Update Software.

Warlow CP, Dennis MS, van Gijn J, Sandercock PAG, Bamford JM, Wardlaw JM (2001). Preventing recurrent stroke and other serious vascular events. In: Warlow CP, Dennis MS, van Gijn J, Sandercock PAG, Bamford JM, Wardlaw JM (eds) *Stroke: a Practical Guide to Management.* Oxford: Blackwell Science, pp. 653–722.

Weir CJ, Murray GD, Dyker AG, Lees KR (1997). Is hyperglycaemia an independent predictor of poor outcome after acute stroke? Results of a long term follow up study. *British Medical Journal* **314**: 1303–6.

Williams B, Poulter NR, Brown MJ *et al.* (2004). Guidelines for management of hypertension: report of the fourth working party of the British Hypertension Society, 2004 – BHS IV. *Journal of Human Hypertension* **18**: 139–85.

Wolf PA, Kannel WB, Verter J (1983). Current status of risk factors for stroke. *Neurologic Clinics* **1**: 330–1.

Woo E, Ma JTC, Robinson JD, Yu YL (1988). Hyperglycemia is a stress response in acute stroke. *Stroke* **19**: 1359–64.

Yano K, Reed DM, MacLean CJ (1989). Serum cholesterol and hemorrhagic stroke in the Honolulu Heart Program. *Stroke* **20**: 1460–5.

8 Diabetes and Peripheral Arterial Disease

Iskandar Idris and Richard Donnelly

8.1 Introduction

Peripheral arterial disease (PAD), defined as lower extremity arterial atherosclerosis, is extremely common in people with diabetes. It is estimated that 1–8% of the diabetic population has PAD at the time of diagnosis (Brand *et al.*, 1989; Premalatha *et al.*, 2000; Adler *et al.*, 2002) and after 20 years approximately 12–45% of patients are affected (Brand *et al.*, 1989; Adler *et al.*, 2002). In the Framingham Study, the presence of diabetes increased the risk of intermittent claudication by 3.5-fold in men and 8.6-fold in women (Brand *et al.*, 1989). Diabetes confers a 10- to 16-fold increase in the lifetime risk of lower limb amputation and is the leading cause of non-traumatic lower limb amputation (Uusitupa *et al.*, 1990; Fowkes, 2001). Diabetes also increases the risk of PAD progression, and among patients with PAD those with diabetes tend to have longer hospital stays and consume a greater percentage of healthcare resources in managing the complications of PAD (Currie *et al.*, 1998). The incidence and outcomes from critical limb ischaemia are significantly worse among patients with diabetes, e.g higher amputation rates (Lehto *et al.*, 1996) and less successful outcomes from revascularisation procedures (angioplasty or bypass grafting) (Faries *et al.*, 2001).

Risk factors for amputation

Studies have looked at various risk factors that contribute to lower extremity amputation in patients with diabetes. Poor glycaemic control is a major factor in the development of lower extremity amputation (Lehto *et al.*, 1996) and seems to be

Diabetic Cardiology Editors Miles Fisher and John J. McMurray
© 2007 John Wiley & Sons, Ltd.

more strongly associated with PAD than coronary artery disease (Adler *et al.*, 2002). High HbA1c and high fasting plasma glucose are associated with a twofold higher risk of amputation compared with well-controlled diabetes (Lehto *et al.*, 1996). Even moderately poor metabolic control of diabetes contributes to a significantly higher risk of amputation. Age is also an important risk factor and in most studies the majority of lower extremity amputations occur in patients over the age of 45 years (Bild *et al.*, 1989). Race may also play an important role, where Blacks with diabetes have been shown to have a 1.4–2.3 times greater incidence of amputation compared to Whites (Bild *et al.*, 1989), although the increased prevalence of hypertension and smoking among Blacks may be contributing factors. The association between amputation risk and smoking is surprisingly weak in most published studies (Lehto *et al.*, 1996), but this is thought to be due to the relatively small number of smokers among patients with diabetes as well as the observation that many patients with symptomatic PAD are likely to have stopped smoking before the baseline study assessments. Smoking and diabetes are such a malignant combination that survival is reduced (Hirsch *et al.*, 1997). Diabetes increases the risk of PAD more in women than in men, resulting in an equal ratio between men and women in the rate of PAD and amputation (Abbott *et al.*, 1990; Uusitupa *et al.*, 1990; Adler *et al.*, 2002).

8.2 Pathogenesis

Clinical differences between diabetic and non-diabetic PAD

Although histologically identical, specific differences exist in the clinical presentation of PAD in patients with diabetes compared to those without diabetes, as listed in Table 8.1. These differences relate to the distribution and morphology of occlusive atherosclerotic lesions in the lower limb. Specifically, diabetes tends to cause more diffuse and more distal (i.e infrapopliteal and tibial) atherosclerotic disease, often associated with vascular calcification (Levin and Bowker, 1993).

Table 8.1 Peripheral Arterial Disease: Differences between patients with and without diabetes. Adapted from Levin ME, Bowker JH (1993). The diabetic foot: Pathophysiology, evaluation and treatment. In: Levin ME, O'Neal LW (eds). *The Diabetic Foot*, 5th edn. St Louis, MO: Mosby Yearbook, p.17.

Clinical	Diabetic	Non-diabetic
Prevalence	~ Higher	~ Lower
Age	Younger	Older
Male : Female	M = F	M > F
Occlusion	Multisegmental	Single segment
Vessels adjacent to occlusion	Affected	Not affected
Collaterals	Affected	Not affected
Lower extremities affected	Both	Often unilateral
Vessels involved	Tibials	Aortic
	Peroneals	Iliac
		Femoral

Table 8.2 Multivariate model of incident PAD at 6 years among 61 of 2,398 patients in the UKPDS. Adapted from Adler *et al.* (2002) UKPDS 59: Hyperglycaemia and other potentially modifiable risk factors for peripheral arterial disease in type 2 diabetes. *Diabetes Care* **25**: 894–9.

Risk factor	Comparison	Odds ratio
Age	Each year older at diagnosis of diabetes	1.10
HbA1c	Each 1% increase	1.28
Systolic blood pressure	Each 10 mmHg increase	1.25
HDL-cholesterol	Each 0.1 mmol/l decrease	1.22
Current smoker	Never smoked	2.90
Cardiovascular disease	None	3.00
Retinopathy	Presence of retinopathy	1.64
Sensory neuropathy	Doubling of voltage threshold	1.31

Risk factors for PAD in patients with diabetes (Table 8.2)

The high PAD risk in patients with diabetes is due to the complex interplay between the various haemodynamic and metabolic components of the metabolic syndrome. Diabetes is no longer considered to be a disease confined to hyperglycaemia but rather part of a syndrome comprising various risk factors, all of which confer an increased risk of atherosclerosis and cardiovascular events (see also Chapter 2). Hence, although the diagnosis and symptoms of diabetes are still defined by hyperglycaemia, other features of the syndrome, especially hypertension and dyslipidaemia, are equally if not more important in the pathogenesis of diabetes-related macrovascular complications such as PAD. Thus, the development of atherothrombotic complications in larger lower limb arteries is multifactorial, reflecting interactions between high glucose, lipids and blood pressure. For example, hypercholesterolaemia and hypertriglyceridaemia have been associated with the increased risk of intermittent claudication and PAD in both cross-sectional and prospective studies of type 2 diabetes (Lehto *et al.*, 1996; Adler *et al.*, 2002). High-density-lipoprotein (HDL)-cholesterol appears to be inversely related to PAD (Adler *et al.*, 2002). Hypertension, both systolic and diastolic, also has a significant impact on the development and progression of PAD in the diabetic population (Murabito *et al.*, 1997; Adler *et al.*, 2000, 2002).

Smoking meanwhile is believed to be the most important risk factor in lower limb arteriopathy both in patients with and without diabetes, conferring nearly a threefold increased risk of PAD (Jonason and Ringqvist, 1985; Hirsch *et al.*, 1997). Epidemiological studies have identified insulin resistance and hyperinsulinaemia, independent of glucose levels, as independent risk factors for PAD in both diabetic and non-diabetic subjects (Price *et al.*, 1996; Matsumoto *et al.*, 1997). An additional risk factor for PAD and amputation is renal transplantation, an effect that is more prevalent in diabetic subjects than in the non-diabetic population (Lemmers and Barry, 1991). The exact mechanism for this remains unclear.

Hyperglycaemia and PAD

There is a positive correlation between hyperglycaemia and the risk of developing PAD (Figure 8.1). In the UK Prospective Diabetes Study (UKPDS), for example, a

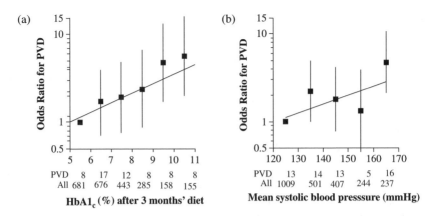

Figure 8.1 Odds ratio for HbA1c (A) and SBP (B) by category adjusted for age, HDL cholesterol, previous cardiovascular disease, smoking, retinopathy, and peripheral sensory neuropathy in 61 patients with incident PVD at 6 years of a total 2,398 patients. A: Adjusted also for SBP. B: Adjusted also for HbA1c. Reference groups are HbA1c <6% and SBP <130 mmHg. Adapted from Adler *et al.* (2002) UKPDS 59: Hyperglycaemia and other potentially modifiable risk factors for peripheral arterial disease in type 2 diabetes. *Diabetes Care* **25**: 894–9.

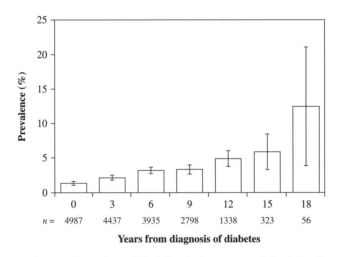

Figure 8.2 Prevalence of PAD (95% CIs) defined as any two of the following: ABPI <0.8, absence of both DP and PT pulses to palpation in at least one leg, intermittent claudication at diagnosis of diabetes, and at 3-year intervals to 18 years. Adapted from Adler *et al.* (2002) UKPDS 59: Hyperglycaemia and other potentially modifiable risk factors for peripheral arterial disease in type 2 diabetes. *Diabetes Care* **25**: 894–9.

1% increase in HbA1c was associated with a 28% increased risk of PAD (95% CI 12–46), independent of other factors including age, systolic blood pressure, smoking and prior cardiovascular disease (Adler *et al.*, 2002). The incidence of PAD increases steadily with duration of diabetes, a reflection of prolonged exposure to high glucose concentrations (Figure 8.2) (Jude *et al.*, 2001). Hyperglycaemia is well recognised to be an important pathogenic factor in the development of peripheral neuropathy, and several studies have shown that peripheral neuropathy, defined as the absence of Achilles tendon reflexes and impaired vibration sense in the great toe, is an independent predictor of amputation even after adjustment for age, sex and duration of diabetes (Nelson *et al.*, 1988; Lehto *et al.*, 1996). Thus, neuropathy compounds the problem of PAD by adding to the risk of amputation. Patients with peripheral neuropathy often fail to notice minor trauma resulting in foot ulceration, infection and gangrene. Hyperglycaemia contributes to small-vessel disease and probably impairs host defences against infection.

Pathophysiology of glycaemic vascular injury

Molecular mechanisms (Figure 8.3)

The abnormal metabolic state associated with type 2 diabetes is associated with chronic low-grade inflammation, endothelial dysfunction, dyslipidaemia and insulin resistance (see also Chapter 2). These factors confer an increased risk of atherosclerosis and PAD, and have led to new hypotheses about the pathogenesis of macrovascular complications and the interactions between metabolic, endocrine and haemodynamic mechanisms. Four pathways have been proposed to explain how hyperglycaemia specifically affects vascular structure and function in the lower limbs:

- increased oxidative stress and free-radical-mediated damage (Baynes and Thorpe, 1999);

- formation of advanced glycosylation end-products (Schmidt *et al.*, 1999);

- diversion of glucose into the aldose reductase pathway (Baynes and Thorpe, 1999; Idris *et al.*, 2001);

- activation of one or more isozymes of protein kinase C (PKC) (Idris *et al.*, 2001).

Hyperglycaemia increases oxidative stress through the generation of reactive oxygen species, and by reducing intracellular levels of natural antioxidants such as vitamins C and E (Baynes and Thorpe, 1999). Insulin-resistant states, via excess liberation of free fatty acids from adipose tissue, also cause an increase in the production of reactive oxygen species (Hennes *et al.*, 1996). Reactive oxygen species such as the superoxide anions directly quench nitric oxide (NO) by forming toxic peroxynitrite ions and reduce the bioavailability of endothelium-derived NO in diabetes (Beckman *et al.*, 2002). Reduced endothelial-derived NO causes failure of endothelium-mediated vasodilatation, enhances platelet activation, increases vascular smooth-muscle proliferation and migration and increases leucocyte adhesion. In addition, reactive oxygen species increase oxidation and facilitate the deposition of low-density-lipoprotein (LDL)-cholesterol in the vessel wall. These pathways are responsible for the accelerated atherosclesosis seen in diabetes (Beckman *et al.*, 2002).

Hyperglycaemia causes non-enzymatic glycosylation of a variety of proteins and lipoproteins in the blood vessel wall to form advanced glycosylation end-products (AGEs). These AGEs accelerate the structural and functional abnormalities associated with atherosclerosis, in part by binding to receptors for AGE and promoting LDL

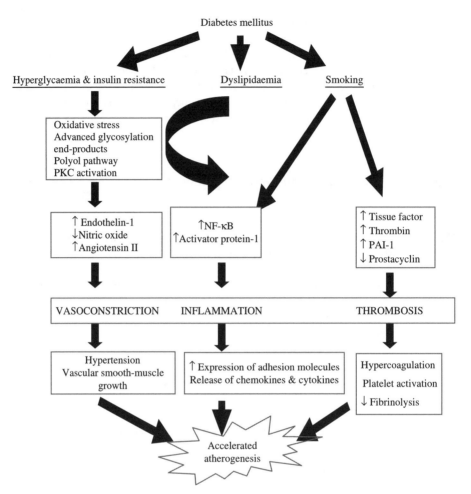

Figure 8.3 Multifactorial pathogenic process involved in the development of accelerated atherosclerosis in patients with diabetes. Complex interaction between hyperglycaemia, adverse metabolic profile, insulin resistance, dyslipidaemia and smoking promotes endothelial dysfunction and increased pro-inflammatory and pro-atherogenic factors.

oxidation and uptake by macrophages, leading to the formation of characteristic foam cells (Schmidt *et al.*, 1999). The receptors for AGEs are up-regulated in diabetes, and coupled to activation of NF-κβ and activator protein-1. These signalling events regulate the expression of various pro-atherogenic genes, which encode for a number of mediators of atherogenesis such as leucocyte and vascular cell adhesion molecules (V-CAM) on the endothelial surface, monocyte chemoattractant proteins that recruit lymphocytes and monocytes into the vascular wall and many pro-inflammatory mediators, including interleukin-1 and tumour necrosis factor (Rosen *et al.*, 2001).

There is increasing evidence that PKC activation is important in hyperglycaemia-related vascular and endothelial dysfunction (Idris *et al.*, 2001). Glucose is transported into vascular cells by GLUT-1 transporters and then metabolised mainly through glycolysis (<5% of intracellular glucose is metabolised by the aldose reductase pathway). In conditions of hyperglycaemia, glycolytic flux increases and stimulates *de novo* synthesis of diacylglycerol (DAG), which in turn activates PKC, a family of 12 structurally and functionally related proteins derived from multiple genes. Activation of one or more of the PKC isoenzymes leads to a variety of biological responses, including changes in cell proliferation and differentiation, glucose and lipid metabolism, smooth-muscle contraction and pro-atherosclerotic gene expression. The PKC activation impairs NO-mediated vasodilatation, increases expression of the vasoconstrictor endothelin-1, enhances monocyte binding to endothelial cells, augments vascular smooth-muscle contractility and growth and enhances vascular endothelial permeability. Pathophysiological studies have implicated the isoenzymes PKC-β and PKC-δ in hyperglycaemia-induced vascular dysfunction (Ishii *et al.*, 1996). The clinical importance of this pathway has been highlighted by the ongoing phase III clinical trials with a specific PKC-β inhibitor, ruboxistaurin, that ameliorates diabetes-induced vascular dysfunction.

8.3 Clinical Features of PAD in Patients with Diabetes

The Fontaine scoring system divides chronic lower limb ischaemia into four stages, namely asymptomatic PAD (Stage I), chronic stable intermittent claudication (Stage II), rest pain due to critical ischaemia (Stage III) and finally those patients with trophic changes such as gangrene and ulceration (Stage IV).

Intermittent claudication

The term claudication is derived from the Latin word for *limping*. In the Framingham Study, diabetes was associated with two- to threefold excess risk of intermittent claudication for both sexes (Brand *et al.*, 1989). Diabetics with intermittent claudication were at especially high risk for cardiovascular events. Claudicants present with a history of exercise-induced pain in the leg, typically affecting the calves, thighs or buttocks, depending on the location of occlusive arterial disease in the lower limb. Superficial femoral artery (SFA) lesions tend to cause calf pain, whereas common femoral artery lesions cause thigh pain and common iliac artery lesions cause buttock pain. Claudication is a cramp-like pain that comes on with exercise; it is usually static and does not radiate. The pain is characteristically relieved by cessation of walking without the need to sit down.

Symptoms of intermittent claudication must be distinguished from pain resulting from other causes such as degenerative arthritic changes, disc disease, thrombophlebitis or even tumours of the spinal cord. One can usually differentiate ischaemic claudication from non-ischaemic claudication by taking a thorough history. Patients with intermittent claudication often only need to stop walking for a couple of minutes before they are able to proceed. Patients with non-ischaemic claudication usually require 15–20 min of rest, having to sit down, change position and or flex/extend their back to get relief. In patients with spinal stenosis, for example, a major differential diagnosis of intermittent claudication, patients report a relatively short walking distance before they get symptoms of back pain, often associated with neurological symptoms in the leg such as paraesthesia, numbness or weakness. Like true claudicants, these patients find that by resting for 5–10 min the symptoms resolve, but unlike patients with claudication they find walking up hill or pushing a trolley much more comfortable as spinal flexion increases the diameter of the spinal canal. The key differentiating feature for spinal stenosis is back pain, which is very unusual in patients with pure vascular disease.

Some patients with diabetes, however, may not have symptoms of intermittent claudication because of the loss of pain sensation. This emphasises the need for frequent routine examination of the patient's feet for signs of PAD and peripheral neuropathy, even in the absence of any symptoms.

Natural history of intermittent claudication

Two-thirds of patients with intermittent claudication either improve spontaneously or remain stable with fixed exercise limitation, while the remaining one-third have progressively deteriorating symptoms. Only 2% of patients with intermittent claudication will eventually require some sort of amputation. There is no easy method of identifying which patients will get worse, but a poor outcome is closely linked to smoking and suboptimal risk factor control. These patients may also have coronary heart disease or cerebrovascular disease; 20% of patients with intermittent claudication will suffer a myocardial infarct over a 5-year period (Weitz et al., 1996).

Clinical signs

The signs in the leg are usually subtle. The affected leg may be cooler to touch and there may be a loss of palpable pulses in the lower limb. Often, however, both femoral and pedal pulses are present, but not the popliteal. The presence of pedal pulses reflects the development of collaterals around the knee. However, after a short walk, the foot will become pale and pulseless. If skin changes are present, e.g. ulceration, by definition this reflects critical ischaemia.

Investigations

The ankle-brachial pressure index (ABPI) is a simple test involving measurement of the ankle systolic blood pressure with an ordinary blood pressure cuff around the calf and a hand-held doppler over the dorsalis pedis or posterior tibial pulses (Feigelson et al., 1994). The ankle pressure is then divided by the systolic pressure in the arm to calculate ABPI; an ABPI value of > 0.9 is normal while an ABPI value of < 0.8 indicates vascular insufficiency. Patients with intermittent claudication typically have an ABPI of 0.6–0.8. A cut-off of 0.8 for ABPI is often used in various epidemiological studies of diabetes and has been shown to be highly specific (99%) for PAD in the general population (Feigelson et al., 1994), while claudication and absence of pulses has a 95% specificity for PAD in the diabetic population (Carter, 1968). Patients with diabetes may have falsely high ABPI readings due to calcified vessels. A small proportion of patients will have a normal resting ABPI that falls to < 0.9 after a period of brief exercise. Thus, measuring the ABPI is a simple way to identify patients with leg symptoms who have occlusive lower limb arterial disease.

In patients with a good history of intermittent claudication but detectable peripheral pulses, treadmill testing may be indicated. Exercise will lead to reduction or loss of peripheral pulses with symptoms of intermittent claudication, and the ABPI often falls to below 0.75. More advanced techniques to assess vascular insufficiency include the use of transcutaneous monitoring of the partial pressure of oxygen and carbon dioxide at the foot using an electrode placed just proximal to the second and third metatarsal heads (Carrington *et al.*, 2001). A partial pressure of oxygen of <30 mmHg is considered abnormal. All patients with PAD should also have routine investigations to detect other treatable risk factors such as blood lipids, glycated haemoglobin and serum creatinine.

Management

The mainstay of treatment for intermittent claudication is smoking cessation and regular exercise. A meta-analysis of randomised controlled trials of physical exercise has shown that regular exercise improves walking distance, but the walking programme should be supervised and involve 30 min per session, at least three times per week for 6 months (Gardner and Poehlman, 1995). The mechanism for the benefit may be derived from improved cardiovascular fitness, increased production of nitric oxide and/or modification of cardiovascular risk factors. In the exercise programme, patients should be told to 'walk through the pain' rather than to stop at the point when the pain begins since this helps to increase the collateral blood supply. Raising the heel of the shoe by 1 cm will also increase the walking distance by reducing the workload on calf muscles. Bicycle riding is probably less beneficial because it exercises the thigh muscles and not the calf muscles.

Oral medications including antiplatelet drugs such as aspirin and clopidogrel are useful adjuvants. Aspirin has been shown to decrease mortality by 20%, and the PAD subgroup of the CAPRIE study has shown a statistically beneficial effect of 75 mg/day of clopidogrel over aspirin on cardiovascular outcomes (CAPRIE Steering Committee, 1996). Cilostazol (a phosphodiesterase III inhibitor), which also has effects on platelet function, vasodilation and lipid levels, has been approved in the UK for improvement in pain-free and maximum walking distances. Double-blind, placebo-controlled trials in over 2000 patients have shown that cilostazol improves exercise tolerance (Reilly and Mohler, 2001). There is evidence from subgroup analyses of multicentre trials that patients with diabetes also respond favourably to cilostazol.

Criteria for surgical referral

Patients with a history of symptoms that are not typical of claudication, or those who have disabling limitation despite medical management, should be referred for vascular surgical assessment. Tests that may be performed in hospital include treadmill testing (or a simple walk test) with postexercise ABPI measurements, duplex scanning (which is a non-invasive method for identifying the location of arterial lesions using real-time ultrasound and Doppler techniques) and occasionally angiography. The majority of claudicants are treated conservatively; only a relatively small proportion are suitable for a revascularisation procedure such as angioplasty with stenting.

Rest pain and critical ischaemia

When PAD worsens, there is insufficient blood to supply the tissues of the leg even at rest and this often presents as continuous pain in the most distal part, namely the forefoot. Nerve ischaemia, manifesting as nocturnal rest pain and a form of neuritis, often precedes the onset of rest pain. It occurs at night when perfusion of the extremities is reduced. Patients often gain relief by hanging their foot over the side of the bed or walking for a few steps. This increases cardiac output, improving perfusion of the lower extremities and providing partial relief of ischaemic neuritis.

Critical ischaemia occurs when the blood supply falls to a critical level at which the viability of distal tissues or the limb is at risk. Critical ischaemia is defined in the European Consensus Document as 'persistently recurring rest pain requiring regular analgesia for more than 2 weeks, or ulceration or gangrene of the foot and toes in combination with an ankle systolic pressure less than 50 mmHg'. Patients with diabetes and severe PAD may not, however, experience rest or night pain due to peripheral neuropathy and loss of sensation. A much higher proportion of these patients will require a surgical procedure such as an amputation. The prognosis for these patients is poor: 50% of those with critical ischaemia will die of atherosclerotic disease within 5 years (Cheng *et al.*, 2000).

Gangrene

Gangrene is tissue death with the appearances of pallor and mottling, progressing to purple and then the characteristic black appearance due to haemoglobin breakdown forming iron sulphide. Traditionally, it can be classified either as dry or wet gangrene. Dry gangrene is the result of a chronic decrease in blood supply leaving a dry, wrinkled appearance. Wet gangrene usually occurs in diabetics, those patients in whom the arterial supply is suddenly occluded or when there is mixed venous and arterial disease. Infection is also usually present.

Ischaemic ulcers are typically painful, and are located at pressure areas such as the heel and in between toes. These areas should always be examined in a routine leg examination. Ulceration in the leg is, however, most commonly due to venous disease and only about 10% are purely secondary to arterial insufficiency. Venous ulcers tend to be located in the gaiter region and have signs of venous hypertension.

Clinical signs

The limb is often cold and pale, and hair loss from the medial aspect of the leg is a characteristic sign. There is poor capillary refill and impaired venous filling of superficial veins, which may even empty to form venous guttering if the blood supply is severely impaired. When critically ischaemic legs are elevated to an angle of 30°, they will turn pale. Buerger's test will also be positive: elevate the leg and then in the dependent position the microvasculature becomes dilated with blood rushing into the foot to give the appearance of hyperaemia. Evidence of trophic changes such as ulceration on pressure points or gangrene at the extremities are common and may be compounded by the presence of neuropathy and infection. The ankle and foot will likely be oedematous due to the ischaemia and a neuropathy affecting sensation or motor function may be present.

Treatment

Critical ischaemia is a much higher priority for vascular surgical assessment. These patients should be seen swiftly by a vascular specialist for further investigations, e.g. duplex and/or angiography, and for urgent treatment. The preferred option is angioplasty or surgical bypass grafting with either autologous saphenous vein or an artificial graft. Angioplasty is ideal if the stenotic lesions are short and proximal, with surgical bypass as the next solution if angioplasty fails. Critical ischaemia threatens the viability of the limb and therefore some attempt at improving blood flow surgically is justified.

Sympathectomy no longer has a role for providing symptomatic control for patients with critical ischaemia. Sclerosed arteries in diabetic patients have very little capacity to dilate after a sympathectomy. Prostacyclin infusions, however, may prolong the survival of critically ischaemic legs (Marchesi *et al.*, 2003).

Acute limb ischaemia

This is due to sudden complete occlusion of the blood supply to the lower limb, most commonly as a result of an embolus or thrombosis in situ. This can stem from a mural thrombus from the heart following a myocardial infarct, valve disease, cardiac arrhythmias such as atrial fibrillation and/or from a left ventricular aneurysm. An acute arterial occlusion by an embolus presents with a very sudden and short history of pain, pulselessness, paraesthesia, paralysis, perishing cold and pallor (the six 'P's, although not all need to be present for the diagnosis and the paraesthesia may actually be anaesthesia). The acute ischaemia may either affect one or both limbs and the patient may not have had a previous history of PAD. The patient will lose the ability to move their toes but sometimes one can still feel a femoral pulse if the occlusion is below this level. The other presentation is when a thrombus has dislodged itself in a limb with PAD. The patient will not have any obvious source of an embolus and the symptoms of claudication, for example, will worsen suddenly rather than presenting with the 6 'P's.

Management

Immediate referral to hospital is mandatory. In cases of an acute embolus, an embolectomy with a Fogarty catheter is the treatment of choice and can be done either with a local anaesthetic or with general anaesthesia. This is followed by anticoagulation. If the ischaemia is not severe and if the clot is more likely to be a thrombus, intra-arterial thrombolysis with tPA may be the best method of treatment.

8.4 Lower Extremity Revascularisation in Patients with Diabetes

Open surgical reconstructions for lower limb ischaemia are divided into supra- and infrainguinal reconstructions. Suprainguinal vascular reconstructions in the form of aorta-bifemoral bypass with Dacron grafts often achieve high patency rates in the presence of a patent superficial femoral artery. The standard procedure for infrainguinal occlusive disease is femoral-popliteal bypass or bypass to the crural arteries. The latter may be preferred for patients with diabetes since arterial occlusion in this group is often located more distally.

Outcomes of percutaneous revascularisation procedures depend on various factors, including the location and length of the lesion, stenosis and the presence of a collateral circulation (Beckman *et al.*, 2002). Patients with diabetes tend to have more severe arterial occlusive disease below the knee, and with reduced distal collateral supply. The results of percutaneous interventions in patients with diabetes may be worse than in non-diabetics. Iliac artery stenting in patients with diabetes achieves a 90% patency rate at 1-year (Dormandy and Rutherford, 2000), although some groups have shown lower patency rates. The 1-year patency rates after femoral artery interventions range from 29% to 80%, with diabetes associated with a less favourable outcome (Stokes *et al.*, 1990). This may be due to poor collateral circulation in patients with diabetes, because in those with good collaterals the patency rates were comparable to that of non-diabetic patients. For infrainguinal ischaemia, the outcomes of surgical revascularisation in diabetes are similar to those without diabetes in terms of limb salvage (Panneton *et al.*, 2000). Overall, it appears that in patients with severe claudication or critical limb ischaemia, surgery seems to be superior to percutaneous revascularisation procedures in the femoral, popliteal and infrapopliteal vessels, but with higher risks of cardiovascular morbidity and mortality (Dormandy and Rutherford, 2000).

8.5 Medical Therapy of PAD in Diabetes

Evidence for secondary prevention

It is important to consider the medical management of patients with PAD not only in the context of lower limb salvage but also in terms of cardiovascular risk protection. This is because patients with PAD have a decreased life expectancy when compared with the general population, explained almost entirely by the high incidence of cardiovascular events. The relative risk of dying from coronary heart disease is 5–6 times that of the normal population over 10 years and after that period of time only half of claudicants are still alive (Criqui *et al.*, 1992). Not surprisingly, most of the evidence pertaining to patients with diabetes and PAD has been extrapolated from large secondary prevention studies undertaken primarily in patients with symptoms of coronary heart disease (CHD), some of whom also had PAD. Given that PAD indicates widespread atherosclerotic disease – e.g. heart and brain – it is important to consider a multifactorial intervention package that targets the lower limb as well as the vasculature (Table 8.3).

Smoking cessation

Cigarette smoking is the single most important risk factor for the development of PAD. Continued smoking is associated with a greater likelihood of developing

Table 8.3 Multi-interventional package for the treatment of PAD in patients with diabetes.

Symptoms/risk factors	Intervention
Intermittent claudication	Exercise, smoking cessation, drugs (e.g. cilostazol and pentoxifylline), angioplasty, vascular surgery for severe symptoms
Smoking cessation	Behavioural therapy, nicotine replacement therapy, bupropion
Hypercoagulability	Aspirin, clopidogrel, warfarin (if in atrial fibrillation)
Hyperglycaemia	Insulin, sulphonylurea, metformin, glitazones
Insulin resistance	Glitazones, metformin
Dyslipidaemia	Statins, fibrate
Hypertension	ACE inhibitor, angiotensin-1 receptor blockers, diuretics (and other agents including beta-blockers)
'At-risk foot'	Foot examination for peripheral vascular disease and peripheral neuropathy, education on foot care, foot ulcer management

disabling claudication, limb-threatening ischaemia, amputation and the need for surgical intervention (Jonason and Ringqvist, 1985; Hirsch *et al.*, 1997). In addition, patency rates and survival are much lower among patients who smoke following a revascularisation procedure (Ameli *et al.*, 1989).

Unlike the increased cancer risk from smoking and the adverse effects on lung function that persist for many years after a long-term smoker gives up cigarettes, the excess risk of cardiovascular disease (i.e. death and non-fatal myocardial infarction) diminishes relatively quickly after smoking cessation, e.g. within 2–4 years (Rosenberg *et al.*, 1990). It is therefore likely that patients with intermittent claudication may accrue the vascular benefits of smoking cessation almost immediately, even though the carcinogenic risk lingers on for at least another decade. The recognition that cigarette smoking is a primary disorder in which addiction to nicotine plays a primary role has resulted in a change to the approach to smoking cessation. The UK guidelines on smoking cessation suggest a specific action plan that integrates behavioural and pharmacological support to aid in cessation as well as preventing relapse (West *et al.*, 2000).

Spontaneous quit rates are low even among patients who want to give up (< 5% per year) whereas most intensive programmes report cessation rates of about 20% with behavioural support alone (Schwartz, 1987). Pharmacological support should therefore be provided for all smokers who are willing to use medication. Quit rates are doubled among motivated patients given various forms of nicotine replacement therapy (NRT) in combination with educational support (Silagy *et al.*, 1994). Nicotine is metabolised quickly with a half-life of 2 h (Henningfield and Kennan, 1993). The concept behind NRT to facilitate smoking cessation is therefore to provide steady-state nicotine levels to prevent withdrawal symptoms while avoiding the reinforcing peaks associated with smoking. After achieving abstinence, NRT can be tapered off and eventually discontinued. The transdermal systems (nicotine patches) provide a slow and steady release of nicotine with low addiction potential. The use of nicotine polacrilex (nicotine gum) should be associated with education on effective chewing strategies. It is essential, for example, to chew the gum to release the nicotine and then allow the saliva to facilitate buccal absorption. The antidepressant bupropion has also been shown to be effective in smoking cessation and can be combined with NRT to further increase cessation rates (Hurt *et al.*, 1997). Adverse effects include a lowered seizure threshold, and bupropion is therefore contraindicated in those with high seizure risk. The weight of evidence, however, favours NRT as the preferred first-line option for smoking cessation. Other therapies where a meta-analysis supports their efficacy in smoking cessation include the antihypertensive clonidine and the antidepressant nortriptylline (Gourlay *et al.*, 2000).

Antiplatelet therapy and warfarin

Although there is no evidence to suggest that aspirin improves walking distance or symptom status, aspirin does modify the clinical course of PAD. Large randomised trials have shown that aspirin, either as monotherapy or in combination with dipyridamole, delays the progression of established PAD, as assessed by serial angiography, and decreases the need for surgical revascularisation (Goldhaber *et al.*, 1992; Hirsh *et al.*, 1992). Aspirin also improves patency rates following revascularisation (Claggett *et al.*, 1992). The standard dose of aspirin for secondary prevention is usually 75–150 mg daily; higher doses of aspirin provide no clear therapeutic advantage but the incidence of gastrointestinal side-effects is much higher. There is some evidence that patients with diabetes require slightly higher doses of aspirin to achieve similar antiplatelet effects (Evangelista *et al.*, 2005).

There is also evidence that newer antiplatelet agents may be preferred instead of aspirin for secondary prevention in patients with PAD. Clopidogrel is an ADP receptor antagonist with superior efficacy in terms of potency and a better adverse effect profile compared to aspirin or ticlopidine. The CAPRIE study included 19 185 patients with atherosclerotic vascular disease (ischaemic stroke, myocardial infarction or symptomatic PAD) and in the subgroup with PAD clopidogrel seems to have a more impressive effect (CAPRIE Steering Committee, 1996). Studies in patients with unstable angina suggest that the benefits of clopidogrel and aspirin are additive, implying that combination antiplatelet therapy may become more widely established (Clopidogrel in Unstable Angina to Prevent Recurrent Events (CURE) Trial Investigators, 2001). Previous combination strategies found only a marginal advantage in adding dipyridamole to aspirin following TIA, but clopidogrel + aspirin seems to be significantly more effective, at least following an episode of unstable angina (relative risk reduction was 20% vs. aspirin alone for the composite primary endpoint of cardiovascular death, myocardial infarction and stroke at 1 year) (Clopidogrel in Unstable angina to prevent Recurrent Events (CURE) Trial Investigators, 2001). Combination antiplatelet therapy may be preferred in those PAD patients who undergo an intervention such as angioplasty or stenting.

It is now recognised from prospective studies and meta-analyses that antithrombotic therapy using warfarin confers significant benefit over aspirin when given to patients with non-valvular atrial fibrillation (NVAF) in whom there is a particular risk of acute embolic lower limb ischaemia and stroke (Stroke Prevention in Atrial Fibrillation Investigators, 1994). Elderly patients, however, are often denied anticoagulation therapy due to fears of increased bleeding risk when the benefits of anticoagulation are in fact greater for elderly patients due to their higher absolute thromboembolic risk.

Conversely, young patients with lower absolute thromboembolic risk are often offered full-dose anticoagulation. Risk stratification is therefore necessary using other clinical, biochemical and even social criteria when determining which patients with NVAF should be offered anticoagulation. There is no evidence to support the routine use of warfarin (instead of aspirin or in addition to aspirin) for secondary prevention in patients in sinus rhythm, although in some patients short-term anticoagulation may be considered surgically beneficial to avoid lower limb complications postoperatively.

Tight glycaemic control

Hyperglycaemia precedes the development of PAD, peripheral neuropathy and lower extremity amputation in patients with diabetes (Adler et al., 2002). In a study involving elderly Dutch patients, a 1% increase in HbA1c was associated with a 35–42% increased risk for ABPI <0.9 or obstructed crural arteries (Beks et al., 1995; Hoogeveen et al., 2000). In the UKPDS, the effect of intensive blood glucose control was investigated in 3867 patients with newly diagnosed type 2 diabetes. Patients who were allocated to the tight glycaemic control group showed a clear trend towards a reduction in deaths from PAD (relative risk 0.26, P = 0.12) and fewer amputations (relative risk 0.61, P = 0.099), although neither endpoint achieved statistical significance (UK Prospective Diabetes Study (UKPDS) Group, 1998a). Treatment of obese patients with metformin had a favourable effect on cardiovascular outcomes overall, but there was no evidence of a specific effect of metformin on amputation rates (UK Prospective Diabetes Study (UKPDS) Group, 1998b). Nevertheless hyperglycaemia in the UKPDS seems to be more strongly linked with PAD than coronary heart disease. (Figure 8.1)

In the Diabetes Control and Complications trial (DCCT), tight glucose control (mean HbA1c 7.2% vs. 9.1%) resulted in a 22% relative risk reduction in major lower limb complications and a 42% relative risk reduction for the combined endpoint of coronary and peripheral arterial events, neither of which reached statistical significance (Diabetes Control and Complications Trial (DCCT) Research Group, 1995). Thus, in large randomised clinical trials, tight glycaemic control seems to have a more profound impact in the prevention of small-vessel rather than large-vessel disease. Increasingly, PAD is also thought to have a significant microvascular component. Microvascular disease, for example, has been shown to increase peripheral resistance and accelerate atherosclerosis. Data from the UKPDS support the likelihood of a shared pathogenesis of PAD with retinopathy (UK Prospective Diabetes Study (UKPDS) Group, 1998a). In addition, a histological study of lower limb small vessels from patients with diabetes and PAD showed that 80% had proliferative changes, with only 5% having atheromatous changes (Blumenthal et al., 1966).

Treating dyslipidaemia

Large randomised placebo-controlled clinical trials that included patients with diabetes and CHD have clearly demonstrated that cholesterol lowering with statins significantly reduces the risk of cardiovascular events. Evidence has also accrued on the benefit of statins on primary prevention of cardiovascular events in patients with diabetes.

The recent CARDS trial, for example, randomised 2338 patients with type 2 diabetes without high LDL-cholesterol to placebo or atorvastatin, 10 mg daily (Colhoun *et al.*, 2004). While this trial excluded patients with severe PAD (defined as warranting surgery), stroke risk was reduced by 48% suggesting that the statins had extra-cardiac effects on the progression of atherosclerotic disease elsewhere in the circulation.

Data are also available in the subgroup of patients with PAD in the Scandinavian Simvastatin Survival (4S) study. Although only 4% of the participants in 4S had intermittent claudication at baseline, the number of cases of new or worsening claudication during the trial was significantly less in the statin treatment group (Pederson *et al.*, 1998). The trial did not report data specific to patients with diabetes. The Heart Protection Study (HPS) included 20 000 patients with coronary or non-coronary arterial disease who were randomised to 40 mg of simvastatin or placebo. A 24% reduction in vascular events was reported with simvastatin and this was consistent in all subgroups, including patients with PAD, irrespective of baseline cholesterol. Included in the HPS study were 5963 patients with diabetes and simvastatin resulted in a significant reduction in macrovascular complications in this subgroup (5.2% vs. 6.5%, P = 0.03) (Heart Protection Study Collaborative Group, 2003). The endpoint included any peripheral artery surgery, angioplasty, lower limb amputation or ischaemic leg ulcer. A Cochrane meta-analysis of lipid-lowering therapy in patients with PAD showed that active therapy reduced disease progression, the severity of claudication and mortality (Leng *et al.*, 1998). This adds further support to the notion that statins have disease-modifying effects on atherosclerosis in the lower limb.

Patients with type 2 diabetes are associated with a more atherogenic lipid profile, in particular a higher fraction of small dense LDL particles and low HDL-cholesterol levels. Reduced levels of HDL-cholesterol were identified as an independent risk factor for PAD in the UKPDS and are characteristic of the insulin resistance syndrome. The VA-HIT study included 769 patients with diabetes (with normal LDL-cholesterol but low HDL-cholesterol) and the use of gemfibrozil, an agent that specifically increases HDL-cholesterol but with less impact on LDL-cholesterol levels, was associated with a 39% reduction in CHD (Robins *et al.*, 2001). This supports evidence from various statin trials, which have shown that treatment with statins did not seem to eliminate the excess CHD risk associated with a low baseline level of HDL-cholesterol. Relatively few data are available on the effect of raising HDL in the subgroups of patients with PAD, but it is unlikely that the favourable and protective effect of raising HDL levels is confined to the coronary circulation.

Thus, patients with symptomatic PAD and hypercholesterolaemia (total cholesterol > 5 mmol/l), as well as those with overt CHD, should be treated with a statin to achieve target LDL-cholesterol levels of < 3 mmol/l. The benefits apply equally to men and women, to those above and below 65 years of age and especially patients with diabetes. Large outcome data targeting HDL-cholesterol in patients with diabetes are awaited.

Treatment of hypertension

Management of hypertension as part of an aggressive overall treatment strategy to reduce cardiovascular risk in patients with diabetes is clearly important (see also

Chapter 6). Data are also available on the impact of hypertension specifically in patients with diabetes associated with PAD. The Framingham epidemiological study provides observational evidence that patients with high blood pressure are at greater risk of developing intermittent claudication (Murabito et al., 1997). Isolated systolic hypertension, in particular, is very common in the elderly and is closely associated pathophysiologically with increased arterial stiffness, pressure-wave reflection and an increased systolic blood pressure load on the heart causing left ventricular hypertrophy. The UKPDS showed that a 10 mmHg increase in systolic blood pressure was associated with a 25% increase in risk whereas a 10 mmHg lowering in systolic blood pressure translated into a non-significant 16% reduction in risk of lower limb amputation or peripheral vascular disease-related mortality (Figure 8.1) (Adler et al., 2000). The Edinburgh Artery Study even suggested that patients with diabetes no longer had a significantly higher risk of PAD after adjustment for systolic blood pressure and lipid levels (MacGregor et al., 1999).

The Appropriate Blood Pressure Control in Diabetes (ABCD) study showed that in a small subgroup of patients with type 2 diabetes and established PAD and a baseline diastolic blood pressure of 80–89 mmHg ($n = 53$), intensive antihypertensive treatment with either enalapril or nisoldipine produced a significant reduction in the number of major cardiovascular events from 12 to 3 (P = 0.046). Further analysis of this subgroup suggested that intensive blood pressure control (mean blood pressure over 4 years 128/75 mmHg) effectively cancelled out the excess risk of a cardiovascular event associated with PAD (Mehler et al., 2003).

Beta-blockers have traditionally been considered a relative contraindication in patients with intermittent claudication. However, many controlled studies have found that beta-blockers do not adversely affect walking capacity or symptoms of intermittent claudication (Radack and Deck, 1991). It is therefore thought that beta-blockers can be used safely in this group of patients particularly if strong indication exists, such as previous myocardial infarction, heart failure or resistant hypertension. Similarly, when considering treatments that block the renin–angiotensin system, the risk of underlying renovascular disease should always be considered in patients with PAD, treatment-resistant hypertension and mild renal impairment, especially smokers.

Evidence from more recent trials has advocated lower thresholds for blood pressure treatment as well as lower blood pressure targets among 'high risk' patients with diabetes (Williams et al., 2004) (see also Chapter 6). This includes patients with existing cardiovascular disease and diabetic renal disease. However, the success rates in achieving current targets for blood pressure control among treated hypertensive patients with diabetes are relatively low even in specialist centres (Andrade et al., 2004). This partly reflects the difficulty in lowering systolic blood pressure, especially in the elderly, and it also reflects issues of tolerability and compliance with multiple antihypertensive therapies that are increasingly necessary in patients with diabetes. Many patients develop postural symptoms or other drug-related side effects that limit the capacity to up-titrate medication in pursuit of target blood pressure levels. Nevertheless, even modest blood pressure reductions confer large clinical benefits and clinicians should strive for lower levels of treated blood pressure within the context of what is acceptable and tolerable therapy for individual patients.

Renin–angiotensin system inhibition in patients with diabetes and PAD

Recent trials have highlighted the benefits of agents that block the renin–angiotensin – system in reducing cardiovascular events independent of their effects on blood pressure lowering. The HOPE study showed that long-term treatment with ramipril (compared to placebo) as add-on to other cardiovascular therapies confers significant reductions in morbidity and mortality among patients with CHD (and asymptomatic patients with diabetes plus one other risk factor) who do not have left ventricular dysfunction. Secondary endpoints included significantly fewer ramipril-treated patients needing cardiac and lower extremity revascularisation procedures (HOPE Study Investigators, 2000). A subgroup analysis of 4046 subjects with PAD in the HOPE trial suggests that this particular subgroup gains even more benefit from ramipril compared with those without PAD (Figure 8.4) (Heart Outcomes Prevention Evaluation Study Investigators, 2000).

The notion of non-blood-pressure-mediated benefits of ACE inhibitors in secondary prevention is also supported by the PROGRESS study, in which both hypertensive and non-hypertensive patients showed a reduction in the risk of recurrent strokes and all major vascular events using ACE inhibitor-based therapy (perindopril) that could not be solely attributable to the antihypertensive effect (PROGRESS Collaborative Group, 2001). Similar findings are also emerging with the use of angiotensin-1 receptor blockers (ARBs), particularly for renoprotection, although these later trials did not report data specific to patients with diabetes and PAD (see Chapter 6).

These well-conducted clinical trials provide persuasive evidence that any patient with symptomatic atherosclerotic disease (or asymptomatic diabetics with one other risk factor), including those with intermittent claudication, should be offered an ACE inhibitor or an ARB as part of secondary prevention, irrespective of other background medical therapies and even if they are normotensive with normal left ventricular function. It seems likely that these agents confer protective effects on the atherosclerotic process

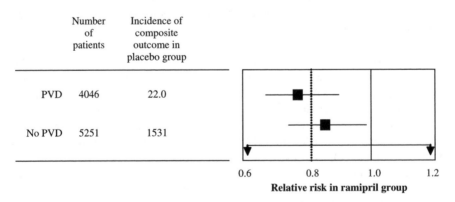

Figure 8.4 The results of the HOPE study according to whether patients had PVD or not at baseline. The benefits of ramipril 10mg/day were at least as good (if not better) in the peripheral vascular disease (PVD) subgroup. Reproduced from the Heart Outcomes Prevention Evaluation (HOPE) Investigators (2000). Effects of an angiotensin converting enzyme inhibitor, ramipril, on cardiovascular events in high-risk patients. *New England Journal of Medicine* **342:** 145-53.

that are clinically important via improved endothelial function, over and above the benefits attributable to blood pressure reduction. ACE inhibitors and ARBs, however, are contraindicated in patients with bilateral renal artery stenosis (RAS), or unilateral RAS in a single functioning kidney. Because the incidence of RAS is quite high in the PAD population, it is therefore essential to use a low starting dose and to check the serum electrolytes 7–10 days after starting or increasing ACE inhibitor therapy.

8.6 Future Therapy for PAD

Therapeutic angiogenesis in patients with diabetes

Advances in molecular and vascular biology have increased our understanding on the pathogenesis of micro- and macrovascular complications of diabetes. Interesting research studies have identified the effects of angiogenic growth factors to promote collateral vessel formation for the treatment of myocardial and lower limb ischaemia.

It is recognised that the severity of symptoms in PAD and the treatment outcomes are related not only to the degree of occlusive arterial disease but also to the extent of collateral vessel formation. For example, the patency rate after femoral artery interventions is lower in patients with diabetes, but in those with good collaterals the patency rates were comparable to that of patients without diabetes (Stokes *et al.*, 1990). Therapeutic angiogenesis seeks to improve tissue perfusion through the growth and proliferation of new blood vessels via local administration of angiogenic growth factors in the form of recombinant protein or gene transfer using viral or plasmid vectors (Collinson and Donnelly, 2004). Gene transfer may have several advantages over protein delivery by virtue of allowing prolonged expression of the protein, reduced systemic exposure to growth factors and ease of delivery to peripheral tissues. Preclinical studies of vascular endothelial growth factor (VEGF) delivered via gene transfer have been able to induce collateral blood flow and arteriogenesis, but results from phase 1 and phase II 'proof of concept' clinical studies have produced inconsistent results. A large placebo-controlled human adenoviral gene transfer study, for example, showed that a single intramuscular injection of VEGF had no effect on walking times and quality of life measures when compared to placebo (Rajagopalan *et al.*, 2003). The inconsistent treatment effect in human studies may be a reflection of differences in VEGF isoforms (e.g. $VEGF_{121}$ and $VEGF_{165}$), utilisation of non-optimal doses and duration of VEGF expression, as well as uncertainties about the efficiency of gene transfer in adult skeletal muscles due to low concentrations of adenoviral receptors (Tomko *et al.*, 1997) and physical barriers to transfection (O'Hara *et al.*, 2001).

8.7 Conclusions

Peripheral arterial disease is a common and disabling symptom associated with increased cardiovascular mortality. Diabetes is a syndrome of multiple pro-atherogenic risk factors that requires a multiple intervention approach. The overall management of patients with PAD should therefore include treatments that improve lower limb symptoms and functional performance, and should be combined with evidence-based therapies to prevent secondary vascular complications. Smoking cessation is essential in patients with PAD, and large randomised clinical trials have shown that statin therapy, tight blood pressure and glycaemic control, antiplatelet agents and ACE inhibitors slow the progression of PAD, promote plaque stabilisation and regression, and protect against acute limb and life-threatening thrombotic events. Emerging therapies include therapeutic angiogenesis to facilitate improvements in symptoms and lower limb outcomes in patients with PAD, and such technology might be especially appropriate for those patients with diabetes.

References

Abbott RD, Brand FN, Kannel WB (1990). Epidemiology of some peripheral arterial findings in diabetic men and women: experiences from the Framingham Study. *American Journal of Medicine* **88**: 376–81.

Adler AI, Stratton IM, Andrew H *et al.* (2000). Association of systolic blood pressure with macrovascular and microvascular complications of type 2 diabetes (UKPDS 36): prospective observational study. *British Medical Journal* **321**: 412–9.

Adler A, Stevens R, Neil A, Stratton I, Boulton A, Holman R (2002). UKPDS 59: Hyperglycaemia and other potentially modifiable risk factors for peripheral arterial disease in type 2 diabetes. *Diabetes Care* **25**: 894–9.

Ameli FM, Stein M, Provan JL, Prosser R (1989). The effect of postoperative smoking on femoropopliteal bypass grafts. *Annals of Vascular Surgery* **3**: 20–25.

Andrade SE, Gurwitz JH, Field TS, Kelleher M, Majumdar SR, Reed G, Black R (2004). Hypertension management: the care gap between clinical guidelines and clinical practice. *American Journal of Managed Care* **10**: 481–6.

Baynes JW, Thorpe SR (1999). Role of oxidative stress in diabetic complications: a new perspective on an old paradigm. *Diabetes* **48**: 1–9.

Beckman JA, Creager MA, Libby P (2002). Diabetes and atherosclerosis: epidemiology, pathophysiology, and management. *Journal of the American Medical Association* **287**: 2570–81.

Beks PJ, Mackaay AJ, de Neeling JN, de Vries H, Bouter LM, Heine RJ (1995). Peripheral arterial disease in relation to glycaemic level in an elderly Caucasian population: the Hoorn study. *Diabetologia* **38**: 86–96.

Bild DE, Selby JV, Sinnock P, Browner WS, Braveman P, Showstack JA (1989). Lower-extremity amputation in people with diabetes. Epidemiology and prevention. *Diabetes Care* **12**: 24–31.

Blumenthal HT, Berns AW, Goldenberg S, Lowenstein PW (1966). Etiologic considerations in peripheral vascular diseases of the lower extremity with special reference to diabetes mellitus. *Circulation* **33**: 98–106.

Brand FN, Abbott RD, Kannel WB (1989). Diabetes, intermittent claudication, and risk of cardiovascular events. The Framingham Study. *Diabetes* **38**: 504–9.

CAPRIE Steering Committee (1996). A randomised, blinded, trial of clopidogrel versus aspirin in patients at risk of ischaemic events. *Lancet* **348**: 1329–39.

Carrington AL, Abbott CA, Griffiths J, Jackson N, Johnson SR, Kulkarni J, Van Ross ER, Boulton AJ (2001). Peripheral vascular and nerve function associated with lower limb amputation in people with and without diabetes. *Clinical Science* **101**: 261–6.

Carter SA (1968). Indirect systolic pressures and pulse waves in arterial occlusive diseases of the lower extremities. *Circulation* **37**: 624–37.

Cheng SW, Ting AC, Lau H, Wong J (2000). Survival in patients with chronic lower extremity ischemia: a risk factor analysis. *Annals of Vascular Surgery* **14**: 158–65.

Claggett GP, Graor RA, Salzman EW (1992). Antithrombotic therapy in peripheral arterial disease. *Chest* **102** (Suppl 4): 516S–28S.

Clopidogrel in Unstable Angina to Prevent Recurrent Events (CURE) Trial Investigators (2001). Effects of clopidogrel in addition to aspirin in patients with acute coronary syndromes without ST-segment elevation. *New England Journal of Medicine* **345**: 494–502.

Colhoun HM, Betteridge DJ, Durrington PN, Hitman GA, Neil HA, Livingstone SJ, Thomason MJ, Mackness MI, Charlton-Menys V, Fuller JH; CARDS Investigators (2004). Primary prevention of cardiovascular disease with atorvastatin in type 2 diabetes in the Collaborative Atorvastatin Diabetes Study (CARDS): multicentre randomised placebo-controlled trial. *Lancet* **364**: 685–96.

Collinson DJ, Donnelly R (2004). Therapeutic angiogenesis in peripheral arterial disease: can biotechnology produce an effective collateral circulation? *European Journal of Vascular and Endovascular Surgery* **28**: 9–23.

Criqui M, Langer P, Fronek A, Feigelson HS, kaluber MR, McCann TJ, Browner D (1992). Mortality over a period of 10 years in patients peripheral arterial disease. *New England Journal of Medicine* **326**: 381–5.

Currie CJ, Morgan CL, Peters JR (1998). The epidemiology and cost of inpatient care for peripheral vascular disease, infection, neuropathy, and ulceration in diabetes. *Diabetes Care* **21**: 42–8.

Diabetes Control and Complications Trial (DCCT) Research Group (1995). Effect of intensive diabetes management on macrovascular events and risk factors in the Diabetes Control and Complications Trial. *American Journal of Cardiology* **75**: 894–903.

Dormandy JA, Rutherford RB (2000). Management of peripheral arterial disease (PAD): TASC Working Group. *Journal of Vascular Surgery* **31**: S1–296.

Evangelista V, Totani L, Rotondo S, Lorenzet R, Tognoni G, De Berardis G, Nicolucci A (2005). Prevention of cardiovascular disease in type-2 diabetes: How to improve the clinical efficacy of aspirin. *Thrombosis and Haemostasis* **93**: 8–16.

Faries PL, LoGerfo FW, Hook SC, Pulling MC, Akbari CM, Campbell DR, Pomposelli FB Jr (2001). The impact of diabetes on arterial reconstructions for multilevel arterial occlusive disease. *American Journal of Surgery* **181**: 251–5.

Feigelson HS, Criqui MH, Fronek A, Langer RD, Molgaard CA (1994). Screening for peripheral arterial disease: the sensitivity, specificity, and predictive value of noninvasive tests in a defined population. *American Journal of Epidemiology* **140**: 526–34.

Fowkes FG (2001). Epidemiological research on peripheral vascular disease. *Journal of Clinical Epidemiology* **54**: 863–8.

Gardner AW, Poehlman ET (1995). Exercise Rehabilitation Programs for the treatment of claudication pain. A meta analysis. *Journal of the American Medical Association* **274**: 975–80.

Goldhaber SZ, Manson JE, Stampfer MJ, LaMotte F, Rosner B, Buring JE, Hennekens CH (1992). Low-dose aspirin and subsequent peripheral arterial surgery in the Physician's Health Study. *Lancet* **340**: 143–5.

Gourlay SG, Stead LF, Benowitz NL (2000). Clonidine for smoking cessation (Cochrane Review). *The Cochrane Library*, Issue 2. Oxford: Oxford Update Software.

Heart Outcomes Prevention Evaluation (HOPE) Study Investigators (2000). Effects of an angiotensin converting enzyme inhibitor, ramipril, on cardiovascular events in high-risk patients. *New England Journal of Medicine* **342**: 145–53.

Heart Protection Study Collaborative Group (2003). MRC/BHF Heart Protection Study of cholesterol-lowering with simvastatin in 5963 people with diabetes: a randomised placebo-controlled trial. *Lancet* **361**: 2005–16.

Hennes MM, O'Shaughnessy IM, Kelly TM, LaBelle P, Egan BM, Kissebah AH (1996). Insulin-resistant lipolysis in abdominally obese hypertensive individuals. *Hypertension* **28**: 120–6.

Henningfield JE, Keenan RM (1993). Nicotine delivery kinetics and abuse liability. *Journal of Consulting and Clinical Psychology* **61**: 743–50.

Hirsch AT, Treat-Jacobson D, Lando HA, Hatsukami DK (1997). The role of tobacco cessation, antiplatelet and lipid-lowering therapies in the treatment of peripheral arterial disease. *Vascular Medicine* **2**: 243–51.

Hirsh J, Dalen JE, Fuster V, Harker LB, Salzman EW (1992). Aspirin and other anti-platelet drugs: the relationship between dose, effectiveness, and side effects. *Chest* **102** (Suppl 4): 327S–36S.

Hoogeveen EK, Kostense PJ, Jakobs C, Rauwerda JA, Dekker JM, Nijpels G, Bouter LM, Heine RJ, Stehouwer CD (2000). Hyperhomocysteinaemia is not associated with isolated crural arterial occlusive disease: The Hoorn Study. *Journal of Internal Medicine* **247**: 442–8.

Hurt RD, Sachs DPL, Glover ED *et al.* (1997). A comparison of sustained-release bupropion and placebo for smoking cessation. *New England Journal of Medicine* **337**: 1195–202.

Idris I, Gray S, Donnelly R (2001). Protein Kinase C activation: isozyme-specific effects on metabolism and cardiovascular complications in Diabetes. *Diabetologia* **44**: 659–73.

Ishii H, Jirousek MR, Koya D, Takagi C, Clermont A, Xia P, Bursell SE, Kern TS, Ballas LM, Heath WF, Stramm LE, Feener EP, King GL (1996). Amelioration of vascular dysfunctions in diabetic rats by an oral PKC-β inhibitor. *Science* **272**: 728–31.

Jonason T, Ringqvist I (1985). Factors of prognostic importance for subsequent rest pain in patients with intermittent claudication. *Acta Medica Scandinavica* **218**: 27–33.

Jude EB, Oyibo SO, Chalmers N, Boulton AJ (2001). Peripheral arterial disease in diabetic and nondiabetic patients: a comparison of severity and outcome. *Diabetes Care* **24**: 1433–7.

Lehto S, Ronnemaa T, Pyorala K, Laakso M (1996). Risk factors predicting lower extremity amputations in patients with NIDDM. *Diabetes Care* **19**: 607–12.

Lemmers MJ, Barry JM (1991). Major role for arterial disease in morbidity and mortality after kidney transplantation in diabetic recipients. *Diabetes Care* **14**: 295–301.

Leng GC, Price JF, Jepson RG (1998). Cochrane review: lipid-lowering therapy in the treatment of lower limb atherosclerosis. *European Journal of Vascular and Endovascular Surgery* **16**: 5–6.

Levin ME, Bowker JH (1993). The diabetic foot: Pathophysiology, evaluation and treatment. In: Levin ME, O'Neal LW (eds). *The Diabetic Foot*, 5th edn. St Louis, MO: Mosby Yearbook, p. 17.

MacGregor A, Price J, Hau C, Lee A, Carson M, Fowkes F (1999). Role of systolic blood pressure and plasma triglycerides in diabetic peripheral arterial disease The Edinburgh Artery Study. *Diabetes Care* **22**: 453–8.

Marchesi S, Pasqualini L, Lombardini R, Vaudo G, Lupattelli G, Pirro M, Schillaci G, Mannarino E (2003). Prostaglandin E1 improves endothelial function in critical limb ischemia. *Journal of Cardiovascular Pharmacology* **41**: 249–53.

Matsumoto K, Miyake S, Yano M, Ueki Y, Yamaguchi Y, Akazawa S *et al.* (1997). Insulin resistance and arteriosclerosis obliterans in patients with NIDDM. *Diabetes Care* **20**: 1738–43.

Mehler PS, Coll JR, Estacio R, Esler A, Schrier RW, Hiatt WR (2003). Intensive blood pressure control reduces the risk of cardiovascular events in patients with peripheral arterial disease and type 2 diabetes. *Circulation* **107**: 753–6.

Murabito JM, D'Agostino RB, Silbershatz H, Wilson PWF (1997). Intermittent claudication: A risk profile from The Framingham Heart Study. *Circulation* **96**: 44–9.

Nelson RG, Gohdes DM, Everhart JE, Hartner JA, Zwemer FL, Pettitt DJ, Knowler WC (1988). Lower-extremity amputations in NIDDM. 12-yr follow-up study in Pima Indians. *Diabetes Care* **11**: 8–16.

O'Hara AJ, Howell JM, Taplin RH, Fletcher S, Lloyd F, Kakulas B, Lochmuller H, Karpati G (2001). The spread of transgene expression at the site of gene construct injection. *Muscle and Nerve* **24**: 488–95.

Panneton JM, Gloviczki P, Bower TC, Rhodes JM, Canton LG, Toomey BJ (2000). Pedal bypass for limb salvage: impact of diabetes on long term outcome. *Annals of Vascular Surgery* **14**: 640–7.

Pederson TR, Kjekshus J, Pyorala K, Olsson AG, Cook TJ, Musliner TA, Tobert JA, Haghfelt T (1998). Effect of simvastatin on ischaemic signs and symptoms in the Scandinavian Simvastatin Survival (4S) study. *American Journal of Cardiology* **81**: 333–5.

Premalatha G, Shanthirani S, Deepa R, Markovitz J, Mohan V (2000). Prevalence and risk factors of peripheral vascular disease in a selected South Indian population: the Chennai Urban Population Study *Diabetes Care* **23**: 1295–300.

Price J, Lee A, Fowkes F (1996). Hyperinsulinaemia: a risk factor for peripheral arterial disease in the non-diabetic population. *Journal of Cardiovascular Risk* **3**: 501–5.

PROGRESS Collaborative Group (2001). Randomised trial of a perindopril-based blood pressure-lowering regimen among 6105 individuals with previous stroke or transient ischaemic attack. *Lancet* **358**: 1033–41.

Radack K, Deck C (1991). Beta-adrenergic blocker therapy does not worsen intermittent claudication in subjects with peripheral arterial disease. A meta-analysis of randomized controlled trials. *Archives of Internal Medicine* **151**: 1769–76.

Rajagopalan S, Mohler ER, Lederman RJ, Mendelsohn FO, Saucedo JF, Goldman CK, Blebea J, Macko J, Kessler PD, Rasmussen HS, Annex BH (2003). Regional angiogenesis with vascular endothelial growth factor in peripheral arterial disease. *Circulation* **108**: 1933–8.

Reilly MP, Mohler ER (2001). Cilostazol: Treatment of intermittent claudication. *Annals of Pharmacotherapy* **35**: 48–55.

Robins SJ, Collins D, Wittes JT, Papademetriou V, Deedwania PC, Schaefer EJ, McNamara JR, Kashyap ML, Hershman JM, Wexler LF, Rubins HB; VA-HIT Study Group (2001). Veterans Affairs High-Density Lipoprotein Intervention Trial. Relation of gemfibrozil treatment and lipid levels with major coronary events: VA-HIT: a randomized controlled trial. *Journal of the American Medical Association* **285**: 1585–91.

Rosen P, Nawroth PP, King G, Moller W, Tritschler HJ, Packer L (2001). The role of oxidative stress in the onset and progression of diabetes and its complications *Diabetes / Metababolism Research and Reviews* **17**: 189–212.

Rosenberg L, Palmer JR, Shapiro S (1990). Decline in the risk of myocardial infarction among women who stop smoking. *New England Journal of Medicine* **322**: 214–17.

Schmidt A, Yan S, Wautier J, Stern D (1999). Activation of receptor for advanced glycation end products: A mechanism for chronic vascular dysfunction in diabetic vasculopathy and atherosclerosis. *Circulation Research* **84**: 489–97.

Schwartz JL (1987). *Review and Evaluation of Smoking Cessation Methods: The United States and Canada, 1978–1985.* Bethesda, MD: National Cancer Institute.

Silagy C, Mant D, Fowler G, Lodge M (1994). Meta-analysis on efficacy of nicotine replacement therapies in smoking cessation. *Lancet* **343**: 139–42.

Stokes KR, Strunk HM, Campbell DR, Gibbons GW, Wheeler HG, Clouse ME (1990). Five year results of iliac and femoral poplitel angioplasty in diabetic patients. *Radiology* **174**: 977–82.

Stroke Prevention in Atrial Fibrillation Investigators (1994). Warfarin versus aspirin for prevention of thromboembolism in atrial fibrillation: Stroke prevention in Atrial Fibrillation II study. *Lancet* **343**: 687–91.

Tomko RP, Xu R, Philipson L (1997). HCAR and MCAR: the human and mouse cellular receptors for subgroup C adenoviruses and group B coxsackieviruses. *Proceedings of the National Academy of Sciences of the United States of America* **94**: 3352–6.

UK Prospective Diabetes Study (UKPDS) Group (1998a). Intensive blood-glucose control with sulphonylureas or insulin compared with conventional treatment and risk of complications in patients with type 2 diabetes (UKPDS 33). *Lancet* **352**: 837–53.

UK Prospective Diabetes Study (UKPDS) Group (1998b). Effect of intensive blood–glucose control with metformin on complications in overweight patients with type 2 diabetes (UKPDS 34). UK Prospective Diabetes Study (UKPDS). *Lancet* **352**: 854–65.

Uusitupa M, Niskanen L, Siitonen O, Pyorala (1990). 5-Year incidence of atherosclerotic vascular disease in relation to gender, risk factors, insulin level and abnormalities in lipoprotein composition in non-insulin dependent diabetic and non-diabetic individuals. *Circulation* **82**: 27–36.

Weitz JI, Byrne J, Clagett GP *et al.* (1996). Diagnosis and treatment of chronic arterial insufficiency of the lower extremities: A critical review. *Circulation* **94**: 3026–49.

West R, McNeill A, Raw M (2000). Smoking cessation guidelines for health professionals: an update. Health Education Authority. *Thorax* **55**: 987–99.

Williams B, Poulter NR, Brown MJ, Davis M, McInnes GT, Potter JF, Sever PS, McG Thom S; British Hypertension Society (2004). Guidelines for management of hypertension: report of the fourth working party of the British Hypertension Society, 2004-BHS IV. *Journal of Human Hypertension* **18**: 139–85.

9 Prevention of Cardiovascular Events in Diabetic Patients

Markku Laakso

9.1 Introduction

The incidence of type 2 diabetes is constantly increasing in almost all populations mainly due to the 'epidemic' of obesity and a sedentary lifestyle. There are over 100 million people worldwide with diabetes, and during the next 15 years the number of type 2 diabetic patients will be doubled in the world. The consequences of this 'epidemic' are multiple, ranging from long-term diabetic complications to a heavy financial burden to healthcare systems and societies, not even mentioning the suffering of diabetic patients with micro- and macrovascular complications.

All macrovascular complications, coronary artery disease (CAD), cerebrovascular disease and peripheral vascular disease are considerably more frequent in patients with type 2 diabetes than in non-diabetic subjects (Pyörälä *et al.*, 1987; Haffner *et al.*, 1998). The prevalence of diabetes is particularly high (approximately 20%) among patients with CAD (EUROASPIRE I and II Group, 2001). Most type 2 diabetic patients die of cardiovascular disease, and atherothrombosis accounts for about 8/10 of all cardiovascular deaths (Gu *et al.*, 1998). In spite of a considerable decline in CAD mortality among the overall population, it has not declined consistently among diabetic patients. In fact, among type 2 diabetic women, CAD mortality has even increased (Gu *et al.*, 1999).

9.2 Coronary Artery Disease in Type 2 Diabetes

Epidemiological and clinical findings

Compared to non-diabetic individuals all clinical manifestations of CAD, myocardial infarction (MI), acute coronary syndrome, sudden death and angina pectoris are at

Diabetic Cardiology   Editors Miles Fisher and John J. McMurray
© 2007 John Wiley & Sons, Ltd.

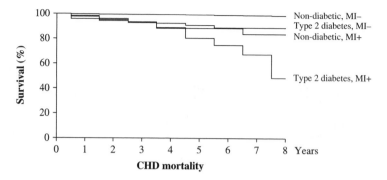

Figure 9.1 Kaplan-Meier estimates of the probability of death from coronary heart disease in 1059 subjects with type 2 diabetes and 1378 nondiabetic subjects with and without prior myocardial infarction. Reproduced from Haffner SM, Lehto S, Rönnemaa T, Pyörälä K, Laakso M (1998). Mortality from coronary heart disease in subjects with type 2 diabetes and in nondiabetic subjects with and without prior myocardial infarction. *New England Journal of Medicine* **339**: 229–34. MI denotes myocardial infarction.

least twofold more common in patients with type 2 diabetes (Laakso and Lehto, 1997) (see also Chapter 3). Type 2 diabetes eliminates the usual female protective advantage for CAD mortality. A 20-year follow-up study of the Nurses' Health Study, including 121 046 diabetic women aged 30–55 years, showed that age-adjusted relative risks of fatal CAD were 8.7 for women with a history of diabetes and no CAD at baseline, 10.6 for women with a history of CAD and no diabetes at baseline, and 25.8 for women with both conditions at baseline compared with women with no diabetes or CAD at baseline (Hu *et al.*, 2001). In our 13-year follow-up study of 835 type 2 diabetic patients without cardiovascular disease at baseline, men had a threefold higher and diabetic women a 9.5-fold higher risk for CAD events (CAD mortality or non-fatal MI) than corresponding non-diabetic individuals (Juutilainen *et al.*, 2004). When we compared the 7-year incidence of CAD mortality among 1373 non-diabetic subjects and 1059 type 2 diabetic subjects, our data demonstrated that type 2 diabetic patients without prior MI had as high a risk of CAD mortality as non-diabetic patients with prior MI (Figure 9.1; Haffner *et al.*, 1998). Similar results were reported from the Organisation to Assess Strategies for Ischaemic Syndromes (OASIS) registry study (Malmberg *et al.*, 2000). These results indicate that type 2 diabetes is a severe disease having a poor prognosis. Also, after an acute MI the mortality rates are high since 44.2% of diabetic men and 36.9% of diabetic women died within 1 year, and a considerable number of patients died even before they reached the hospital (Miettinen *et al.*, 1998).

Several clinical studies show that CAD is more severe and diffuse in type 2 diabetic patients than in non-diabetic subjects (Gu *et al.*, 1999). Furthermore, compared to non-diabetic subjects diabetic patients have a substantially higher prevalence of coronary artery calcification evaluated by electron beam-computed tomography (Wagenknect *et al.*, 2001).

Pathophysiology of coronary artery disease in type 2 diabetes (see also Chapter 2)

Knowledge from basic mechanisms of atherothrombosis to findings from clinical trials are needed to change evidence-based treatment guidelines of cardiovascular disease in patients with type 2 diabetes. Our understanding of the pathophysiology of atherothrombosis has substantially increased during recent years, and potential new mechanisms and risk factors for atherosclerosis and thombosis have been identified. For example, the role of inflammation in atherosclerosis has been officially accepted as an important risk factor for cardiovascular disease (Beckman *et al.*, 2002). However, not all risk factors are easy or even possible to measure, and therefore their impact on CAD is difficult to prove. For example, it is quite easy to assay C-reactive protein (CRP) but more difficult to measure endothelial dysfunction. If a risk factor cannot be measured, it cannot have the status of a 'proven' risk factor for cardiovascular disease. In addition, a cardiovascular risk factor needs to be tested in a controlled trial setting in order to change clinical practice. Furthermore, not only one single trial but several trials are needed to substantiate the changes in clinical practice. To illustrate these several steps in changing clinical practice Table 9.1 lists potential risk factors for cardiovascular disease from lesion initiation to plaque rupture and thrombosis.

It is generally accepted that the endothelium plays a central role in the initiation of early atherosclerosis (De Vriese *et al.*, 2000). Particularly important is nitric oxide, which regulates vascular relaxation and structure. In addition, the endothelium synthesises other bioactive substances: endothelin-1, angiotensin II, prostaglandins and other reactive oxygen species. In type 2 diabetes the production of nitric oxide is impaired because of insulin resistance, hyperglycaemia and elevated levels of free fatty acids (FFA) (Inoguchi *et al.*, 2000). In contrast, the production of endothelin-1 is increased due to hyperglycaemia (Hattori *et al.*, 1991) and hyperinsulinaemia (Ferri *et al.*, 1995).

Table 9.1 Trial evidence in the prevention of cardiovascular disease in patients with type 2 diabetes.

	Positive trial evidence
Single intervention	
Dyslipidaemia	
High LDL-cholesterol	Yes
Low HDL-cholesterol/high triglycerides	Yes
Elevated blood pressure	Yes
Hyperglycaemia	Yes (?)
Insulin resistance	No
Weight loss	No
Increased physical activity	No
Inflammation	No
Multifactorial intervention[a]	Yes

[a]Treatment of dyslipidaemia, elevated blood pressure and hyperglycaemia, cessation of smoking, increased physical exercise, diet change, cardiovascular medication (aspirin, ACE inhibitors/angiotensin II receptor antagonists, vitamins).

The accumulation of low-density lipoprotein (LDL)-cholesterol in subendothelial matrix is the primary initiating event in the process of atherosclerosis. In type 2 diabetes compositional changes in LDL particles are common (small, dense and oxidised LDL). These changes lead to pro-atherogenic LDL particles readily undergoing oxidative modification (Laakso, 1995). In addition, a defect in insulin's antilipolytic effect in adipose tissue leads to a high flux of FFAs into the liver and elevated synthesis rates of very-low-density lipoprotein (VLDL) particles. Low high-density lipoprotein (HDL) level is a typical finding in patients with type 2 diabetes mainly due to an exchange of cholesterol from HDL to VLDL via cholesteryl ester transfer protein (Laakso, 1995).

In type 2 diabetes endothelium produces an excess of pro-inflammatory molecules in response to minimally oxidised LDL and advanced glycosylation end-products (AGEs) (Creager *et al.*, 2003). The AGEs have been implicated in LDL modification, accumulation and inflammatory activation. They are accompanied by oxidative reactions that generate oxygen free radicals and contribute to oxidative stress. Hyperglycaemia activates nuclear factor-κB, leading to an increase in adhesion molecules such as selectin, vascular adhesion molecule-1 and intracellular adhesion molecule-1 (Collins and Cybulsky, 2001). Finally, vascular endothelium regulates the balance between coagulation and fibrinolysis. In type 2 diabetic patients tissue plasminogen activator and plasminogen activator inhibitor type 1 are increased (Vague and Juhan-Vague, 1997).

Formation of fibrous plaques includes an accumulation of lipids (mostly cholesterol) and smooth muscle cells. In type 2 diabetic patients elevated levels of angiotensin II induce an inflammatory response in endothelial cells and smooth muscle cells.

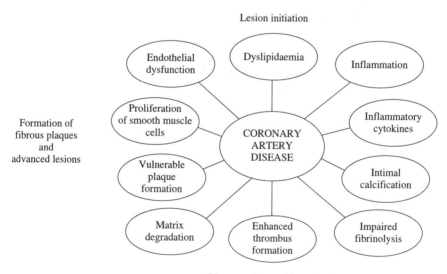

Figure 9.2 Pathogenesis of coronary artery disease in patients with type 2 diabetes. Reproduced from Laakso M, Kubaszek A (2003). Coronary artery disease in type 2 diabetes. *International Diabetes Monitor* **15**: 1–8.

Elevated blood pressure also contributes to the formation of fibrous plaques, which are more vulnerable to rupture in type 2 diabetic patients than in non-diabetic subjects because they have fewer vascular muscle cells (Fukumoto *et al.*, 1998). Coronary tissue from patients with diabetes exhibits a larger content of lipid-rich atheroma, macrophage infiltration and subsequent thrombosis than coronary tissue from patients without diabetes (Moreno *et al.*, 2000). In addition to thin fibrous cap due to decreased collagen production by vascular muscle cells, inflammation increases susceptibility to plaque rupture in type 2 diabetic patients. Diabetic patients who die suddenly show an increased number of fissured atherosclerotic plaques (Davies, 1989). Enhanced coagulation and impaired platelet function contribute to thrombosis.

Figure 9.2 summarises the pathophysiology of CAD in diabetic patients (Laakso and Kubaszek, 2003). Practically all major mechanisms leading to lesion initiation, formation of fibrous plaques and advanced lesions, plaque rupture and thrombosis are abnormal in type 2 diabetes.

9.3 Potential and Proven Risk Factors for Atherothrombosis in Patients with Type 2 Diabetes

All major pathophysiological pathways leading to accelerated atherothrombosis are disturbed in patients with type 2 diabetes. However, to prove that a risk factor is contributing to a higher risk of cardiovascular disease in patients with type 2 diabetes, two conditions must be fulfilled. First, a potential risk factor has to be associated with cardiovascular risk in longitudinal studies. Secondly, evidence from trials is needed to demonstrate that normalisation of a risk factor reduces the cardiovascular event rate. Many potential risk factors from atherothrombosis in patients with type 2 diabetes have been studied in a cross-sectional setting. With respect to endothelial function, previous studies have shown that subjects with insulin resistance or type 2 diabetes have an impairment in their ability to increase blood flow to peripheral insulin-sensitive tissues, at least partly due to their inability to induce NO-mediated vasodilatation (Creager *et al.*, 2003). However, endothelial dysfunction is difficult to measure in large population-based studies, and therefore prospective studies on type 2 diabetic patients are missing.

Dyslipidaemia

Typical diabetic dyslipidaemia includes an elevation in total and VLDL–triglycerides as well as a low HDL-cholesterol level (Laakso and Lehto, 1997). In addition, although the LDL-cholesterol level is normal, LDL particles are small and dense, they easily penetrate the vascular wall and are therefore atherogenic. Several prospective population-based studies have indicated that in type 2 diabetic patients the total and LDL-cholesterol levels are similar risk factors for cardiovascular disease as they are in non-diabetic subjects. Low HDL-cholesterol level and high levels of total triglycerides may be even more important risk factors among type 2 diabetic patients than in non-diabetic individuals (Laakso and Lehto, 1997).

Elevated blood pressure

Elevated blood pressure has been shown to occur more often in type 2 diabetic patients than in non-diabetic individuals. The mechanisms explaining a higher prevalence of hypertension among diabetic patients are largely unknown but might be related to insulin resistance among these individuals (Pyörälä *et al.*, 1987; Laakso and Lehto, 1997). Elevated levels of systolic and diastolic blood pressure are equally important risk factors for CAD in type 2 diabetic patients as they are in non-diabetic subjects (Laakso and Lehto, 1997).

Smoking

Cigarette smoking is less common, or as common among type 2 diabetic patients and normoglycaemic individuals. Similar to non-diabetic subjects the risk of CAD in patients with type 2 diabetes depends on the number of cigarettes smoked (Laakso and Lehto, 1997). Smoking may act directly or adversely influence risk factors contributing to the development of CAD (Tsiara *et al.*, 2003). Smoking can cause endothelial dysfunction, dyslipidaemia (low HDL-cholesterol, high total triglycerides) and impaired platelet function. Smoking also increases insulin resistance and induces changes in growth factors and adhesion molecules.

Obesity and central obesity

Most of type 2 diabetic patients are obese, and centrally obese. Although obesity contributes to disturbances in almost all cardiovascular risk factors, there is no consensus based on prospective studies to demonstrate that obesity is an independent risk factor for cardiovascular disease in type 2 diabetic patients.

Insulin resistance and hyperglycaemia

Insulin resistance (hyperinsulinaemia) is a characteristic finding in patients with type 2 diabetes. It often clusters with obesity, central obesity, elevated blood pressure, elevated levels of total triglycerides, haemostatic abnormalities and low-grade inflammation (Laakso, 1996). This clustering of cardiovascular risk factors (the metabolic syndrome) predicts CAD events in non-diabetic subjects (Lempiäinen *et al.*, 1999) and in patients with type 2 diabetes (Lehto *et al.*, 2000). Prospective studies are still missing to show that insulin resistance is an independent risk factor for CAD in patients with type 2 diabetes. Several population-based prospective studies have shown a positive association between hyperglycaemia and cardiovascular disease in type 2 diabetic patients (Laakso, 1999). However, this risk is not particularly strong for CAD.

Low-grade inflammation

Type 2 diabetic subjects are more prone to inflammation than are non-diabetic subjects (Biondi-Zoccai *et al.*, 2003). In addition, inflammatory cytokines are elevated in insulin-resistant states and type 2 diabetes (Schmidt *et al.*, 1999). Although CRP has been shown to predict cardiovascular events in non-diabetic individuals (Koenig *et al.*, 1999), long-term prospective studies are missing concerning type 2 diabetic patients. In addition to CRP, tumor necrosis factor-α and interleukin-6 have been shown to be associated with cardiovascular complications in non-diabetic subjects (Jager *et al.*, 2000).

Intimal calcification

Intimal calcification is a typical finding in people with either type 1 or type 2 diabetes, but unfortunately there are no data to show that it predicts cardiovascular disease among diabetic individuals.

Coagulation defects

Impaired fibrinolysis and enhanced thrombus formation are shown to be frequent findings in diabetic patients. Increased platelet adhesiveness and aggregability are characteristic findings in type 2 diabetes. In addition, increased levels of fibrinogen, von Willebrand factor, Factors VII and VIII and PAI-1 are found. Unfortunately, prospective studies are almost missing to demonstrate that impaired fibrinolysis and enhanced thrombus formation predict CAD in type 2 diabetes (Vague and Juhan-Vague, 1997; Biondi-Zaoccai *et al.*, 2003).

Other potential risk factors

There are multiple potential risk factors for CAD in patients with type 2 diabetes. An early marker for atherothrombosis in type 2 diabetes is impaired vasodilatation. Oxidative stress and the formation of AGEs are typical findings in people with type 2 diabetes, and hyperglycaemic state is associated with a high concentration of vasoconstrictors, cellular adhesion molecules, PAI-1 and cytokines (Beckman *et al.*, 2002). Unfortunately, data from prospective population-based studies or from clinical trials are almost completely missing on these potential risk factors to predict CAD, probably because many of these risk factors are difficult to measure in a large sample of patients. Mechanisms related to the formation of fibrous plaques and advanced lesions are difficult to test *in vivo*, and data are missing to prove that those mechanisms are operative in a cross-sectional or longitudinal setting in people with type 2 diabetes.

9.4   Treatment Effects of Cardiovascular Risk Factors on the Risk of CAD in Type 2 Diabetes

Dyslipidaemia

Both primary and secondary lipid-lowering trials aiming to prevent coronary heart disease in patients with type 2 diabetes have been conducted, but in these trials diabetic patients have usually formed only a small subset of study subjects. The best evidence available is from statin trials. In primary prevention trials lovastatin (Downs *et al.*, 1998) but also gemfibrozil (Koskinen *et al.*, 1992) have been shown to reduce the risk of CAD considerably. However, due to a small number of diabetic patients included in these trials the risk reductions were not statistically significant. In the Antihypertensive and Lipid-Lowering Treatment to Prevent Heart Attack Trial – Lipid Lowering Trial (ALLHAT-LLT) pravastatin did not reduce CAD events significantly in 3638 hypertensive patients with type 2 diabetes (ALLHAT Officers and Coordinators for the ALLHAT Collaborative Research Group, 2002). In the primary prevention arm of the Heart Protection Study (HPS) simvastatin led to reduced risk (26%) from CAD events (Heart Protection Study Group, 2002) in 3982 patients with diabetes. In the Ango-Scandinavian Cardiac Outcomes Trial – Lipid Lowering Arm (ASCOT-LLA) atorvastatin (10 mg/day) did not significantly reduce the risk of CAD events in 2532 patients with diabetes (Sever *et al.*, 2003). In the FIELD study fenofibrate did not reduce the risk of CAD events in 9795 patients with diabetes, most of whom had no previous cardiovascular disease (FIELD Study Investigators, 2005).

Several statin trials on the secondary prevention of CAD have been carried out. The Scandinavian simvastatin Survival Study (4S) (Pyörälä *et al.*, 1997) and the HPS (Heart Protection Study Group, 2002) with simvastatin treatment, the Cholesterol and Recurrent Events (CARE) trial (Goldberg *et al.*, 1998) and the LIPID trial (Long-term Intervention with Pravastatin in Ischaemic Disease (LIPID) Study Group, 1998) with pravastatin treatment and the Post Coronary Artery Bypass Graft Trial (Hoogwerf *et al.*, 1999) with lovastatin treatment have shown that these drugs reduce the risk of CAD events. The reduction of the risk of CAD in the HPS (Heart Protection Study Group, 2002) was independent of the baseline LDL-cholesterol indicating that the beneficial effect of LDL reduction is present throughout the range of LDL-cholesterol concentration and also at low LDL-cholesterol levels. The Lescol Intervention Prevention Study (LIPS) showed that fluvastatin in 202 diabetic patients who had undergone percutaneous coronary intervention was effective in preventing CAD events (Serruys *et al.*, 2002). In the secondary prevention arm of the PROSPER trial pravastatin did not significantly reduce the risk of CAD events (Vijan and Hayward, 2004). The Veterans Affairs High-Density Lipoprotein Cholesterol Intervention Trial (VA-HIT) randomised patients with a history of CAD and normal LDL- and low HDL-cholesterol levels to gemfibrozil or placebo. A 24% reduction in death from CAD, non-fatal MI and stroke was observed both in diabetic and non-diabetic subjects (Rubins *et al.*, 1999). The Diabetes Atherosclerosis Intervention Study (DAIS) with fenofibrate treatment (the first lipid-lowering study completed solely in diabetic patients) demonstrated that fibrate therapy reduced the progression of coronary atherosclerosis evaluated by angiography (Diabetes Atherosclerosis Intervention Study Investigators, 2001).

A meta-analysis of primary prevention trials showed that the pooled relative risk for cardiovascular events with lipid-lowering therapy was 0.78 (95% CI 0.67–0.89). The corresponding relative risk in secondary prevention trials was 0.76 (95% CI 0.59–0.93) (Vijan and Hayward, 2004). This analysis did not include a recent primary prevention trial, the Collaborative Atorvastatin Diabetes Study (CARDS) (Colhoun *et al.*, 2004), which included 2838 diabetic patients aged 40–72 years who were randomised to receive placebo or atorvastatin (10 mg/day). The trial was terminated two years earlier than expected because the prespecified early stopping rule for efficacy had been met. Acute CAD events were reduced by 31% (−59 to 16) and rate of stroke by 48% (−69 to −11). Atorvastatin reduced the death rate by 27% (−48 to 1, $P = 0.059$).

Elevated blood pressure

Several trials have shown that aggressive management of elevated blood pressure decreases the risk of CAD events in diabetic patients (see also Chapter 6). Until 1999 all trials published were based on subgroup analyses of larger trials. The first of these, the Systolic Hypertension in the Elderly Programme (SHEP) (Curb *et al.*, 1996), showed beneficial effects of chlorthalidone on cardiovascular events among elderly diabetic hypertensive patients with isolated systolic hypertension. The Systolic Hypertension in Europe (SYST-EUR) trial (Tuomilehto *et al.*, 1999) also showed that nitrendipine reduced macrovascular events in elderly diabetic hypertensive subjects. More recently, the angiotensin-converting enzyme (ACE) inhibitors and angiotensin II receptor blockers have been shown to be effective in the prevention of progressive nephropathy (EUCLID Study Group, 1997; Brenner *et al.*, 2001; Lewis *et al.*, 2001; Parving *et al.*, 2001) and cardiovascular events in type 2 diabetic patients. Captopril treatment was beneficial in diabetic hypertensive patients in the reduction of cardiovascular events in the Captopril Prevention Project (CAPPP) (Hansson *et al.*, 1999) and ramipril treatment in the MICRO-HOPE study (Heart Outcomes Prevention Evaluation (HOPE) Study Investigators, 2000).

In the Losartan Intervention for Endpoint Reduction in Hypertension (LIFE) study, losartan reduced total and cardiovascular mortality compared to atenolol in hypertensive diabetic patients with left ventricular hypertension (Lindholm *et al.*, 2002). Despite an equivalent decrease in blood pressure, losartan was more effective than atenolol in the reduction of macrovascular complications. Losartan reduced the combined endpoint (cardiovascular death, stroke or MI) by 24%, total mortality by 39% and the incidence of diabetes by 25% compared to atenolol. In the Swedish Trial in Old Patients with Hypertension 2 (STOP-2), three drugs were compared for the treatment of hypertension: calcium channel blockers, ACE inhibitors and beta-blockers plus diuretics (Lindholm *et al.*, 2000). In type 2 diabetic patients no differences in the risks of total cardiovascular events or total mortality were found. Similarly in the ALLHAT study no differences were found in CAD events or all-cause mortality when comparing treatments with chlorthalidone, enalapril or amlopidine in 12 063 diabetic patients (ALLHAT Officers and Coordinators for the ALLHAT Collaborative Research Group, 2002). In the Nordic Diltiazem (NORDIL) trial, comparing treatment with diltiazem and treatment with beta-blockers or diuretics or both, no differences in combined cardiovascular endpoints or total mortality were found in 727 diabetic patients (Hansson *et al.*, 2000). Similarly, in the International Nifedipine GITS Study Intervention as a Goal in Hypertension Treatment (INSIGHT) trial, comparing treatment with long-acting nifedipine and with coamilozide, no differences in the risk for cardiovascular endpoints or total mortality were found in 1302 diabetic patients (Brown *et al.*, 2000).

The first hypertension trial including type 2 diabetic patients only was the United Kingdom Prospective Diabetes Study (UK Prospective Diabetes Study Group, 1998). Tight control with antihypertensive medication (atenolol or captopril) reduced significantly both cardiovascular and microvascular complications. On the basis of all evidence published, it can be concluded that no mode of antihypertensive treatment is superior compared to others in the treatment of elevated blood pressure in type 2 diabetic patients. However, for diabetic patients with albuminuria or proteinuria an ACE inhibitor or an angiotensin II receptor antagonist should be used as a first-line therapy, or included in the combination therapy.

Hyperglycaemia

Although the treatment of hyperglycaemia is effective in the prevention of microvascular complications (retinopathy, nephropathy), limited evidence exists that the treatment of hyperglycaemia prevents CAD events in patients with type 2 diabetes. The UKPDS study included a large number of type 2 diabetic patients ($n = 3867$) (UK Prospective Diabetes Study (UKPDS) Group, 1998a). Over 10 years, the intensively treated group (sulphonylurea or insulin) had 0.9% lower glycosylated haemoglobin A1c than did the conventional group treated with diet only (7.0 vs. 7.9%). Although microvascular complications reduced significantly (25%, $P = 0.0099$), there was only a 16% reduction in MI, which was not statistically significant ($P = 0.052$). Intensive treatment did not decrease the risk of death, stroke or amputation. In a subgroup analysis metformin decreased cardiovascular events but this analysis was based on quite a small number of subjects ($n = 342$). Surprisingly, the combination of metformin with sulphonylureas increased mortality (UK Prospective Diabetes Study (UKPDS) Group, 1998b). However, in the Swedish Diabetes Mellitus and Insulin–Glucose Infusion in Acute Myocardial Infarction (DIGAMI) study, intensive insulin treatment during an acute MI and during the following months reduced mortality (Malmberg *et al.*, 1999) (see also Chapter 4, p. 84). In the recent PROactive study the effects of 45 mg of pioglitazone were examined in patients with type 2 diabetes and existing cardiovascular disease (Dormandy *et al.*, 2005). Compared with placebo there was an insignificant reduction in the primary composite endpoint that included cardiac, stroke and peripheral vascular clinical and procedural outcomes. There was, however, a significant reduction in a predefined main secondary endpoint comprising all-cause mortality, MI and stroke. The main side-effect of pioglitazone was an increase in reported heart failure, but this was not centrally adjudicated and is more likely to represent fluid retention and ankle oedema (see also Chapter 5). More information from ongoing trials is needed to establish the role of the improvement of glycaemic control as an efficient way to improve the cardiovascular prognosis in patients with type 2 diabetes.

Multifactorial intervention

As reviewed above several randomised clinical trials have been carried out to investigate the effects of intensified intervention involving a single risk factor in patients with type 2 diabetes. In the Steno-2 Study (Gaede *et al.*, 2003), the investigators compared the effects of a targeted, intensified, multifactorial intervention with that of conventional treatment on modifiable risk factors for cardiovascular disease in patients with type 2 diabetes and microalbuminuria.

Eighty patients were randomly assigned to receive conventional treatment and 80 to receive intensive treatment, with a stepwise implementation of behavioural modification and pharmacological therapy that targeted hyperglycaemia, dyslipidaemia and microalbuminuria, along with secondary prevention of cardiovascular disease with aspirin. The goal of dietary intervention was a total daily intake of fat $< 30\%$ of the daily energy intake. Light-to-moderate exercise for at least 30 min 3–5 times weekly was recommended. Smoking cessation was encouraged. All patients were prescribed an ACE inhibitor or angiotensin II receptor antagonist, and a daily vitamin–mineral supplementation. All patients received aspirin therapy, if not contraindicated. Hypoglycaemic agents were introduced if a patient was unable to maintain glycosylated haemoglobin A1c values below 6.5%. If a patient had hypertension, thiazides, calcium channel blockers and beta-blockers were added as needed on ACE inhibitor (or angiotensin II receptor blockade) therapy. Raised cholesterol concentration was treated with statins.

For the primary composite endpoint (death from cardiovascular causes, non-fatal MI, coronary-artery bypass grafting, percutaneous coronary intervention, non-fatal stroke, amputation as a result of ischaemic or vascular surgery for peripheral atherosclerosis artery disease) the unadjusted hazard ratio for the intensive therapy group as compared with the conventional therapy group was 0.47 (95% CI 0.24–0.73; $P = 0.008$) during a mean of 7.8 years' follow-up. Adjustment for confounding variables had no substantial effect.

The changes in lifestyle were moderate; the only significant differences between the groups were in relative intake of carbohydrate and fat. The changes in body mass index were not different between the groups. The groups differed significantly with respect to glycosylated haemoglobin A1c values (changes in conventional and intensive therapy groups of 0.2% and -0.5%, $P < 0.001$, respectively) and LDL-cholesterol (-0.33 and -1.22 mmol/l, $P < 0.001$, respectively). Intensive treatment decreased systolic and diastolic blood pressure by 10 and 5 mmHg, respectively ($P < 0.001$).

Compared to conventional therapy, patients in the intensive treatment group reached the treatment goals with respect to total cholesterol (< 4.53 mmol/l, $P < 0.001$) and systolic blood pressure (< 130 mmHg, $P < 0.001$) whereas with respect to

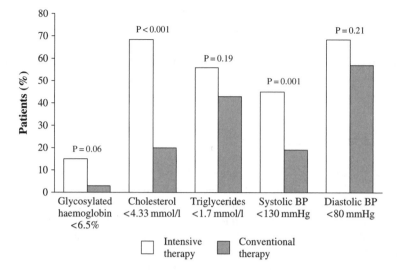

Figure 9.3 Percentage of patients with type 2 diabetes who reached the intensive-treatment goals at a mean of 7.8 years of follow-up in the Steno-2 Trial. Reproduced from Gaede P, Vedel P, Larsen N, Jensen GVH, Parving HH, Pedersen O (2003). Multifactorial intervention and cardiovascular disease in patients with type 2 diabetes. *New England Journal of Medicine* **348:** 383–93.

glycosylated haemoglobin A1c ($< 6.5\%$, $P = 0.06$), total triglycerides ($< 1.7\,\text{mmol}/1$, $P = 0.19$) and diastolic blood pressure ($< 80\,\text{mmHg}$, $P = 0.21$) the goals were not reached (Figure 9.3). The study design did not allow conclusions to be drawn about which treatment component was the most crucial one in producing diabetes-related complications. However, the Steno-2 trial proves the principle that focused, multifactorial intervention reduces substantially the risk of both cardiovascular and microvascular events in patients with type 2 diabetes and microalbuminuria.

9.5 Summary

Type 2 diabetes is a continuously growing health problem, and therefore prevention of CAD remains a challenge for the future. Accumulating information on the pathophysiology of CAD in type 2 diabetes offers hope for the prevention of cardiovascular disease (Gaede *et al.*, 2003). Since classic risk factors are also operative in patients with type 2 diabetes, the treatment of hyperglycaemia is not enough in the prevention of diabetes-associated cardiovascular disease. In particular, the treatment of dyslipidaemia and elevated blood pressure results in large cardiovascular benefits for patients with type 2 diabetes (Table 9.1). In fact, all major cardiovascular risk factors should be equally and simultaneously treated to prevent macrovascular complications in patients with type 2 diabetes, as shown recently by the Steno-2 trial (Gaede *et al.*, 2003). However, we are still missing trial evidence that weight loss, increased physical activity and improved insulin sensitivity reduce the risk of CAD in type 2 diabetic patients. Results from these ongoing trials should be available soon to give answers to these important questions.

Acknowledgements

Our research projects referred to in this review have been financially supported by grants from the Academy of Finland and the Kuopio University Hospital (EVO grant nos 5019 and 5123).

References

ALLHAT Officers and Coordinators for the ALLHAT Collaborative Research Group (2002). Major outcomes in high-risk hypertensive patients randomized to angiotensin-converting enzyme inhibitor or calcium channel blocker vs. diuretic. The antihypertensive and lipid-lowering treatment to prevent heart attack trial (ALLHAT). *Journal of American Medical Association* **288**: 2981–97.

Beckman JA, Creager MA, Libby P (2002). Diabetes and atherosclerosis. Epidemiology, pathophysiology, and management. *Journal of American Medical Association* **287**: 2570–81.

Biondi-Zoccai GGL, Abbate A, Liuzzo G, Biasucci LM (2003). Atherothrombosis, inflammation, and diabetes. *Journal of American College of Cardiology* **41**: 1071–7.

Brenner BM, Cooper ME, de Zeeuw D, Keane WF, Mitch WE, Parving HH, Remuzzi G, Snapinn SM, Zhang Z, Shahinfar S for the RENAAL Study Investigators (2001). Effects of losartan on renal and cardiovascular outcomes in patients with type 2 diabetes and nephropathy. *New England Journal of Medicine* **345**: 861–9.

Brown MJ, Palmer CR, Castaigne A, de Leeuw PW, Mancia G, Rosenthal T, Ruilope LM (2000). Morbidity and mortality in patients randomised to double-blind treatment with a long-acting calcium-channel blocker or diuretic in the International Nifedipine GITS study: Intervention as a Goal in Hypertension Treatment (INSIGHT). *Lancet* **356**: 366–72.

Colhoun HM, Betteridge J, Durrington PN, Hitman GA, Neil HAW, Livingstone SJ, Thomason MJ, Mackness M, Charlton-Menys V, Fuller JN on behalf of the CARDS investigators (2004). Primary prevention of cardiovascular disease with atorvastatin in type 2 diabetes in the Collaborative Atorvastatin Diabetes Study (CARDS): multicentre randomised placebo-controlled trial. *Lancet* **364**: 685–96.

Collins T, Cybulsky MI (2001). NF-kappaB: pivotal mediator or innocent bystander in atherogenesis? *Journal of Clinical Investigation* **107**: 255–64.

Creager MA, Luscher TF, Cosentino F, Beckman JA (2003). Diabetes and vascular disease. Pathophysiology, clinical consequences, and medical therapy: part I. *Circulation* **108**: 1527–32.

Curb DJ, Pressel SL, Cutler JA, Savage PJ, Applegate WB, Black H, Camel G, Davis BR, Frost PH, Gonzales N, Guthrie N, Guthrie G, Oberman A, Rutan GH, Stamler J for the Systolic Hypertension in the Elderly Program Cooperative Research Group (1996). Effect of diuretic-based antihypertensive treatment on cardiovascular disease risk in older diabetic patients with isolated systolic hypertension. *Journal of American Medical Association* **276**: 1886–92.

Davies MJ (1989). The pathological basis of angina pectoris. *Cardiovascular Drugs and Therapy* **3** (Suppl 1): 249–55.

De Vriese AS, Verbreuen TJ, Van de Voorde J, Lameire NH, Vanhoutte PM (2000). Endothelial dysfunction in diabetes. *British Journal of Pharmacology* **130**: 963–74.

Diabetes Atherosclerosis Intervention Study Investigators (2001). Effect of fenofibrate on progression of coronary artery disease in type 2 diabetes: The Diabetes Atherosclerosis Intervention Study, a randomised study. *Lancet* **357:** 905–10.

Dormandy JA, Charbonnel B, Eckland DJ *et al.* on behalf of the PROactive Investigators (2005). Secondary prevention of macrovascular events in patients with type 2 diabetes in the PROactive study (PROspective pioglitAzone Clinical Trial in macroVascular Events): a randomised controlled trial. *Lancet* **366**: 1279–89.

Downs JR, Clearfield M, Weis S, Whithney E, Shapiro DR, Beere PA, Langendorfer A, Stein EA, Kruyer W , Gotto AM Jr for the AFCAPS/TexCAPS Research Group (1998). Primary prevention of acute coronary events with lovastatin in men and women with average cholesterol levels: results of AFCAPS/TexCAPS. Air Force/Texas Coronary Atherosclerosis Prevention Study.*Journal of American Medical Association* **279**: 1615–22.

EUCLID Study Group (1997). Randomised placebo-controlled trial of lisinopril in normotensive patients with insulin-dependent diabetes and normoalbuminuria or microalbuminuria. *Lancet* **349**: 1787–92.

EUROASPIRE I and II Group (2001). Clinical reality of coronary prevention guidelines: a comparison of EUROASPIRE I and II in nine countries. *Lancet* **357**: 995–1001.

Ferri C, Pittoni V, Piccoli A, Laurenti O, Cassone MR, Bellini C, Properzi G, Valensini G, De Mattia G, Santucci A (1995). Insulin stimulates endothelin-1 secretion from human endothelial cells and modulates its circulating levels in vivo. *Journal of Clinical Endocrinology and Metabolism* **80**: 829–35.

FIELD Study Investigators (2005). Effects of long-term fenofibrate therapy on cardiovascular events in 9795 people with type 2 diabetes (the FIELD study): randomised controlled trial. *Lancet* **366**: 1849–61.

Fukumoto H, Naito Z, Asano G, Aramaki T (1998). Immunohistochemical and morphometric evaluations of coronary atherosclerotic plaques associated with myocardial infarction and diabetes mellitus. *Atherosclerosis and Thrombosis* **5**: 29–35.

Gaede P, Vedel P, Larsen N, Jensen GVH, Parving HH, Pedersen O (2003). Multifactorial intervention and cardiovascular disease in patients with type 2 diabetes. *New England Journal of Medicine* **348**: 383–93.

Goldberg RB, Mellies MJ, Sacks FM, Moye LA, Howard BV, Howard WJ, Davis BR, Cole TG, Pfeffer MA, Braunwald E for the CARE Investigators (1998). Cardiovascular events and their reduction with pravastatin in diabetic and glucose-intolerant myocardial infarction survivors with average cholesterol levels. Subgroup analyses in the Cholesterol And Recurrent Events (CARE) Trial. *Circulation* **98**: 2513–9.

Gu K, Cowie CC, Harris MI (1998). Mortality in adults with and without diabetes in a national cohort of the U.S. population, 1971–1993. *Diabetes Care* **21:** 1138–45.

Gu K, Cowie CC, Harris MI (1999). Diabetes and decline in heart disease mortality in US adults. *Journal of American Medical Association* **281**: 1291–7.

Haffner SM, Lehto S, Rönnemaa T, Pyörälä K, Laakso M (1998). Mortality from coronary heart disease in subjects with type 2 diabetes and in nondiabetic subjects with and without prior myocardial infarction. *New England Journal of Medicine* **339**: 229–34.

Hansson L, Lindholm LH, Niskanen L, Lanke J, Hedner T, Niklason A, Luomanmäki K, Dahlöf B, de Faire U, Morlin C, Karlberg BE, Wester P, Björck JE for the CAPPP Study Group (1999). Effect of angiotensin-converting-enzyme inhibition compared with conventional therapy on cardiovascular morbidity and mortality in hypertension: the Captopril Prevention Project (CAPPP) randomised trial. *Lancet* **353**: 611–6.

Hansson L, Hedner T, Lund-Johansen P, Kjeldsen SE, Lindholm LH, Syvertsen JO, Lanke J, de Faire U, Dahlöf B, Karlberg BE (2000). Randomised trial of effects of calcium antagonists compared with diuretics and beta-blockers on cardiovascular morbidity and mortality in hypertension: the Nordic Diltiazem (NORDIL) study. *Lancet* **356**: 359–65.

Hattori Y, Kasai K, Nakamura T, Emoto T, Shimoda S (1991). Effect of glucose and insulin on immunoreactive endothelin-1 release from cultured porcine aortic endothelial cells. *Metabolism* **40**: 165–70.

Heart Outcomes Prevention Evaluation (HOPE) Study Investigators (2000). Effects of ramipril on cardiovascular and microvascular outcomes in people with diabetes mellitus: results of the HOPE study and MICRO-HOPE substudy. *Lancet* **355**: 253–9.

Heart Protection Study Group (2002). MRC/BHF Heart Protection Study of cholesterol lowering with simvastatin in 20 536 high-risk individuals: a randomised placebo-controlled trial. *Lancet* **360**: 7–22.

Hoogwerf BJ, Waness A, Cressman M, Canner J, Campeau L, Domanski M, Geller N, Herd A, Hickley A, Hunninghake DB, Knatterud GL, White C (1999). Effects of aggressive cholesterol lowering and low-dose anticoagulation on clinical and angiographic outcomes in patients with diabetes. The Post Coronary Artery Bypass Graft Trial. *Diabetes* **48**: 1289–94.

Hu FB, Stampfer MJ, Solomon CG, Liu S, Willett WC, Speizer FE, Nathan DM, Manson JE (2001). The impact of diabetes mellitus on mortality from all causes and coronary heart disease in women. *Archives of Internal Medicine* **161**: 1717–23.

Inoguchi T, Li P, Umeda F, Yu HY, Kakimoto M, Imamura M, Aoki T, Etoh T, Hashimoto T, Naruse M, Sano H, Utsumi H, Nawata H (2000). High glucose level and free fatty acid stimulate reactive oxygen species production through protein kinase C-dependent activation of NAD(P)H oxidase in cultured vascular cells. *Diabetes* **49**: 1939–45.

Jager A, van Himsbergh VW, Kostense PJ, Emeis JJ, Nijpels G, Dekker JM, Heine Rj, Bouter LM, Stehouwer CD (2000). Increased levels of soluble vascular cell adhesion molecule-1 are associated with the risk of cardiovascular mortality in type 2 diabetes: the Hoorn Study. *Diabetes* **49**: 485–91.

Juutilainen A, Kortelainen S, Lehto S, Rönnemaa T, Pyörälä K, Laakso M (2004). Gender difference in the impact of type 2 diabetes on coronary heart disease. *Diabetes Care* **27**: 2898–904.

Koenig W, Sund M, Fröhlich M, Fischer HG, Lowel H, Doring A, Hutchinson WL, Pepys MB (1999). C-reactive protein, a sensitive marker of inflammation, predicts future risk of coronary heart disease in initially healthy middle-aged men. Results from the MONICA (Monitoring Trends and Determinants in Cardiovascular Disease) Augsburg Cohort Study, 1984 to 1992. *Circulation* **99**: 237–42.

Koskinen P, Mänttäri M, Manninen V, Huttunen JK, Heinonen OP, Frick MH (1992). Coronary heart disease incidence in NIDDM patients in the Helsinki Heart Study. *Diabetes Care* **15**: 820–5.

Laakso M (1995). Epidemiology of diabetic dyslipidemia. *Diabetes Reviews* **3**: 408–22.

Laakso M (1996). Insulin resistance and coronary heart disease. *Current Opinion of Lipidology* **7**: 217–26.

Laakso M (1999). Hyperglycemia and cardiovascular disease in type 2 diabetes. *Diabetes* **48**: 937–42.

Laakso M, Kubaszek A (2003). Coronary artery disease in type 2 diabetes. *International Diabetes Monitor* **15**: 1–8.

Laakso M, Lehto S (1997). Epidemiology of macrovascular disease in diabetes. *Diabetes Reviews* **5**: 294–315.

Lehto S, Rönnemaa T, Pyörälä K, Laakso M (2000). Cardiovascular risk factors clustering with endogenous hyperinsulinaemia predict death from coronary heart disease in patients with type II diabetes. *Diabetologia* **43**: 148–55.

Lempiäinen P, Mykkänen L, Pyörälä K, Laakso M, Kuusisto J (1999). Insulin resistance syndrome predicts coronary heart disease events in elderly nondiabetic men. *Circulation* **100**: 123–8.

Lewis EJ, Hunsicker LG, Clarke WR, Berl T, Pohl MA, Lewis JB, Ritz E, Atkins RC, Rohde R, Raz I (2001). Renoprotective effect of the angiotensin-receptor antagonist irbesartan in patients with nephropathy due to type 2 diabetes. *New England Journal of Medicine* **345**: 851–60.

Lindholm LH, Hansson L, Ekblom T, Dahlöf B, Lanke J, Linjer E, Schersten B, Wester PO, Hedner T, de Faire U (2000). Comparison of antihypertensive treatments in preventing cardiovascular events in elderly diabetic patients: results from the Swedish Trial in Old Patients with Hypertension-2. *Journal of Hypertension* **18**: 1671–5.

Lindholm LH, Ibsen H, Dahlöf B, Devereux RB, Beevers G, de Faire U, Fyhrquist F, Julius S, Kjeldsen SE, Kristiansson K, Lederballe-Pederson O, Nieminen MS, Omvik P, Oparil S, Wedel H, Aurup P, Edelman J, Snapinn S for the LIFE Study Group (2002). Cardiovascular morbidity and mortality in patients with diabetes in the Losartan Intervention For Endpoint reduction in hypertension study (LIFE). *Lancet* **359**: 1004–10.

Long-term Intervention with Pravastatin in Ischaemic Disease (LIPID) Study Group. Prevention of cardiovascular events and death with pravastatin in patients with coronary heart disease and a broad range of initial cholesterol levels. *New England Journal of Medicine* **339**: 1349–57.

Malmberg K, Norhammar A, Wedel H, Ryden L. (1999). Glycometabolic state at admission: important risk marker of mortality in conventionally treated patients with diabetes mellitus and acute myocardial infarction: long-term results from the Diabetes and Insulin-Glucose Infusion in Acute Myocardial Infarction (DIGAMI) study. *Circulation* **99**: 2626–32.

Malmberg K, Yusuf S, Gerstein HC, Brown J, Zhao F, Hunt D, Piegas L, Calvin J, Keltai M, Budaj A (2000). Impact of diabetes on long-term prognosis in patients with unstable angina and non-Q-wave myocardial infarction: results of the OASIS (Organization to Assess Strategies for Ischemic Syndromes) registry. *Circulation* **102**: 1014–9.

Miettinen H, Lehto S, Salomaa V, Mähönen M, Niemelä M, Haffner SM, Pyörälä K, Tuomilehto J (1998). Impact of diabetes on mortality after the first myocardial infarction. The FINMONICA Myocardial Infarction Register Study Group. *Diabetes Care* **21**: 69–75.

Moreno PR, Murcia AM, Palacios IF, Leon MN, Bernardi VH, Fuster V, Fallon JT (2000). Coronary composition and macrophage infiltration in atherectomy specimens from patients with diabetes mellitus. *Circulation* **102**: 2180–4.

Parving HH, Lehnert H, Brochner-Mortenson J, Gomis R, Andersen S, Arner P for the Irbesartan in Patients with Type 2 Diabetes and Microalbuminuria Study Group (2001). The effect of irbesartan on the development of diabetic nephropathy in patients with type 2 diabetes. *New England Journal of Medicine* **345**: 870–8.

Pyörälä K, Laakso M, Uusitupa M (1987) Diabetes and atherosclerosis:an epidemiologic view. *Diabetes Metabolism Reviews* **3**: 463–524.

Pyörälä K, Pedersen TR, Kjekshus J, Faergeman O, Olsson AG, Thorgeirsson G, for the Scandinavian SImvastatin Survival Study (4S) Group (1997). Cholesterol lowering with simvastatin improves prognosis of diabetic patients with coronary heart disease: a subgroup analysis of the Scandinavian Simvastatin Survival Study (4S). *Diabetes Care* **20**: 614–20.

Rubins HB, Robins SJ, Collins D, Fye CL, Anderson JW, Elam MB, Faas FH, Linares E, Schaefer EJ, Schectman G, Wilt TJ, Wittes J for the Veterans Affairs High-density Lipoprotein Cholesterol Intervention Trial Study Group (1999). Gemfibrozil for the secondary prevention of coronary heart disease in men with low levels of high-density lipoprotein cholesterol. *New England Journal of Medicine* **341**: 410–8.

Schmidt MI, Duncan BB, Sharrett AR, Lindberg G, Savage PJ, Offenbacher S, Azambuja MI, Tracy RP, Heiss G (1999). Markers of inflammation and prediction of diabetes mellitus in adults (Atherosclerosis Risk in Communbities Study): a cohort study. *Lancet* **353**: 1649–52.

Serruys PW, de Feyter P, Macaya C, Kokott N, Puel J, Vrolix M, Branzi A, Bertolami MC, Jackson G, Strauss B, Meier B for the Lescol Intervention Prevention Study (LIPS) Investigators (2002). Fluvastatin for prevention of cardiac events following successful first percutaneous coronary intervention: a randomized controlled trial. *Journal of American Medical Association* **287**; 3215–22.

Sever PS, Dahlöf B, Poulter NR, Wedel H, Beevers G, Caufield M, Collins R, Kjeldsen SE, Kristinsson A, McInnes GT, Mehlsen J, Nieminen M, O'Brien E, Östergren J for the ASCOT Investigators (2003). Prevention of coronary and stroke events with atorvastatin in hypertensive patients who have average or lower-than-average cholesterol concentrations, in the Anglo-Scandinavian Cardiac Outcomes Trial – Lipid Lowering Arm (ASCOT-LLA): a multicentre randomised controlled trial. *Lancet* **361**: 1149–58.

Tsiara S, Elisaf M, Mikhailidas DP (2003). Influence of smoking on predictors of vascular disease. *Angiology* **54**: 507–30.

Tuomilehto J, Rastenyte D, Birkenhäger WH, Thijs L, antikainen R, Bulpitt CJ,Fletcher AE, Forette F, Goldhaber A, Palatini P, Sarti C, Fagard R (1999). Effects of calcium-channel blockade in older patients with diabetes and systolic hypertension. *New England Journal of Medicine* **340**: 677–84.

UK Prospective Diabetes Study Group (1998). Tight blood pressure control and risk of macrovascular and microvascular complications in type 2 diabetes (UKPDS 38). *British Medical Journal* **317**: 703–13.

UK Prospective Diabetes Study (UKPDS) Group (1998a). Intensive blood-glucose control with sulphonylureas or insulin compared with conventional treatment and risk of complications in patients with type 2 diabetes (UKPDS 33). *Lancet* **352**: 837–53.

UK Prospective Diabetes Study (UKPDS) Group (1998b). Effect of intensive blood glucose control with metformin on complications in overweight patients with type 2 diabetes (UKPDS 34). *Lancet* **352**: 854–65.

Vague P, Juhan-Vague I (1997). Fibrinogen, fibrinolysis and diabetes mellitus: a comment. *Diabetologia* **40**: 738–40.

Vijan S, Hayward RA (2004). Pharmacological lipid-lowering therapy in type 2 diabetes mellitus: background paper for the American College of Physicians. *Annals of Internal Medicine* **140**: 650–8.

Wagenknect LE, Bowden DW, Carr JJ, Langefeld CD, Freedman BI, Rich SS (2001). Familial aggregation of coronary artery calcium in families with type 2 diabetes. *Diabetes* **50**: 861–6.

10 Prevention of Diabetes as a Means of Preventing Cardiovascular Disease

Stephen J. Cleland and Jonathan Shaw

10.1 Hyperglycaemia as a Risk Factor for Cardiovascular Disease

Our understanding of the role of traditional risk factors for cardiovascular disease (CVD), such as hypertension, hypercholesterolaemia, smoking and diabetes, has evolved significantly over the last decade. Rather than viewing these risk factors as 'all or nothing' phenomena with pathogenic thresholds at particular levels, we now regard them as continuous variables, each contributing to overall CVD risk. In this paradigm, 'targets' for risk factor reduction are artificial, since they do not describe a clinically relevant threshold, and should vary depending on the cumulative risk for individual patients. However, this method of approaching CVD risk assessment runs into difficulties when one considers diabetes and hyperglycaemia. Unlike type 1 diabetes, where chronic hyperglycaemia is the hallmark of the disease process, type 2 diabetes (T2D) exhibits much more complex pathophysiology: while glucose levels still define the diagnosis, hyperglycaemia is only one of several metabolic abnormalities, many of which are also established or potential CVD risk markers (see also Chapter 2).

Epidemiological studies

In an attempt to understand the significance of chronic hyperglycaemia in the context of T2D and CVD, we first need to consider the evidence (from both epidemiological and mechanistic studies) that blood glucose is directly related to accelerated atherothrombotic disease. A number of studies have proposed a direct association between glycaemic

Diabetic Cardiology   Editors Miles Fisher and John J. McMurray
© 2007 John Wiley & Sons, Ltd.

control and incidence of cardiovascular events in diabetic populations (Kuusisto *et al.*, 1994; Moss *et al.*, 1994; Andersson and Svardsudd, 1995). Coutinho and colleagues performed a meta-regression analysis of 20 studies, pooling data from over 95 000 individuals (94% male), predominantly without diabetes, followed for over 12 years (Coutinho *et al.*, 1999). They demonstrated a positive association between glycaemia (both fasting and post-glucose load) and cardiovascular events (Figure 10.1). The findings supported the notion that glucose is a continuous risk factor for CVD with no obvious pathogenic threshold. Compared with a glucose level of 4.2 mmol/l (75 mg/dl), a fasting level of 6.1 mmol/l (110 mg/dl) and a 2-h glucose level of 7.8 mmol/l (140 mg/dl) were associated with a relative cardiovascular event risk of 1.33 (95% CI 1.06–1.67) and 1.58 (95% CI 1.19–2.10), respectively. In those studies included in the meta-regression analysis where adjustment for other CVD risk factors was performed, the effects of glucose were independent in only the minority. However, the DECODE analysis of European cohort studies showed that, even after adjustment for other CVD risk factors, the 2-h but

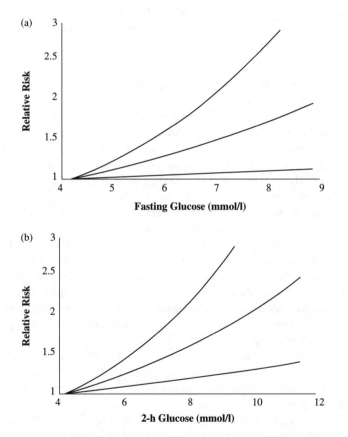

Figure 10.1 The curves and 95% CIs (within which the curve lies) for fasting (A), and 2-h postprandial (B) glucose values demonstrate a smooth positive association with relative risk for cardiovascular events. Reproduced from Coutinho M, Gerstein HC, Wang Y, Yusuf S (1999). The relationship between glucose and incident cardiovascular events: a metaregression analysis of published data from 20 studies of 95,783 individuals followed for 12.4 years. *Diabetes Care* **22**: 233–40.

not the fasting glucose level was an independent predictor of mortality (DECODE Study Group, 1999).

Mechanistic studies

Results from physiological and experimental studies support an important role of glucose in the development of atherothrombotic disease. Endothelial dysfunction is a feature of T2D (Williams *et al.*, 1996) and hyperglycaemia appears to play a specific role (Hogikyan *et al.*, 1998). Glucose-induced oxidative stress has several implications for acceleration of atherosclerotic plaque formation (Giugliano *et al.*, 1996; Ceriello, 2003) and pro-inflammatory cytokine release has been demonstrated in response to hyperglycaemia (Esposito *et al.*, 2002). In addition, glycosylated products including LDL-cholesterol (Graier and Kostner, 1997)) and advanced glycosylation end-products (Vlassara and Palace, 2002) have been shown to disrupt normal macrovascular function. Therefore, hyperglycaemia undoubtedly plays a role in diabetic vascular disease, and it is likely that it behaves as a continuous risk factor even through the spectrum of 'normoglycaemia'.

Hyperglycaemia as a risk for CVD in diabetes

However, questions have been raised about the relative importance of hyperglycaemia as a CVD risk factor in T2D. In the United Kingdom Prospective Diabetes Study (UKPDS), more intensive glycaemic control did not result in significantly fewer CVD events, despite a significant linear association between HbA1c and CVD events on cross-sectional analysis (Stratton *et al.*, 2000). One reason for this anomaly may be related to the difficulty in lowering glucose levels in T2D, and the difference in HbA1c between the two groups was simply insufficient to show significant outcome differences. An alternative explanation is that glycaemia, in the context of T2D, is predominantly a surrogate marker for other more potent CVD risk factors. The most obvious of these is insulin resistance, which is thought to be the main feature underpinning the metabolic syndrome (Figure 10.2). While glucose dysregulation is an integral feature of this syndrome, the cumulative effect of other factors, including vascular endothelial dysfunction, atherogenic dyslipidaemia, hypertension, oxidative stress, pro-inflammation, pro-thrombosis and pro-coagulation, is likely to promote and accelerate atherothrombotic lesions (see also Chapter 2).

If we are to conclude that hyperglycaemia is only one of many risk markers in T2D, and that its apparent direct association with CVD may be confounded by its 'bystander' role, then several questions are raised. For example, is there any justification for using the diagnosis of T2D as a categorical risk factor when calculating CVD risk? Should the diagnosis of T2D be restricted to glycaemic criteria alone? If the majority of pre-diabetes is associated with the metabolic syndrome, should we not be moving away from definitions dependent on glucose alone to identify pre-diabetes? When considering these issues it is important to remember that a threshold (involving current definitions of diabetes: fasting glucose ≥ 7.0 or 2-h post-glucose load ≥ 11.1) does appear to be clinically relevant in terms of microvascular complications (Expert Committee on the Diagnosis and Classification of Diabetes Mellitus, 1997). Therefore,

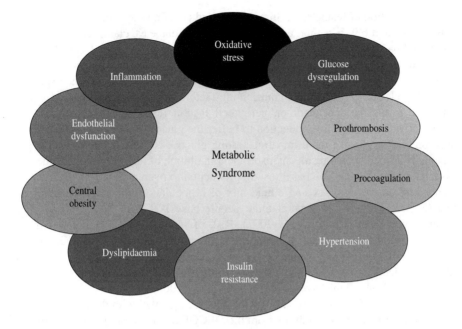

Figure 10.2 Glucose dysregulation is only one of many features of the metabolic syndrome, which is underpinned by insulin resistance.

it is important to record the transition from pre-diabetes to diabetes in order to begin the annual processes of retinal screening, sensory neuropathy assessment and measurement of urinary albumin excretion. In addition, the very fact that glucose is an easily measured surrogate marker for other risk factors associated with the metabolic syndrome promotes it as a useful screening marker in CVD risk assessment. As we will go on to discuss, there are a number of ongoing debates as to the definition and management of pre-diabetes and how this condition should be screened for. In addition, we will summarise a series of intervention studies in pre-diabetes and ask whether preventing or delaying the progress to frank diabetes can simultaneously reduce cardiovascular risk.

10.2 Risk of Cardiovascular Disease in Pre-diabetes

The American Diabetes Association (ADA) has recently introduced the term pre-diabetes in an attempt to simplify what has become an increasingly confusing literature on impaired glucose tolerance (IGT) and impaired fasting glucose (IFG) (see also Chapter 11). In fact, pre-diabetes was introduced as an official term nearly 40 years ago, although with an entirely different definition (World Health Organization, 1965), and some may argue that it may be a misleading label for some subjects with intermediate metabolic states who might never go on to develop frank diabetes. The term IGT has been in use since 1979 and is defined by a fasting plasma venous glucose level of < 7.0 mmol/l and a 2-h post-glucose load level between 7.8 and 11.0 mmol/l. The concept of IFG was introduced more recently (Expert Committee on the Diagnosis and Classification of Diabetes Mellitus, 1997) and is defined by a fasting glucose level between 6.1 and 6.9. Whether, as in the diagnosis of diabetes, classification should be confirmed by repeat testing has not as yet been established in official guidelines.

The terms IGT and IFG are not mutually exclusive, but certainly identify different subgroups of the population with metabolic dysregulation. This is understandable when the relevant physiological contributing factors are examined. Impaired glucose tolerance is mostly dependent on peripheral insulin resistance in association with failure of sufficient insulin production to buffer the glucose excursion associated with absorption of a glucose load. Impaired fasting glucose is more dependent on hepatic insulin resistance, which results in insufficient inhibition of fasting gluconeogenesis, in association with inadequate basal insulin production to overcome hepatic dysfunction. Depending on the age, sex and ethnic mix of a population, the prevalences of IGT and IFG can vary but in general more people have IGT than IFG, with a smaller group having both (Unwin *et al.*, 2002). Risk of future diabetes is greatest if both IGT and IFG are present, and IGT appears to be more predictive than IFG, although if the cut-off for IFG is lowered to the most recent ADA definition ($\geq 5.6\,\mathrm{mmol/l}$) (American Diabetes Association, 2004a) then the sensitivity of IFG rivals that of IGT (Shaw *et al.*, 1999; Gabir *et al.*, 2000; Unwin *et al.*, 2002).

Both IGT and IFG also predict CVD incidence. In parallel with the meta-regression analysis described above, analyses from the DECODE study (combining data from 13 prospective European studies) have demonstrated all-cause mortality hazard ratios of 1.20 (95% CI 1.04–1.38) for IFG and 1.50 (95% CI 1.33–1.69) for IGT when compared with normoglycaemia. However, when the analyses were confined to CVD events and adjusted for body mass index (BMI), systolic blood pressure (SBP), cholesterol and smoking, IGT remained a significant predictor (hazard ratio 1.34; 95% CI 1.14–1.57) whereas the effect of IFG was lost (hazard ratio 1.09; 95% CI 0.90–1.30), implying that a 2-h oral glucose tolerance test (OGTT) level may be the optimal glucose parameter for cardiovascular event prediction. The question remains whether there are mechanistic explanations for these observations – for example, could exaggerated postprandial glucose excursions play a key role in accelerating atheromatous lesions? Or could peripheral insulin resistance, to which IGT is strongly related, be exerting an influence on risk, possibly via circulating factors such as adipocytokines? There is no doubt that measurement of blood glucose (either fasting or post-glucose load) remains a useful tool to identify individuals at risk of both T2D and CVD, but it should be viewed as a continuous risk variable to be interpreted in conjunction with other risk markers associated with the metabolic syndrome. The resulting 'big picture' estimate of risk is important for designing strategies to target certain groups for primary prevention of T2D and CVD.

Of course, we should be able to glean useful information about the relative contribution of hyperglycaemia to cardiovascular risk from intervention studies designed to demonstrate significant delay or prevention of diabetes, defined by glycaemic thresholds. These studies will be summarised in detail in the next section. If an intervention were simply to reduce blood glucose levels then any associated reduction in cardiovascular outcomes could be ascribed to a glucose effect. However, as we will go on to discuss, most of the published studies in pre-diabetic subjects involve interventions that impact on other facets of the metabolic syndrome, potentially resulting in reduced cardiovascular risk via glucose-independent mechanisms.

10.3 Intervention Trials in Pre-diabetes (Table 10.1)

Diet and exercise

While two previous randomised controlled trials (RCT) had suggested beneficial effects of a healthy lifestyle in terms of T2D incidence, they were suboptimal in design (Eriksson and Lindgarde; 1991 Pan *et al.*, 1997). However, more recently, the results of two well-designed lifestyle intervention trials conducted in overweight subjects with IGT have been published.

In the Finnish Diabetes Prevention Study (DPS), 522 middle-aged obese subjects with IGT were randomised to receive the usual brief advice on diet and exercise or intensive individualised instruction on exercise, food intake and weight reduction. After a mean follow-up period of 3.2 years, there was a 58% relative reduction in T2D incidence in the group given the intensive lifestyle instruction (annual incidence 3.2% vs. 7.8% in control group). The number needed to treat (NNT) for 1 year to prevent one case of T2D was 22 (Tuomilehto *et al.*, 2001). In the American Diabetes Prevention Program (DPP), 3234 subjects (slightly younger and more obese than the Finnish subjects) were recruited and randomised to receive either intensive diet and exercise counselling or usual advice. In addition, a third group received metformin, which will be discussed later. After a mean follow-up of 2.8 years, there was an annual T2D incidence of 11% in the control group compared with 4.8% in the lifestyle intervention group, giving a relative risk reduction that was identical to the Finnish study of 58% (NNT = 22) (Knowler *et al.*, 2002). Subjects in the Finnish study have now been followed for a further 4 years, with a median total follow-up of 7 years (Lindstrom *et al.*, 2006). Beneficial lifestyle changes achieved by participants in the intervention group were maintained after the discontinuation of the intervention, and during the total follow-up there was a 43% reduction in relative risk. Longer follow-up of the American subjects is awaited.

Thus, there is no doubt that intensive lifestyle change can at least delay the onset of T2D in subjects who are at high risk for the condition, although the cost and intensity of the intervention may not be realistic outside a clinical trial setting. In addition, it has already been argued that hyperglycaemia is but one of many potential CVD risk factors in obese, sedentary middle-aged subjects, and it is debatable whether crossing a particular (artificial) glycaemic threshold will have any real impact on future risk of macrovascular events, although minimising risk for future development of retinopathy may be a good enough reason in itself to prevent diabetes. There have not been (and are unlikely ever to be) any RCTs of lifestyle intervention with CVD events as the primary endpoint, but it appears highly likely from physiological studies that healthy diet, weight loss and exercise will affect a number of features associated with the metabolic syndrome, resulting in overall CVD risk reduction. For example, exercise has been associated with favourable lipid profiles (mainly increased HDL-cholesterol) (Warner *et al.*, 1995), improvements in endothelium-mediated coronary vasodilation (Hambrecht *et al.*, 2000), changes in body composition (preferential loss of visceral adiposity) (Pratley *et al.*, 2000), diminished insulin resistance (Ryan, 2000; Taniguchi *et al.*, 2000; Wojtaszewski *et al.*, 2000; Kanaley and Weinstock, 2001) and increased fibrinolysis (Stratton *et al.*, 1991), all of which may be mechanisms by which exercise CVD risk is reduced and glucose regulation improved.

Table 10.1 Summary of diabetes prevention trials.

Trial name	Subject number	Inclusion criteria	Mean age	Mean BMI	Trial duration (years)	Intervention	Incidence of diabetes (% p.a.)	Relative risk reduction	NNT (1 year) to prevent one case of diabetes
Diabetes Prevention Program (USA)	3234	IGT	51	34	2.8	Control	11.0		
						Lifestyle	4.8	58%	16
						Metformin	7.8	31%	31
Diabetes Prevention Study (Finland)	522	IGT	55	31	3.2	Control	7.8		
						Lifestyle	3.2	58%	22
TRIPOD (USA)	236	Previous GDM	35	30	2.5	Placebo	12.3		
						Troglitazone	5.4	56%	15
DREAM (multinational)	5269	IGT and/or IFG	55	31	3	Placebo	8.3	62%	21
						Rosiglitazone	3.5		
STOP-NIDDM (multinational)	1429	IGT	55	31	3.3	Placebo	12.7		
						Acarbose	9.7	25%	33
XENDOS (Sweden)	3305	IGT + NGT	44	37	4	Placebo + lifestyle	2.3		
						Orlistat + lifestyle	1.6	37%	142
XENDOS (IGT subgroup)	694	IGT	N/A	N/A	4	Placebo + lifestyle	7.2		
						Orlistat + lifestyle	4.7	45%	40

GDM = gestational diabetes mellitus; NGT = normal glucose tolerance.

If we are to accept the 'common sense' conclusion that intensive diet and lifestyle advice should be offered to those people at risk of developing T2D, who should be selected for this intervention and how should they be identified? If we stick to evidence-based practice, then only middle-aged obese subjects with IGT should be targeted. But it could be argued that waiting until this advanced stage of metabolic dysregulation may be too late to reverse the spiral into T2D and CVD. While it is understandable that this particular group was chosen for the RCTs (because of the high underlying event rate), lifestyle intervention must surely be commenced at a much earlier stage, if necessary at a population level, until long-term prediction of individual risk for T2D and CVD can be more accurately defined. This area will be expanded later when screening is discussed.

Metformin

The annual incidence of T2D in the DPP group randomised to 850 mg of metformin twice a day was 7.8% (Knowler *et al.*, 2002), representing a 31% relative risk reduction and an NNT of 31. Metformin appeared to have no effect in subjects who were older (>60 years) and leaner (BMI < 30), and it is not known whether this effect is additive to that of intensive lifestyle intervention since none of the subjects received both. Despite this positive result, the most recent position statement from the ADA (American Diabetes Association, 2004b) states that 'drug therapy should not be routinely used to prevent diabetes until more information is known about its cost-effectiveness'. Given that metformin is a cheap drug and intensive individualised nutrition and exercise counselling is expensive, this statement appears misguided. In addition, analyses have been published suggesting that both interventions are, indeed, cost-effective (Diabetes Prevention Program Research Group, 2003) and that metformin may, in fact, be superior in this regard (Palmer *et al.*, 2004). From a practical point of view, it is unlikely that the success of intensive lifestyle intervention will be reproduced in typical populations due to lack of subject motivation and adherence and, realistically, metformin prescription may be more efficacious (assuming that the tablets are swallowed!).

While metformin is effective at reducing blood glucose levels in established T2D, it is becoming increasingly apparent that it may affect other CVD risk factors and may even have direct vascular effects. Its main action is to reduce hepatic gluconeogenesis (Hundal *et al.*, 2000) and also to increase peripheral insulin sensitivity, probably by disrupting respiratory chain oxidation in mitochondria (Kirpichnikov *et al.*, 2002). It also has beneficial effects on lipid metabolism (DeFronzo and Goodman, 1995) and decreases coaguability, probably by reducing PAI-1 levels (Charles *et al.*, 1998). In the UK Prospective Diabetes Study (UKPDS) metformin treatment was compared with conventional treatment in a subgroup of overweight diabetic patients. The incidence of myocardial infarction in the metformin group was reduced by 39%, which is more than would have been predicted by the difference in achieved HbA1c (0.6%). In addition, when the metformin group was compared with a group treated with sulphonylurea or insulin, to control for glycaemic control, there was still a significant reduction in incidence of stroke and any diabetes-related endpoint (UK Prospective Diabetes Study (UKPDS) Group, 1998). These results are supported by a cross-sectional study in which mortality rates were significantly reduced in patients on metformin monotherapy compared with sulphonylurea monotherapy (odds ratio 0.60, 95%CI 0.49–0.74) (Johnson *et al.*, 2002). In man, metformin does not appear to alter blood pressure (as it does in some animal models) (Dorella *et al.*, 1996), but there is some evidence in T2D patients for a modest improvement in vascular endothelial function (assessed by forearm plethysmography) after 3 months of metformin compared with placebo, although no attempt was made to control for glycaemia (Mather *et al.*, 2001).

Extrapolation from these data leads us to a serendipitous observation. Metformin may well reduce CVD risk in obese subjects with diabetes and pre-diabetes but by mechanisms that are largely unrelated to the reason for its initial development as a glucose-lowering agent. Of course, by delaying or preventing diabetes, it may have a double action in reducing CVD risk. Certainly, thus far, it shows excellent potential as an adjunct to healthy lifestyle in subjects at increased risk of both T2D and CVD.

Thiazolidinediones

In the TRIPOD study, 236 Hispanic women (mean age 35, BMI 30) with a previous history of gestational diabetes were randomised to receive either placebo or troglitazone. After a median follow-up of 30 months, the annual T2D incidence was 5.4% in the troglitazone group compared with 12.3% in the control group, representing a relative risk reduction of 56% (NNT = 15) (Buchanan *et al.*, 2002) While this is an impressive result, it is a small study in a single subgroup of the population and, in any case, troglitazone has now been withdrawn from clinical use due to serious hepatic side-effects.

The DREAM study tested whether either rosiglitazone or ramipril was superior to placebo in preventing T2D among over 5000 people with IGT and several hundred with IFG. The subjects were overweight with IGT and/or IFG and were followed for 3 years. A 2×2 study design was used, so that subjects could get both drugs, one drug + placebo or double placebo. No subject had evidence of CVD at baseline.

At the end of the study 11.6% of the individuals given rosiglitazone and 26.0% of the placebo group developed the composite primary outcome, which was diabetes or death. Treatment with rosiglitazone reduced the progression to diabetes by 60%, which is almost identical to the reductions seen in DPS and DPP (DREAM Trial Investigators, 2006a), but ramipril treatment did not significantly affect the progression to diabetes (DREAM Trial Investigators, 2006b). There was a significant incidence of cardiac failure with rosiglitazone, which is worrying in subjects who were free of CVD at baseline. Additionally, there was an average increase in weight of 2.2 kg, which is concerning given that the average BMI at baseline was over 30. The results at the end of the study were while the subjects were still taking rosiglitazone, which may have been masking the presence of diabetes rather than delaying the progression to diabetes.

The results when patients have been washed-out of drugs, as well as other important data such as changes in HbA1c and lipids, will be published at a later date. This study may also yield some valuable information about changes in CVD risk factors in pre-diabetes in response to glitazones, but was not powered to compare any differences in CVD event rates. There are increasing amounts of data – excellently summarised in a recent review (Diamant and Heine, 2003) – suggesting that thiazolidinediones have pleiotropic effects that may reduce CVD risk in addition to improving glucose regulation. As well as increasing insulin sensitivity and improving pancreatic beta-cell function, peroxisome proliferator activator receptor-gamma (PPAR-γ) agonists also exert anti-inflammatory effects, lower blood pressure, reduce the atherogenic lipid profile characteristic of the metabolic syndrome, alter body fat distribution and improve vascular endothelial function (Diamant and Heine, 2003). In the PROactive study in patients with T2D and established vascular disease, pioglitazone significantly reduced the main secondary endpoint, which was a composite of cardiovascular death, myocardial infarction and stroke. As expected, glycosylated haemoglobin (HbA1c) was reduced, and there were reductions in blood pressure, triglycerides and LDL-cholesterol and improvements in HDL-cholesterol (Dormandy *et al.*, 2005), but markers of inflammation were not measured. However, there is very little evidence for these effects outside the context of established T2D and many of the studies are small and not adequately controlled with respect to glycaemia. There is a need for good quality research using these drugs in subjects with pre-diabetes and the metabolic syndrome to demonstrate potential cardiovascular benefits over and above effects on glucose regulation.

Acarbose

In the STOP-NIDDM trial, 1429 subjects with IGT (mean age 55, BMI 31) were randomised to receive either an α-glucosidase inhibitor (100 mg of acarbose three times a day) or placebo over a mean follow-up of 3.3 years (Chiasson *et al.*, 2002). A relatively high proportion discontinued the trial early (211 on acarbose, 130 on placebo). Despite this, by 'intention to treat' analysis, there was a significant 25% relative risk reduction in the group assigned to acarbose (annual incidence 9.7% vs. 12.7% in placebo group; NNT = 33). Therefore, it appears that reducing postprandial glucose absorption can delay the progress from IGT to T2D. Whether this is related to blunting of overall glucose absorption, reduction of peak postprandial glucose levels or weight loss due to overall calorie reduction remains unclear. Unfortunately, outwith the context of a clinical trial, this drug class is often poorly tolerated and adherence rates tend to be low in patients with established T2D. This factor is likely to restrict its use in pre-diabetic subjects despite the positive evidence now available.

An *a priori* (but under-powered) secondary objective of the STOP-NIDDM study was to measure the development of cardiovascular events and hypertension (>140/90). Acarbose was associated with a 49% relative risk reduction ($P = 0.03$) in cardiovascular events (incidence over 3.3 years of 4.7% in placebo group vs. 2.2% in acarbose group), resulting in an NNT of 40 to prevent one cardiovascular event over 3.3 years (Figure 10.3) (Chiasson *et al.*, 2003) In addition, only 24% of the acarbose group developed hypertension during the follow-up period compared with 34% in the placebo group ($P = 0.006$), giving an NNT of 19 to prevent one case of hypertension over 3.3 years (Chiasson *et al.*, 2003). These results should be viewed with some caution. The original study was not powered for these secondary endpoints and event numbers were relatively small, raising the possibility of a chance observation during multiple testing. However, support for the potential of acarbose to reduce

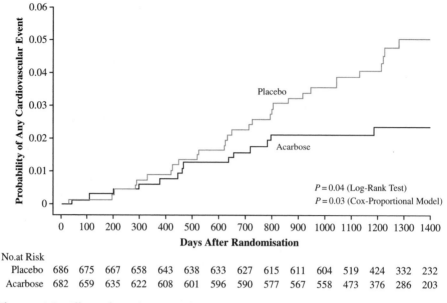

Figure 10.3 Effect of acarbose on the probability of remaining free of cardiovascular disease (coronary heart disease, cardiovascular death, congestive heart failure, cerebrovascular event and peripheral vascular disease). Reproduced from Chiasson JL, Josse RG, Gomis R, Hanefeld M, Karasik A, Laakso M. STOP-NIDDM Trial Research Group (2003). Acarbose treatment and the risk of cardiovascular disease and hypertension in patients with impaired glucose tolerance: the STOP-NIDDM trial. *Journal of the American Medical Association* **290**: 486–94.

CVD is seen in a meta-analysis of seven studies in patients with established T2D (Hanefeld *et al.*, 2004). Cardiovascular events occurred in 6.1% of those on acarbose and 9.4% of those on placebo (relative risk reduction of 35%). The effect remained significant after adjustment for weight, systolic blood pressure and triglycerides, but the magnitude of risk reduction after such adjustments was not given. It is debatable whether studies of acarbose could ever be regarded as double-blind, given the nature of the gastrointestinal side-effects. Again, whether the results reflect specific effects of postprandial glycaemia or generalised negative energy balance remains to be clarified.

Orlistat

In the XENDOS trial, 3305 obese subjects (mean age 44 years, BMI 37), 21% of whom had IGT, were randomised to receive either a gastrointestinal lipase inhibitor (120 mg of orlistat three times a day) or placebo for 4 years (Torgerson *et al.*, 2004). All subjects were given concomitant diet and exercise advice. There was a high dropout rate, although more subjects (52%) on orlistat completed the study than on placebo (34%), suggesting that successful weight loss outweighed potential gastrointestinal side-effects. In the whole group, the annual incidence of T2D was 2.3% on placebo and 1.6% on orlistat. While this represents a significant relative risk reduction of 37%, the low absolute risk reduction means that 142 subjects would have to be treated for 1 year to prevent one case of T2D. On further analysis, it was clear that most of the effect on

T2D prevention was in the 694 subjects with IGT, in whom annual incidence of T2D was 7.2% on placebo and 4.7% on orlistat, giving an equivalent NNT of 40. Mean weight loss was significantly greater with orlistat than placebo (5.8 kg vs. 3.0 kg).

In addition, orlistat treatment conferred significant improvements in a number of CVD risk factors and markers, including blood pressure, lipid profile, waist circumference and PAI-1 (Torgerson et al., 2004). As yet, no data have been published on CVD event rate in this trial. It seems likely that there will be insufficient power to demonstrate any difference, despite the large numbers of subjects recruited. Improvements in CVD risk are most likely related to weight loss, although there is an evolving literature on the importance of postprandial lipaemia in blunting of vascular endothelial function (Vogel et al., 1997; Marchesi et al., 2000; Gaenzer et al., 2001; Nappo et al., 2002; Van Oostrom et al., 2003).

Renin–angiotensin system blockade

The benefits of angiotensin-converting enzyme (ACE) inhibitors in the prevention of CVD and reduction of mortality have been clearly demonstrated (Yusuf et al., 2001; Fox et al., 2003). More recently, it has become apparent that angiotensin II blockers probably have similar effects (Dahlof et al., 2002; Pfeffer et al., 2003). A number of these large studies designed to assess the impact of such agents on CVD have also reported on the incidence of diabetes. The Captopril Prevention Project (CAPPP) involved 10 413 patients without biochemical evidence of diabetes, and compared captopril to beta-blockers and thiazides (Hansson et al., 1999). Those on captopril were 14% less likely to develop diabetes over the 6-year trial. The Heart Outcomes Prevention Evaluation (HOPE) study included 5720 individuals who were at high cardiovascular risk and had no self-reported diabetes (Yusuf et al., 2001). They were randomised to either placebo or ramipril (up to 10 mg per day), and there was a significant reduction of 34% in the incidence of self-reported type 2 diabetes over 4½ years (155 or 5.4% of the subjects on placebo vs. 102 or 3.6% of the subjects assigned to ramipril). The Losartan Intervention for Endpoint reduction study (LIFE) was a large programme designed to compare losartan and atenolol in hypertensive subjects with left ventricular hypertrophy (Dahlof et al., 2002). Over a mean follow-up of 4.8 years, 241 (6%) subjects on losartan and 319 (8%) on atenolol developed diabetes.

These studies carry the tantalising prospect that a group of drugs known to reduce CVD may also prevent diabetes. However, at this stage, it may be premature to draw such a conclusion. The evidence on diabetes prevention comes from studies where diabetes was not a primary endpoint, and in which biochemical diagnosis of glucose intolerance (both at study entry and trial completion) was incomplete. Furthermore, it is unclear whether the observed effects were due to the benefits of the agents themselves or to the withholding of alternative drugs known to increase the risk of diabetes. Both thiazides and beta-blockers have been associated with the development of T2D. In the only prospective trial that was performed with progression to diabetes as the primary endpoint, ramipril did not reduce progression to diabetes, although more subjects regressed to normoglycaemia (DREAM Trial Investigators, 2006b). The authors offered several possible explanations for the negative results, including the facts that subjects were free of vascular disease at baseline, so had little activation of the renin–angiotensin system, and that comparisons were made with placebo rather than a beta-blocker or diuretic.

The NAVIGATOR trial has recruited 7500 subjects with IGT who were randomised to valsartan (an angiotensin II blocker), nateglinide (a short-acting insulin secretagogue), dual therapy or placebo for a minimum duration of 3 years (NAVIGATOR Trial Steering Committee, 2002). It is powered to answer questions on reductions of CVD risk, and should establish whether or not prevention of type 2 diabetes merely reduces the risk of biochemical progression or actually cuts down on serious symptomatic disease. The results will also help to tease out whether it is the reduction in postprandial glycaemia *per se* that helps to delay or prevent T2D, since it is unlikely that the group taking nateglinide will lose weight.

10.4 Screening for Pre-diabetes

There are several good reasons why measurement of blood glucose can be used as an effective screening tool. Firstly, as described above, it can be helpful in predicting risk for two important and common diseases, T2D and CVD, and screening for pre-diabetes will inevitably identify a group of individuals with asymptomatic T2D. Secondly, the mechanisms by which hyperglycaemia is involved in the pathophysiology of these diseases are increasingly well understood, ensuring that the screening test is directly relevant to the disease process. Thirdly, pre-diabetes (and T2D itself) has a prolonged (asymptomatic) preclinical phase during which intervention strategies may be instituted. Fourthly, measurement of blood glucose is an acceptable, reliable and relatively cheap method of identifying this prolonged preclinical phase. Finally, as summarized above, there is now evidence that intervention in the preclinical phase (evidence base predominantly in middle-aged obese subjects with IGT) can delay or prevent disease, although the current evidence is predominantly for T2D rather than CVD.

However, trials have not yet been performed to determine whether or not a screening programme *per se* can reduce the incidence of or complications from T2D, and there is still no clear consensus on who should be screened and how often. Furthermore, a screening programme must be cost-effective but it is not yet known if the costs of earlier identification and intervention will be offset by future reductions in healthcare costs resulting from reduced morbidity and mortality from T2D and CVD. The ADA Position Statement on 'Prevention or Delay of Type 2 Diabetes' published in 2004 (American Diabetes Association, 2004b) concludes that 'men and women ≥ 45, particularly those with BMI ≥ 25, are candidates for screening to detect pre-diabetes (IFG or IGT)'. In addition, it is also acknowledged that screening should be considered in younger individuals with BMI ≥ 25 who have additional risk factors including first-degree relative with T2D, habitual physical inactivity, member of 'high risk' ethnic population, history of gestational diabetes, hypertensive, atherogenic lipid profile, history of vascular disease and history of polycystic ovary syndrome. It is proposed that re-screening at 3-year intervals 'is reasonable' in subjects with normoglycaemia, and that either fasting plasma glucose or 2-h post-glucose load level could be used as screening tools, with confirmatory measurements on a separate day (although fasting plasma glucose would be preferred from a resource viewpoint). If pre-diabetes is confirmed, it is suggested that monitoring for development of T2D should be performed every 1–2 years. While the Position Statement strongly backs the use of lifestyle intervention in pre-diabetes, it falls short of recommending pharmacological treatment, stating that there is insufficient evidence to support the cost-effectiveness of such an approach (this issue is discussed in more detail in previous sections).

While the cost-effectiveness of community screening has yet to be tested, it could be argued that this approach would serve to enhance public awareness about both T2D and CVD and help to encourage healthy living at a population level in terms of diet and exercise. From a commonsense standpoint, there is much to be said in support of population health initiatives with Government backing linked to positive incentives (e.g. cheaper healthy foods, free use of community leisure facilities), but this would require significant investment of time and resources in a relatively healthy generation in an attempt to prevent morbidity and mortality several decades in the future, a concept that is unlikely to be welcomed by politicians whose careers depend on being re-elected at 4-year intervals.

10.5 Summary and Conclusions

We are currently in the midst of a global epidemic of type 2 diabetes, which may well reverse the downward trend in CVD mortality seen in recent decades. The epidemic is being driven by the increasing prevalence of 'unhealthy lifestyle' involving a combination of obesity, physical inactivity and a diet high in saturated fat and refined carbohydrate. While established diabetes has long been regarded as an important cardiovascular risk factor, and hyperglycaemia has been shown to promote vascular dysfunction by a variety of mechanisms, there is increasing awareness that by the time a typical obese middle-aged subject is diagnosed with type 2 diabetes, he has already accrued significant cardiovascular risk in terms of hypertension, endothelial dysfunction, coagulopathy, atherogenic lipid profile and circulating pro-inflammatory adipocytokines. Indeed, there is now evidence that the overlapping conditions of pre-diabetes (encompassing both IFG and IGT) and the metabolic syndrome confer significant risk not only for development of diabetes but also of CVD. In recognition of the need to prevent these serious diseases, a number of trials have been designed to demonstrate delay or prevention of type 2 diabetes in high-risk groups (predominantly obese middle-aged subjects with IGT).

Convincing evidence has now been published for beneficial effects of intensive diet and exercise counselling as well as pharmacological agents such as metformin, rosiglitazone, acarbose and orlistat, although, as yet, the evidence that improvement of glucose dysregulation will translate into cardiovascular benefit is less robust. Interpretation of results from these diabetes prevention studies is complicated by the fact that both lifestyle and drug interventions have beneficial physiological effects not directly related to glucose handling, and it seems likely that they will prevent cardiovascular events more than would be expected by their effect on blood glucose alone. Now that effective interventions have been proven in the prolonged preclinical phase of these common diseases, there is a strong case for screening programmes to identify and target those at high risk. As yet, there is no clear consensus on screening criteria, partly because of the paucity of cost–benefit analyses in this area. However, common sense dictates that much would be gained by a population approach, warning of the future dangers of an unhealthy lifestyle and providing positive incentives for healthy eating and participation in regular physical activity. Governments must be persuaded of the importance of this approach to prevent widespread premature morbidity and mortality in future decades.

References

American Diabetes Association (2004a). Screening for type 2 diabetes. American Diabetes Association Position Statement. *Diabetes Care* **27**: S11–4.

American Diabetes Association (2004b). Prevention or delay of type 2 diabetes. American Diabetes Association Position Statement. *Diabetes Care* **27**: S47–54.

Andersson DKG, Svardsudd K (1995). Long-term glycemic control relates to mortality in type II diabetes. *Diabetes Care* **18**: 1534–43.

Buchanan TA, Xiang AH, Peters RK, Kjos SL, Marroquin A, Goico J, Ochoa C, Tan S, Berkowitz K, Hodis HN, Azen SP (2002). Preservation of pancreatic B-cell function and prevention of type 2 diabetes by pharmacological treatment of insulin resistance in high-risk Hispanic women. *Diabetes* **51**: 2796–803.

Ceriello A (2003). New insights on oxidative stress and diabetic complications may lead to a 'causal' antioxidant therapy. *Diabetes Care* **26:** 1589–96.

Charles MA, Morange P, Eschwege E, Andre P, Vague J, Juhan-Vague I (1998). Effect of weight change and metformin on fibrinolysis and vWF in obese nondiabetic subjects: the BIGPRO1 study. *Diabetes Care* **21:** 1967–72.

Chiasson JL, Josse RG, Gomis R, Hanefeld M, Karasik A, Laakso M for the STOP-NIDDM Trial Research Group (2002). Acarbose for prevention of type 2 diabetes mellitus: the STOP-NIDDM randomised trial. *Lancet* **359**: 2072–7.

Chiasson JL, Josse RG, Gomis R, Hanefeld M, Karasik A, Laakso M for the STOP-NIDDM Trial Research Group (2003). Acarbose treatment and the risk of cardiovascular disease and hypertension in patients with impaired glucose tolerance: the STOP-NIDDM trial. *Journal of the American Medical Association* **290**: 486–94.

Coutinho M, Gerstein HC, Wang Y, Yusuf S (1999). The relationship between glucose and incident cardiovascular events: a metaregression analysis of published data from 20 studies of 95,783 individuals followed for 12.4 years. *Diabetes Care* **22**: 233–40.

Dahlof B, Devereux RB, Kjeldsen SE, Julius S, Beevers G, de Faire U, Fyhrquist F, Ibsen H, Kristiansson K, Lederballe-Pedersen O, Lindholm LH, Nieminen MS, Omvik P, Oparil S, Wedel H for the LIFE Study Group (2002). Cardiovascular morbidity and mortality in the Losartan Intervention For Endpoint reduction in hypertension study (LIFE): a randomised trial against atenolol. *Lancet* **359:** 995–1003.

DECODE Study Group (1999). Glucose tolerance and mortality: comparison of WHO and American Diabetes Association diagnostic criteria. *Lancet* **354**: 617–21.

DeFronzo RA, Goodman AM (1995). Efficacy of metformin in patients with NIDDM – The Multicenter Metformin Study Group. *New England Journal of Medicine* **333**: 541–9.

Diabetes Prevention Program Research Group (2003). Within-trial cost-effectiveness of lifestyle intervention or metformin for the primary prevention of type 2 diabetes. *Diabetes Care* **26:** 2518–23.

Diamant M, Heine RJ (2003). Thiazolidinediones in type 2 diabetes mellitus: current clinical evidence. *Drugs* **63**: 1373–405.

Dorella M, Giusto M, Da Tos V, Campagnolo M, Palatini P, Rossi G, Ceolotto G, Felice M, Semplicini A, Del Prato S (1996). Improvement of insulin sensitivity by metformin treatment does not lower blood pressure of nonobese insulin-resistant hypertensive patients with normal glucose tolerance. *Journal of Clinical Endocrinology and Metabolism* **81:** 1568–74.

Dormandy JA, Charbonnel B, Eckland DJA, Erdmann E, Massi-Benedetti M, Moules IK *et al.* (2005). Secondary prevention of macrovascular events in patients with type 2 diabetes in the PROactive Study (PROspective pioglitAzone Clinical Trial In macroVascular Events): a randomised controlled trial. *Lancet* **366:** 1279–89.

DREAM Trial Investigators (2006a). Effect of rosiglitazone on the frequency of diabetes in patients with impaired glucose tolerance or impaired fasting glucose: a randomised trial. *Lancet* **368:** 1096–105.

DREAM Trial Investigators (2006b). Effect of ramipril on the incidence of diabetes. *New England Journal of Medicine* **355:** 1551–62.

Eriksson KF, Lindgarde F (1991). Prevention of type 2 (non-insulin-dependent) diabetes mellitus by diet and physical exercise: the 6-year Malmo feasibility study. *Diabetologia* **34:** 891–8.

Esposito K, Nappo F, Marfella R, Giugliano G, Giugliano F, Ciotola M, Quagliaro L, Ceriello A, Giugliano D (2002). Inflammatory cytokine concentrations are acutely increased by hyperglycemia in humans: role of oxidative stress. *Circulation* **106:** 2067–72.

Expert Committee on the Diagnosis and Classification of Diabetes Mellitus (1997). Report of the expert committee on the diagnosis and classification of diabetes mellitus. *Diabetes Care* **20**: 1183–97.

Fox KM for the EURopean trial On reduction of cardiac events with Perindopril in stable coronary Artery disease Investigators (2003). Efficacy of perindopril in reduction of cardiovascular events among patients with stable coronary artery disease: randomised, double-blind, placebo-controlled, multicentre trial (the EUROPA study). *Lancet* **362:** 782–8.

Gabir MM, Hanson RL, Dabelea D, Imperatore G, Roumain J, Bennett PH *et al.* (2000). The 1997 American Diabetes Association and 1999 World Health Organization criteria for hyperglycemia in the diagnosis and prediction of diabetes. *Diabetes Care* **23**: 1108–12.

Gaenzer H, Sturm W, Neumayr G *et al.* (2001). Pronounced postprandial lipemia impairs endothelium-dependent dilation of the brachial artery in men. *Cardiovascular Research* **52:** 509–16.

Giugliano D, Ceriello A, Paolisso G (1996). Oxidative stress and diabetic vascular complications. *Diabetes Care* **19:** 257–67.

Graier WF, Kostner GM (1997). Glycated low-density lipoprotein and atherogenesis: the missing link between diabetes mellitus and hypercholesterolaemia? *European Journal of Clinical Investigation* **27:** 457–9.

Hambrecht R, Wolf A, Gielen S *et al.* (2000). Effect of exercise on coronary endothelial function in patients with coronary artery disease. *New England Journal of Medicine* **342:** 454–60.

Hanefeld M, Cagatay M, Petrowitsch T, Neuser D, Petzinna D, Rupp M (2004). Acarbose reduces the risk for myocardial infarction in type 2 diabetic patients: meta-analysis of seven long-term studies. *European Heart Journal* **25:** 10–6.

Hansson L, Lindholm LH, Niskanen L *et al.* (1999). Effect of angiotensin-converting-enzyme inhibition compared with conventional therapy on cardiovascular morbidity and mortality in hypertension: The Captropril Prevention Project (CAPPP) randomised trial. *Lancet* **353:** 611–6.

Hogikyan RV, Galecki AT, Pitt B, Halter JB, Greene DA, Supiano MA (1998). Specific impairment of endothelium-dependent vasodilation in subjects with type 2 diabetes independent of obesity. *Journal of Clinical Endocrinology and Metabolism* **83:** 1946–52.

Hundal RS, Krssak M, Dufour S, Laurent D, Chandramouli V *et al.* (2000). Mechanism by which metformin reduces glucose production in type 2 diabetes. *Diabetes* **49:** 2063–9.

Johnson JA, Majumdar SR, Simpson SH, Toth EL (2002). Decreased mortality associated with the use of metformin compared with sulfonylurea monotherapy in type 2 diabetes. *Diabetes Care* **25:** 2244–8.

Kanaley JA, Weinstock RS (2001). Nonpharmacologic therapy in the treatment of insulin resistance. *Current Opinion in Endocrinology and Diabetes* **8**: 219–25.

Kirpichnikov D, McFarlane SI, Sowers JR (2002). Metformin: an update. *Annals of Internal Medicine* **137**: 25–33.

Knowler WC, Barrett-Connor E, Fowler SE, Hamman RF, Lachin JM, Walker EA *et al.* (2002). Reduction in the incidence of type 2 diabetes with lifestyle intervention or metformin. *New England Journal of Medicine* **346**: 393–403.

Kuusisto J, Mykkanen L, Pyorala K, Laakso M (1994). NIDDM and its metabolic control predict coronary heart disease in elderly subjects. *Diabetes* **43**: 960–7.

Lindstrom J, Ilanne-Parikka P, Peltonen M, Aunola S, Eriksson JG, Hemio K *et al.* (2006). Sustained reduction in the incidence of type 2 diabetes by lifestyle intervention: follow-up of the Finnish Diabetes prevention Study. *Lancet* **368**: 1673–9.

Marchesi S, Lupattelli G, Schillaci G *et al.* (2000). Impaired flow-mediated vasoactivity during post-prandial phase in young healthy men. *Atherosclerosis* **153**: 397–402.

Mather KJ, Verma S, Anderson TJ (2001). Improved endothelial function with metformin in type 2 diabetes mellitus. *Journal of the American College of Cardiology* **37**: 1344–50.

Moss SE, Klein R, Klein BEK, Meuer SM (1994). The association of glycemia and cause-specific mortality in a diabetic population. *Archives of Internal Medicine* **154**: 2473–9.

Nappo F, Esposito K, Cioffi M *et al.* (2002). Postprandial endothelial activation in healthy subjects and in type 2 diabetic patients: role of fat and carbohydrate meals. *Journal of the American College of Cardiology* **39**: 1145–50.

NAVIGATOR Trial Steering Committee (2002). Nateglinide and Valsartan in Impaired Glucose Tolerance Outcomes Research: rationale and design of the NAVIGATOR Trial. *Diabetes* **51** (suppl 2): A116.

Palmer AJ, Roze S, Valentine WJ, Spinas GA, Shaw JE, Zimmet PZ (2004). Intensive lifestyle changes or metformin in patients with impaired glucose tolerance: modeling the long-term health economic implications of the diabetes prevention program in Australia, France, Germany, Switzerland, and the United Kingdom. *Clinical Therapeutics* **26**: 304–21.

Pan XR, Li GW, Hu YH, Wang JX, Yang WY, An ZX, Hu ZX, Lin J, Xiao JZ, Cao HB, Liu PA, Jiang XG, Jiang YY, Wang JP, Zheng H, Zhang H, Bennett PH, Howard BV (1997). Effects of diet and exercise in preventing NIDDM in people with impaired glucose tolerance. The Da Qing IGT and Diabetes Study. *Diabetes Care* **20**: 537–44.

Pfeffer MA, Swedberg K, Granger CB, Held P, McMurray JJ, Michelson EL, Olofsson B, Ostergren J, Yusuf S, Pocock S for the CHARM Investigators and Committees (2003). Effects of candesartan on mortality and morbidity in patients with chronic heart failure: the CHARM-Overall programme. *Lancet* **362**: 759–66.

Pratley RE, Hagberg JM, Dengel DR *et al.* (2000). Aerobic exercise training-induced reductions in abdominal fat and glucose-stimulated insulin responses in middle-aged and older men. *Journal of the American Geriatrics Society* **48**: 1055–61.

Ryan AS (2000). Insulin resistance with aging: effects of diet and exercise. *Sports Medicine* **30**: 327–46.

Shaw J, Zimmet P, de Courten M, Dowse G, Chitson P, Gareeboo H *et al.* (1999). Impaired fasting glucose or impaired glucose tolerance. What best predicts future diabetes in Mauritius? *Diabetes Care* **22**: 399–402.

Stratton J, Chandler WL, Schwartz RS *et al.* (1991). Effects of physical conditioning on fibrinolytic variables and fibrinogen in young and old healthy adults. *Circulation* **83**: 1692–7.

Stratton IM, Adler AI, Neil HAW, Matthews DR, Manley SE, Cull CA, Hadden D, Turner RC, Holman RR on behalf of the UKPDS Group (2000). Association of glycaemia with macrovascular and microvascular complications of type 2 diabetes (UKPDS 35): prospective observational study. *British Medical Journal* **321**: 405–12.

Taniguchi A, Fukushima M, Sakai M *et al.* (2000). Effect of physical training on insulin sensitivity in Japanese type 2 diabetic patients. *Diabetes Care* **23:** 857–8.

Torgerson JS, Hauptman J, Boldrin MN, Sjostrom L (2004). XENical in the Prevention of Diabetes in Obese Subjects (XENDOS) Study: a randomized study of orlistat as an adjunct to lifestyle changes for the prevention of type 2 diabetes in obese patients. *Diabetes Care* **27:** 155–61.

Tuomilehto J, Lindstrom J, Eriksson JG, Valle TT, Hamalainen H, Ilanne-Parikka P *et al.* (2001). Prevention of type 2 diabetes mellitus by changes in lifestyle among subjects with impaired glucose tolerance. *New England Journal of Medicine* **344:** 1343–50.

UK Prospective Diabetes Study (UKPDS) Group (1998). Effect of intensive blood glucose control with metformin on complications in overweight patients with type 2 diabetes (UKPDS 34). *Lancet* **352:** 854–65.

Unwin N, Shaw J, Zimmet P, Alberti KGMM (2002). Impaired glucose tolerance and impaired fasting glycaemia: the current status on definition and intervention. *Diabetic Medicine* **19:** 708–23.

Van Oostrom AJ, Sijmonsma TP, Verseyden C *et al.* (2003). Postprandial recruitment of neutrophils may contribute to endothelial dysfunction. *Journal of Lipid Research* **44:** 576–83.

Vlassara H, Palace MR (2002). Diabetes and advanced glycation endproducts. *Journal of Internal Medicine* **251:** 87–101.

Vogel RA, Corretti MC, Plotnick GD (1997). Effect of a single high-fat meal on endothelial function in healthy subjects. *American Journal of Cardiology* **79:** 350–4.

Warner JG Jr, Brubaker PH, Zhu Y *et al.* (1995). Long-term (5-year) changes in HDL cholesterol in cardiac rehabilitation patients. Do sex differences exist? *Circulation* **92:** 773–7.

Williams SB, Cusco JA, Roddy M-A, Johnstone MT, Creager, MA (1996). Impaired nitric oxide-mediated vasodilation in patients with non-insulin-dependent diabetes mellitus. *Journal of the American College of Cardiology* **27:** 567–74.

Wojtaszewski JFP, Hansen BF, Gade J *et al.* (2000). Insulin signaling and insulin sensitivity after exercise in human skeletal muscle. *Diabetes* **49:** 325–31.

World Health Organization (1965). *Expert Committee on Diabetes Mellitus: First Report.* Technical Report Series 310. Geneva: World Health Organization.

Yusuf S, H Gerstein, B Hoogwerf *et al.* for the HOPE Study Investigators (2001). Ramipril and the development of diabetes. *Journal of the American Medical Association* **286:** 1882–5.

11 Diabetes for Cardiologists

David Macfarlane, Colin Perry and Miles Fisher

11.1 Introduction

We are in the midst of a worldwide epidemic of diabetes mellitus that appears to be driven largely by obesity and westernisation of diet and lifestyle. While there are clear associations between diabetes and the development of cardiovascular disease, individuals without diabetes *per se* but who have the clinical phenotype of insulin resistance also have an increased risk of developing cardiovascular disease (see Chapter 2). Recent changes in the diagnostic criteria for diabetes and the development of criteria for diagnosis of the metabolic syndrome have highlighted the extent of these metabolic abnormalities in both the developed and developing world. In this chapter we will briefly review the epidemiology of diabetes and the metabolic syndrome, and will discuss the criteria on which diagnostic categories are based in more detail. We will review the treatments of type 1 and type 2 diabetes, and discuss the evidence that supports the micro- and macrovascular benefits of good glycaemic control.

11.2 Epidemiology of Diabetes Mellitus

It has been estimated that there are approximately 150 million people with diabetes worldwide and that this number may rise to well over 200 million by the end of this decade (Figure 11.1) (Zimmet, 2000). The vast majority of these patients will have type 2 diabetes, which is characterised by resistance to insulin action in liver, skeletal muscle and fat, and is linked closely with obesity and a sedentary lifestyle (Chapter 2). The prevalence of type 2 diabetes (diagnosed and undiagnosed cases) in a recent UK study was estimated to be approximately 4% (Forouhi *et al.*, 2006), however the dramatic increase in the prevalence of diabetes in the developing world is of greater concern from a global and a public health perspective; in some Arab and Chinese communities where there has been rapid westernisation of diet and lifestyle, the prevalence of diabetes is between 14% and 20% (Hossain *et al.*, 2007).

Diabetic Cardiology Editors Miles Fisher and John J. McMurray
© 2007 John Wiley & Sons, Ltd.

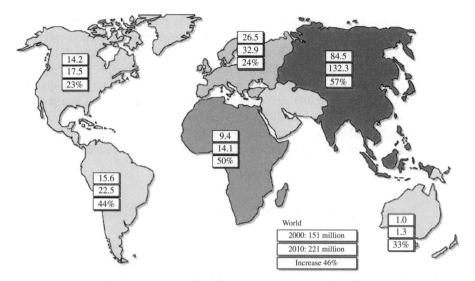

Figure 11.1 Numbers of people with diabetes in millions for 2000 and 2010 and the percentage increases. Reproduced from Zimmet P, Alberti KG, Shaw J (2001). Global and societal implications of the diabetes epidemic. *Nature* **414**: 782-7.

The prediction of these large increases in the prevalence of diabetes is based on observations suggesting that there may be as many as 200 million people worldwide with impaired glucose tolerance (Zimmet *et al.*, 2001), 30–40% of whom will go on to develop diabetes over the next 5–10 years. In addition, while type 2 diabetes has been traditionally thought of as a disease of older adults, and was previously termed 'maturity onset diabetes', there is an emerging epidemic of type 2 diabetes in young adults and even children. Recent population figures suggest an incidence of 0.53/100 000 new cases of type 2 diabetes per year in UK children under the age of 17 years (Haines *et al.*, 2007), while type 2 diabetes represents between 8% and 45% of all newly reported cases of diabetes in children and young adults (Ehtisham and Barrett, 2004).

The epidemiology of coronary heart disease in diabetes mellitus is described in detail in Chapter 1. People with diabetes have a higher prevalence of coronary heart disease (CHD), and those with no history of vascular disease are at increased risk of suffering a first vascular event earlier than those without diabetes. Twenty per cent of people with diabetes have evidence of cardiovascular disease at the time diabetes is diagnosed, and 65–75% of patients will eventually die from cardiovascular causes. From a cardiological perspective, one-quarter to one-third of patients with CHD will be previously diagnosed as having diabetes, and two-thirds of patients with acute coronary syndromes will have either diabetes or some form of impaired glycaemia if detailed testing is performed (Norhammar *et al.*, 2002).

Both the Framingham Heart Study (Kannel and McGee, 1979) and the Multiple Risk Factor Intervention Trial (MRFIT) (Stamler *et al.*, 1993) have demonstrated that diabetes is an independent cardiovascular risk factor with increases in age-adjusted prevalence and mortality from cardiovascular disease. Indeed, the National Cholesterol Education Programme (NCEP) considers that a diagnosis of diabetes is equivalent to the diagnosis of CHD; this assumption is based largely on data from a study by

Haffner (Haffner *et al.*, 1998), which suggested that in patients with type 2 diabetes and no history of cardiovascular disease the risk of myocardial infarction (MI) was comparable to that seen in patients without diabetes but with a previous MI. While subsequent studies have suggested that this may overestimate the CV risk in patients with diabetes (Evans *et al.*, 2002), there is no doubt that all patients with diabetes should have their cardiovascular risk carefully evaluated, and that there is a pressing need for better methods of risk stratification (Stephens *et al.*, 2004) that use data from large epidemiological studies containing high numbers of patients with diabetes, in order that those at greatest risk are targeted for the most aggressive lifestyle and pharmacological interventions.

11.3 New Diagnostic Criteria for Diabetes Mellitus

The diagnosis of diabetes is based on the risk in the longer term of developing microvascular complications such as retinopathy, nephropathy and neuropathy. It was apparent that some patients who did not fulfil the previous diagnostic criteria for diabetes were at risk of developing subsequent microvascular disease, while those diagnosed on the basis of fasting hyperglycaemia were not at equivalent risk of developing microvascular endpoints as those diagnosed on postprandial values. In 1997 the American Diabetes Association suggested lowering the diagnostic fasting glucose threshold from 7.8 to 7.0 mmol/l, and no longer suggested the use of the oral glucose tolerance test. Four years later, the World Health Organization, while endorsing the reduction in the fasting plasma glucose threshold, recommended retaining the oral glucose tolerance test, especially for further testing of subjects with a new diagnostic category of 'impaired fasting glucose' (6.1–6.9 mmol/l).

The reason for changing these criteria was based largely on observations of the significance of a fasting plasma glucose level of >7.8 mmol/l versus a postprandial glucose level of >11.1 mmol/l (the previous diagnostic thresholds). Furthermore, data from the Framingham offspring study have shown that there is a continuous relationship between fasting glucose and risk of subsequent development of cardiovascular disease, even at plasma glucose concentrations below the diagnostic range for diabetes. As such these new criteria were an attempt to better identify those at risk of developing micro- and macrovascular complications. This change in the criteria appears to have identified more young and obese patients as having diabetes. The additional category of impaired fasting glucose highlights those who are at risk of developing diabetes in the longer term and also those who have an elevated macrovascular risk. This diagnostic category has also been proposed as one of the criteria in the identification of patients who have the metabolic syndrome (see below). It is suggested that in patients with impaired fasting glucose, oral glucose tolerance testing continues to be undertaken as this may identify patients who satisfy the postprandial criteria for type 2 diabetes or impaired glucose tolerance, both of which are 'higher up' the diagnostic hierarchy than impaired fasting glucose.

Patients with impaired glucose tolerance are therefore at an increased risk of developing diabetes and of cardiovascular events. The effects on cardiovascular outcomes of interventions to reduce the development of diabetes in patients with impaired glucose tolerance are discussed in detail in Chapter 10.

Changes in nomenclature were also introduced. The previous categories of 'insulin-dependent' and 'non-insulin-dependent' diabetes have been discarded and replaced with 'type 1' and 'type 2' diabetes, which reflect disease aetiology rather than treatment. This is particularly relevant in light of the high number of patients (as many as 40% according to the United Kingdom Prospective Diabetes Study (UKPDS); Turner *et al.*, 1999) with type 2 diabetes who go on to require insulin as their disease progresses, although fundamentally they have a relative rather than an absolute insulin deficiency.

The impact of new diagnostic criteria on the prevalence of diabetes

Publications by the Diabetes Epidemiology Collaborative Analysis of Diagnostic Criteria in Europe (DECODE) study group have used the new criteria for the diagnosis of diabetes and applied them to European populations in an attempt to define the prevalence of all three diagnostic categories. In the UK, data from Newcastle have suggested a prevalence of diabetes of 17.1% and 13.9% in males and females, respectively, in the 60–69-year age range. The prevalence of diagnosed diabetes in these age groups, however, is recorded at 3.3%. Clearly the application of these new criteria will have a significant impact on the prevalence of diabetes. In the same population the prevalence of isolated impaired glucose tolerance was calculated as 7.9% in men and 8.5% in females. Isolated impaired fasting glucose was found in 13.8% of males and 10.6% of females. Across Europe, impaired glucose tolerance in 60–69-year-olds was identified in 8.1% of males and 11.1% of females, while isolated impaired fasting glucose was found in 8.9% of males and 4.7% of females. Type 2 diabetes, including undiagnosed cases, is anticipated to be present in 15.5% of males and 16.1% of females in this age range.

11.4 Metabolic Syndrome

Definition and classification

The association of insulin resistance, dysglycaemia, hypertension, obesity and dyslipidaemia was first described formally by Reaven in 1988 in his Banting lecture (Reaven, 1988). Since then this syndrome has been referred to as the 'insulin resistance syndrome' and the 'metabolic syndrome' as well as 'syndrome X'. More recently there have been attempts to assemble diagnostic criteria for what has become known as the 'metabolic syndrome' and apply these criteria to populations so that prevalence figures may be obtained. The World Health Organization (WHO) (World Health Organization, 1999), the National Cholesterol Education Programme (NCEP)/Adult Treatment Panel (ATP) III (NCEP/ATPIII, 2001) and the International Diabetes Federation (IDF) (Alberti *et al.*, 2006) have disseminated similar although not identical criteria that are based on the presence of several core metabolic and cardiovascular criteria such as hypertension, dyslipidaemia, obesity and elevation of either fasting insulin or fasting glucose (Table 11.1). Clearly the introduction of formal criteria for this syndrome has highlighted the extent to which cardiovascular risk factors coexist. It has also

Table 11.1 Definitions of the metabolic syndrome.

IDF 2005 (abdominal obesity plus two or more risk factors)	NCEP/ATPIII 2001 (at least three risk factors)	WHO 1999 (diabetes/impaired glucose tolerance/insulin resistance plus any two or more risk factors)
Waist circumference ≥ 90 cm (m), ≥ 80 cm (f)	Waist circumference ≥ 102 cm (m), ≥ 88 cm (f)	BMI $\geq 30\,kg/m^2$, and/or waist to hip ratio > 0.9 (m), 0.85 (f)
Blood pressure ≥ 130/ ≥ 85 mmHg	Blood pressure ≥ 130/ ≥ 85 mmHg	Blood pressure ≥ 140/ ≥ 90 mmHg, or on medication
Fasting glucose ≥ 5.6 mmol/l or pre-existing diabetes	Fasting glucose ≥ 6.1 mmol/l or on medication for diabetes	Diabetes, impaired glucose tolerance or insulin resistance
Triglycerides ≥ 1.7 mmol/l	Triglycerides ≥ 1.7 mmol/l	Triglycerides ≥ 1.7 mmol/l and/or HDL-cholesterol < 0.91 mmol/l (m), < 1.01 mmol/l (f)
HDL-cholesterol < 1.04 mmol/l (m) < 1.3 mmol/l (f)	HDL-cholesterol < 1.04 mmol/l (m) < 1.3 mmol/l (f)	Urinary albumin excretion rate ≥ 20 μg/min

shifted the focus from purely glycaemic control in the treatment of patients with type 2 diabetes to a more generalised approach in order to address treatment of cardiovascular risk factors with agents such as ACE inhibitors, statins and aspirin.

Prevalence of the metabolic syndrome

As is the case for the diagnosis of diabetes, the application of different diagnostic criteria for the metabolic syndrome results in differing figures of prevalence and the identification of different individuals. It is still too early to see how the new IDF definition of the metabolic syndrome will fare, but application of the NCEP/ATPIII and WHO diagnostic criteria to individuals aged > 20 years in the National Health and Nutritional Examination Survey (NHANES) cohort resulted in an age-adjusted prevalence of 23.9% and 25.1%, respectively. Particular differences were noted in the prevalence for certain subgroups, such as African-American males, in whom the WHO estimates were higher (Ford and Giles, 2003). An earlier study by the same authors, using the NCEP/ATPIII criteria, had estimated similar overall prevalence figures (though as high as 43.5% in the 60–69-year age group), and suggested that this translated to 47 million US residents using the 2000 census data (Ford *et al.*, 2002). It is also anticipated that the prevalence will continue to increase; in a recent publication from the US Centers for Disease Control and Prevention, the prevalence of the metabolic syndrome was compared between 1988–1994 and 1999–2000 using the NCEP definition. The age-adjusted prevalence was 24.1% in 1988–1994 and 27.0% in 1999–2000. The most striking figure was of a 23.5% increase in the prevalence in females across this time-frame, largely explained by increases in blood pressure, waist to hip ratio and hypertriglyceridaemia (Ford *et al.*, 2004).

The metabolic syndrome and cardiovascular risk

The DECODE study group have undertaken similar studies in the metabolic syndrome in an attempt to clarify its prevalence and also to define its relationship with cardiovascular mortality. Using a modification of the WHO definition of the metabolic syndrome and excluding patients with diabetes, the non-diabetic adult prevalence of metabolic syndrome in Europeans was found to be 15.7% in males and 14.2% in females. Over a median follow-up of 8.8 years the hazard ratio for all-cause and cardiovascular mortality was 1.44 and 2.26 in men and 1.38 and 2.78 in women, respectively, after adjustment for age, cholesterol and smoking status (Hu *et al.*,2004).

Interesting comparisons between the cardiovascular risk associated with the diagnosis of the metabolic syndrome have been made. While there is no doubt that the application of both sets of criteria identifies at-risk individuals, there remains debate about the best method of factoring insulin resistance as a discrete variable. Insulin resistance is best measured using the euglycaemic hyperinsulinaemic clamp, which is labour and time intensive. Clearly this is not suitable for inclusion as a key criterion in diagnostic criteria because it is only measured in certain specialised centres. The NCEP criteria include fasting plasma glucose ≥ 6.1 mmol/l, whereas the WHO criteria allow this or hyperinsulinaemia (fasting insulin in the upper quartile for patients without diabetes), which may mean that this favours the inclusion of patients who are insulin resistant. The application of the NCEP criteria to 443 individuals with formal measurements of insulin sensitivity identified only 46% of the most insulin-resistant tertile of individuals (Cheal *et al.*, 2004). Thus, many insulin-resistant individuals will not be identified using these criteria. The question of the importance of insulin resistance as an isolated cardiovascular risk factor remains as yet unanswered, however the results of the European Group for the study of Insulin Resistance Relationship between Insulin Resistance and Cardiovascular disease (EGIR/RISC) study, a Europe-wide prospective study of the relationship between insulin resistance (measured using the euglycaemic hyperinsulinaemic clamp) and development of atherosclerosis (measured by carotid intima medial thickness, will shed important light on this (Hills *et al.*, 2004).

In the last two years several senior diabetologists (Gale, 2005; Kahn *et al.*, 2005) have expressed concern about the clinical usefulness of the various definitions of the metabolic syndrome. There is strong epidemiological evidence to support the observation that these risk factors cluster together, however little progress has been made in determining the pathophysiological reason for this. While screening for and treating cardiovascular risk factors is now a cornerstone of modern medicine, it is less clear whether there is any benefit in considering these risk factors as part of a syndrome, certainly in terms of pharmacological management.

11.5 Treatment of Diabetes Mellitus

The benefits of good glycaemic control in type 1 diabetes

The landmark Diabetes Control and Complications Trial (DCCT), which reported in 1993, was the first large study to demonstrate that intensified glucose-lowering treatment in type 1 diabetes was associated with reduction in the development of microvascular endpoints (Diabetes Control and Complications Trial Research Group, 1993). While this had been assumed for many years previously, the findings of this study were extremely important in setting glycaemic targets and defining 'good' glycaemic control. The DCCT was designed to test the hypothesis that improved glycaemic control, as a result of intensified insulin therapy, would reduce the development of microvascular complications. The goal of the intensive therapy arm was to maintain blood glucose values as near to the non-diabetic range as possible and this was achieved using either multiple daily injections of subcutaneous insulin or treatment with a subcutaneous insulin pump. Conventional therapy consisted of one or two insulin injections per day. The mean duration of follow-up was 6.5 years. In the intensive therapy group the mean capillary blood glucose was 8.6 ± 1.7 mmol/l as against 12.8 ± 3.1 mmol/l in the conventional therapy group. In those without microvascular disease at the outset there was a 76% reduction in the adjusted mean risk for the development of retinopathy during follow-up in the group receiving intensified compared to conventional therapy. In the secondary intervention cohort, patients had microvascular disease at randomisation, and retinopathy, microalbuminuria and neuropathy were all shown to have a slower rate of progression in association with intensified insulin therapy. As the patients in this study were relatively young, the first report of the DCCT in 1993 was unable to demonstrate any change in the incidence or progression of macrovascular disease.

Following the DCCT, however, the Epidemiology of Diabetes Interventions and Complications (EDIC) trial has continued to study the patients who were initially included in the DCCT, although they are all now treated according to conventional guidelines and targets. Patients who were randomised to intensified insulin therapy in the DCCT underwent ultrasound of internal and common carotid arteries to measure intima medial thickness in 1994–1996 and again in 1999–2000. In patients who had received intensified therapy during the DCCT, progression of intima medial thickness was significantly less than in those who received conventional therapy (Nathan *et al.*, 2003). Subsequent analysis was of participants who were followed up for 17 years in total (11 years following discontinuation of the DCCT). At completion of the DCCT all participants were offered intensive insulin therapy (given the benefits that were noted in the intensively treated group) and so, not surprisingly, 11 years later there was very little difference in the mean HbA1c between the groups originally assigned to intensive or conventional therapy (mean HbA1c $7.9\% \pm 1.3$ vs. $7.8\% \pm 1.3$, respectively). Lower albumin excretion, total cholesterol and triglycerides did persist in the group that originally received intensive therapy. At the 17-year follow-up, this group had a 42% (95% CI 9–63%) relative risk reduction in a composite endpoint of cardiovascular mortality, non-fatal MI, silent MI, coronary revascularisation, angina and stroke (Diabetes Control and Complications Trial/Epidemiology of Diabetes Interventions and Complications (DCCT/EDIC) Study Research Group, 2005). This translated to a number needed to treat to prevent one event of 23 (95% CI 12–352). Thus a period of improved metabolic control 11 years earlier seemed to reduce the risk of macrovascular disease. This has raised the concept of 'metabolic memory' in which there may be a residual risk attached to a previous period of poor control, despite there being a subsequent improvement, and has prompted others to consider that even more aggressive management in young patients with type 1 diabetes may be appropriate (Gerstein, 2006).

Achieving good glycaemic control: risks and side-effects

In the DCCT patients randomised to intensified insulin therapy had treatment regimes based either on a basal bolus regime of insulin, consisting of one or two long-acting insulin injections in combination with short-acting insulin injections at mealtimes, or the use of a continuous subcutaneous infusion of insulin. Pump devices delivering continuous insulin infusions have been more popular in the USA than in Europe, presumably as a result of these findings in the DCCT, however they remain expensive and suitable only for patients who are highly motivated. Even basal bolus therapy requires a considerable amount of effort from patients to achieve good diabetic control. Table 11.2 outlines the main insulin regimens that are currently used in the treatment of type 1 and 2 diabetes. The fundamental problems of insulin delivery (i.e. that insulin is injected subcutaneously and absorbed into the

Table 11.2 Common insulin regimes.

	Basal bolus regime	Twice-daily premixed insulin	Once-daily insulin
Description	Consists of soluble human insulin or rapid-acting analogue with meals and long-acting human insulin or analogue at night	Consists of two (or occasionally three) premixed insulin injections, usually at breakfast and dinner	Insulin injected only once daily. Only suitable in patients with type 2 diabetes
Advantages and disadvantages	Offers flexibility and the most physiological approach to insulin delivery, however requires good compliance and commitment in order to achieve good control	Twice-daily regime may improve compliance, however it is inflexible and difficult to achieve tight glycaemic control. Difficult to control fasting blood glucose without risk of overnight hypoglycaemia	Once-daily regime that may offer adequate control of symptoms in the elderly and is easy to administer. Unlikely to achieve good glycaemic control and is very inflexible
Example	Insulin Aspart or Lispro with meals, insulin Glargine or Detemir at night	Twice-daily Humalog Mix 25/Novomix 30	Once-daily Insulatard or Glargine

systemic rather than portal circulation over a prolonged period) have limited our ability to achieve improved glycaemic targets. Improved glycaemic control with minimisation of side-effects must be the fundamental goal of all novel glucose-lowering strategies. The main important side-effects of insulin therapy are weight gain and hypoglycaemia.

Weight gain and improved glycaemic control

Weight gain is associated with improved glycaemic control, and is a complication of therapy with both insulin and oral insulin secretagogues, such as the sulphonylureas. This is a major problem when considered in terms of the poor compliance with medication that is known to be prevalent in patients with diabetes (Morris *et al.*, 1997). Often weight gain following improved glycaemic control is a reflection of the previous poor glycaemic control and associated weight loss, secondary to the catabolism of adipose tissue and protein, however this is seen by many patients as a major disadvantage of the treatment of diabetes, particularly in the young. In the main DCCT study, intensified therapy was associated with an increase in the risk of becoming overweight, and at 5 years the mean weight gain was 4.6 kg greater in those receiving intensified than conventional therapy. In an ancillary study of the DCCT, it was observed that patients who gained most weight on the intensified treatment arm had associated blood pressure and circulating lipid changes that worsened the cardiovascular risk profile and were greater than those seen in the patients randomised to conventional control who also gained weight (Purnell *et al.*, 1998). These observations have given rise to the notion that while improved glycaemic control undoubtedly reduces microvascular risk, the effects on macrovascular risk remain less clear and detailed analysis of the DCCT/EDIC cardiovascular endpoints with regard to changes in other cardiovascular risk factors is keenly awaited.

11.6   Hypoglycaemia

Most patients with insulin-treated diabetes will say that their greatest short-term fear is of hypoglycaemia. Unfortunately, improved glycaemic control is associated with an increased risk of hypoglycaemia. In the DCCT, all subjects were asked about hypoglycaemic effects throughout the mean 6.5-year follow-up period. The rates of severe hypoglycaemia in the intensified group were 61.2 per 100 patient-years vs. 18.7 per 100 patient-years in the conventional group (relative risk 3.28). The greatest predictors of hypoglycaemia were a past history of hypoglycaemia and a lower level of HbA1c (Diabetes Control and Complications Trial Research Group, 1997). The reason for the increase in hypoglycaemia associated with insulin regimes that are as close to physiological as practicable reflect the differences between administered and secreted insulin. Whereas in healthy individuals the ingestion of a meal is associated with a short-lived burst of pancreatic insulin secretion, patients with diabetes who are treated with subcutaneous human soluble insulin injected (as recommended) 30 min before a meal will have a non-physiological elevation in circulating insulin some hours after they have stopped eating. Thus there is the risk of hypoglycaemia when approaching the preprandial state, accentuated by the fact that this is often when exercise is undertaken. Similarly, following a 10 p.m. injection of subcutaneous isophane insulin (e.g. Insulatard), there will be a peak of insulin action in the middle of the night, when anti-insulins such as cortisol and growth hormone are at their nadir, often resulting in nocturnal hypoglycaemia and morning (rebound) hyperglycaemia. It has been suggested that the use of the newer insulin analogues may reduce the risk of hypoglycaemia (Bolli *et al.*, 1999). Rapid-acting analogues have a short duration of action, reducing late hypoglycaemia, while long-acting analogues such as insulin Glargine and Detemir have smoother profiles that may reduce peaks and troughs of insulin action and in particular reduce overnight hypoglycaemia.

Cardiovascular effects of hypoglycaemia

The counter-regulatory response to hypoglycaemia includes activation of the autonomic nervous system and the release of large amounts of adrenaline. In a healthy individual there is an increase in heart rate (although this is rarely above 100 beats per minute), widening of the pulse pressure and an increase in cardiac output. In a patient with CHD this profound autonomic activation may have serious consequences, and there are several case reports of provocation of angina, MI and arrhythmias such as atrial fibrillation. Indeed, it is surprising that there are not more documented cardiovascular consequences of hypoglycaemia, and this may be because of a failure to consider hypoglycaemia as a precipitant of an acute event, and the difficulties of confirming hypoglycaemia at postmortem because of continuing changes in blood glucose following death.

There is a well-described, but poorly understood, syndrome of sudden death seen in young patients with type 1 diabetes, often referred to as the 'dead in bed' syndrome. In 1991, a series of 22 sudden deaths in young patients with type 1 diabetes was published (Tattersall and Gill, 1991). These were characterised by sudden unexpected death and were not thought to be associated with seizure activity. Several other groups have gone on to describe similar findings in such patients (Sartor and Dahlquist, 1995; Thordarson and Sovik, 1995). Clearly hypoglycaemia is a strong candidate as a provoking factor, and there is considerable speculation as to the precise mechanism. It has been proposed that hypoglycaemia is associated with abnormalities of cardiac repolarisation, often detected in the clinical setting as lengthening of the corrected QT interval and an increase in QT dispersion. These abnormalities, which predispose to potentially fatal arrhythmias, may occur as a result of sympatho-adrenal activation, perhaps causing catecholamine-mediated stimulation of the myocardium, or reductions in serum potassium secondary to the release of adrenaline. Other potential causes of sudden death, such as undiagnosed coronary artery disease, non-hypoglycaemic arrhythmias and severe hypoglycaemia, have also been implicated. With the falling number of postmortem examinations and the relative rarity of these events, it may be some time before the true mechanism(s) underlying these events is elucidated.

11.7 Treatment of Type 2 Diabetes

In the past decade there has been a significant increase in the number of drugs available to treat type 2 diabetes, and several different types of oral anti-diabetic agents are now currently available. They can be classified according to their mechanism of action as those that: increase insulin secretion, e.g. *sulphonylureas* and *meglitinide analogues*; reduce insulin resistance, e.g. *metformin* and *the thiazolidinediones (TZDs)*; and delay absorption of glucose, e.g. α-*glucosidase inhibitors* (Bailey and Day, 2003). With the exception of the α-glucosidase inhibitors and the meglitinide analogue nateglinide, all of the above medications have a similar efficacy in improving glycaemic control: reducing glycosylated HbA1c by 1–2%.

Sulphonylureas

In the presence of glucose, sulphonylureas (SUs) act to close potassium ATPase channels in pancreatic beta cells, leading to depolarisation and insulin secretion (Kennedy *et al.*, 1988; Ashcroft and Rorsman, 1989). Their efficacy is therefore dependent on sufficient beta-cell function, which, given the progressive nature of the disease, tends to reduce with time leading to beta-cell failure, which has previously been misleadingly referred to as 'SU failure' (Matthews *et al.*, 1998).

The first generation of SUs included tolbutamide and chlorpropamide, and these were later followed by newer second-generation SUs in the 1970s and 1980s, such as glibenclamide and gliclazide (Kennedy *et al.*, 1988; Gerich, 1989). As described above, troublesome side-effects of SUs include weight gain (on average 1–4 kg) and hypoglycaemia, the latter occurring more frequently with the longer acting SUs, e.g. glibenclamide (Rendell, 2004). They do not lead to an improvement in blood pressure and have no consistent effect on lipids (Bailey and Day, 2003).

The UK Prospective Diabetes Study (UKPDS) was a landmark trial examining the effects of tight glycaemic control on macrovascular and microvascular disease in 4209 patients recently diagnosed with type 2 diabetes (UK Prospective Diabetes Study (UKPDS) Group, 1998a). After a 3-month run-in period, patients were randomised to either conventional therapy (diet/exercise) versus intensive therapy with oral anti-diabetic agents or insulin. Follow-up was for a mean of 10 years. In the cohort randomised to intensive therapy with SUs (chlorpropamide, glibenclamide or glipizide) there was a significant reduction in the incidence of retinopathy, micoalbuminuria and peripheral neuropathy. However, despite a trend towards a 16% reduction in fatal and non-fatal MI, this was not statistically significant ($P = 0.052$). Review of the epidemiological data suggests that a fall in HbA1c should be associated with less macrovascular disease, and this has led some to speculate that the benefits of improved glycaemic control may be partially offset by the negative cardiovascular effects of the oral agents used in the management of type 2 diabetes (Stratton *et al.*, 2000).

In particular, though still controversially, it has been proposed that patients receiving treatment with SUs are at increased risk of macrovascular disease as suggested in the University Group Diabetes Project in patients receiving tolbutamide therapy (Goldner *et al.*, 1971). One explanation for this is the non-selective effect of first- and second-generation SUs on pancreatic and cardiac K-ATPase channels. It is hypothesised that inhibition of cardiac K-ATPase channels prevents opening of these channels, blocking calcium influx and so preventing 'ischaemic preconditioning' where the myocardium is protected from ischaemic reperfusion injury via prior brief exposure to sublethal ischaemia (Nichols *et al.*, 1991; Gross and Auchampach, 1992; Toombs *et al.*, 1993). There is also a proposed protective effect on mitochondria through shortening of the cardiac action potential. Glimepiride, a third-generation SU, has a greater selectivity for pancreatic K-ATPase channels, but whether this selectivity leads to improvements in cardiovascular risk is not known (Langtry and Balfour, 1998).

Meglitinide analogues

Also known as 'non-SU secretagogues' or 'postprandial glucose regulators', the first meglitinide analogue repaglinide was developed from the non-SU portion of glibenclamide and introduced in the UK in 1998. It was followed later by nateglinide, a derivative of D-phenylalanine. They have a similar mechanism of action to SUs in closing K-ATPase channels in pancreatic beta cells, and the side-effect profiles are also similar (Dornhorst, 2001). Their effects on ATP-dependent potassium channels in the myocardium are largely untested. Postprandial hyperglycaemia is reduced in a dose-related manner, but their effect on fasting glycaemia is less pronounced than with the SUs (Rosenstock *et al.*, 2004). Their place in the management of type 2 diabetes is unclear and there is as yet no published evidence that the use of these agents leads to improvements in cardiovascular outcomes. In the UK the license for nateglinide is limited, and it can only be prescribed in combination with metformin.

The NAVIGATOR (Nateglinide and Valsartan in Impaired Glucose Tolerance Outcomes Research) study is a multinational, randomised, double-blind, placebo-controlled, forced-titration, 2×2 factorial design trial involving around 7500 patients with impaired glucose tolerance, aged greater than 50 years. It is currently under way to assess whether treatment with either nateglinide or valsartan can prevent the development of type 2 diabetes and/or reduce the risk of developing cardiovascular disease, and is due to report in 2008.

Metformin

The mode of action of metformin, the only available biguanide, is complex and not fully understood, but its principal antihyperglycaemic effect is thought to be reduction of hepatic gluconeogenesis, as a result of increased hepatic insulin sensitivity. It is dependent on the presence of circulating insulin and adequate beta-cell function. Unless combined with SUs, metformin is unlikely to cause severe hypoglycaemia as it is an 'insulin sensitiser' and does not stimulate insulin secretion (Bailey and Turner, 1996). In fact, metformin leads to a reduction in hyperinsulinaemia, a factor proposed to be involved in the pathogenesis of macrovascular disease (Ruige *et al.*, 1998) (see Chapter 2).

Metformin is the first-line oral anti-diabetic agent in the obese because, unlike the SUs, it does not lead to significant weight gain (Hermann *et al.*, 1994). Given the risk of lactic acidosis, metformin is contraindicated in congestive cardiac failure, renal failure, liver disease, patients undergoing general anaesthesia and suspected tissue hypoxia (MI, sepsis). It has also been advised that it should be withheld in those receiving contrast media, e.g. coronary angiography, although there is no evidence of a harmful effect. From a practical point of view metformin should be discontinued in the short term in patients presenting with acute coronary syndromes. If the patient subsequently shows no signs of shock, heart failure or renal impairment then metformin can be cautiously re-introduced.

In the UKPDS a cohort of 342 obese patients were randomised to monotherapy with metformin (UK Prospective Diabetes Study (UKPDS) Group, 1998b). In addition to the similar improvements in microvascular disease as those receiving intensive therapy with insulin or SU, those receiving metformin had a significant reduction in macrovascular disease, including MI and stroke. This reduced risk could not be explained by improved glycaemic control alone, as HbA1c levels were similar between the different treatment groups. Furthermore, the effect was not seen in those on combination therapy with metformin and SU. A 32% risk reduction was demonstrated for any diabetes-related endpoint ($P = 0.002$), with a 39% risk reduction for MI ($P = 0.01$) and a 36% reduction in all-cause mortality ($P = 0.011$) in those receiving metformin monotherapy.

Other benefits of metformin, which may contribute to its cardiovascular effects, include stabilisation of weight, improvement in lipid profile, increased fibrinolysis and reduced plasminogen activator inhibitor-1 (PAI-1) (Grant et al., 1991). Classically patients with type 2 diabetes and the metabolic syndrome have high triglycerides, high LDL-cholesterol and low HDL-cholesterol, and metformin may improve all of these parameters (Buse et al., 2004), as well as having a beneficial effect on endothelial dysfunction (Mather et al., 2001), a factor closely linked to the development of atherosclerosis . These findings, and in particular the reduction in MIs, have led to an increase in the use of metformin as first-line treatment in non-obese patents with type 2 diabetes.

Thiazolidinediones

Thiazolidinediones (TZDs) are also known as peroxisome proliferator activated receptor-gamma (PPAR-γ) agonists after the nuclear receptor strongly expressed in adipose tissue on which they exert their effect. They improve insulin sensitivity by increasing transcription of various insulin-sensitive genes, including those encoding lipoprotein lipase, GLUT 4 and fatty acid transport protein. As a result of this mechanism of action, their maximal antihyperglycaemic effect can take up to 3 months (Yki-Jarvinen, 2004; Boden and Zhang, 2006).

The first TZD – troglitazone – was withdrawn due to reports of hepatotoxicity (Murphy et al., 2000). In retrospect this may have been related to a vitamin E part of the compound, as the newer drugs pioglitazone and rosiglitazone appear to have a much safer side-effect profile, with current guidance recommending that liver function is tested at baseline and intermittently thereafter. The main side-effect of the PPAR-γ agonists is fluid retention. This can lead to significant weight gain, a dilutional anaemia and obvious problems with fluid overload in patients with heart failure, in whom they are contraindicated (Higgs and Krentz, 2004).

A recent meta-analysis of randomised controlled trials involving TZDs showed that while the TZDs currently available have similar effects on glycaemic control, they have differing outcomes on lipid profiles. Pioglitazone had a neutral or beneficial effect on lipids whereas, interestingly, rosiglitazone appeared to have more complex effects and potentially less beneficial effects with an associated increase in both LDL-cholesterol and total cholesterol and a neutral effect on TGs. Both drugs increased levels of HDL-cholesterol. Both drugs cause a modest but significant reduction in systolic and diastolic blood pressure (Chiquette *et al.*, 2004; Derosa *et al.*, 2004).

As described in Chapter 2, insulin resistance, endothelial dysfunction and chronic inflammation appear to be closely related in the pathogenesis of atherosclerosis. The TZDs exert a number of complex metabolic effects in addition to the effects on lipids described above and, like metformin, reduce insulin resistance. Initial studies showed an improvement in endothelial dysfunction, with associated reduction in microalbuminuria – a known marker of cardiovascular risk. Furthermore, they have shown regression of intima media thickness of carotid arteries measured by ultrasound. This is proposed to be via a reduction in vascular smooth-muscle cell growth and intimal hyperplasia. In relation to this, the TZDs appear to have a number of anti-atherosclerotic properties, including reduction in CRP, PAI-1, TNF-α and reactive oxygen species, which makes them attractive candidates to improve macrovascular disease (Nesto, 2004).

PROactive (Prospective pioglitazone Clinical Trial in Macrovascular Events) (Dormandy *et al.*, 2005) was a large multicentre European randomised, placebo-controlled outcome trial of over 5000 patients with type 2 diabetes and known cardiovascular disease, assessing the affect of pioglitazone on macrovascular mortality and morbidity. In this high-risk study population, already on modern secondary prevention agents, a forced dose titration of pioglitazone or placebo was used as 'add on' therapy to current treatment regimes (including insulin in one-third of patients), which could be optimised throughout the course of the trial to ensure best possible glycaemic control. Mean follow-up was 34.5 months, and an HbA1c reduction of 0.5% ($P < 0.001$) was achieved versus placebo. A 10% reduction in the primary composite endpoint was observed, although this failed to reach statistical significance ($P = 0.095$). However, a significant reduction in the prespecified secondary composite endpoint of all-cause mortality, non-fatal MI and stroke was observed (hazard ratio 0.84, 95% CI 0.72–0.98, $P = 0.027$). Despite an increased number of admissions for suspected heart failure in the pioglitazone group, no differences in mortality rates from heart failure were observed between the treatment groups.

ADOPT (A Diabetes Outcome Progression Trial) (Kahn *et al.*, 2006) was a randomised, double-blind, parallel group study of more than 4000 drug-naive patients with recently diagnosed type 2 diabetes (within 3 years), comparing rosiglitazone, metformin or glibenclamide and examining time to treatment failure (plasma glucose $\geq$ 10 mmol/l after an overnight fast). The study was designed prior to the standardisation of glycosylated haemoglobin assays, when treatment targets were based on fasting glucose measurements. Rosiglitazone therapy was associated with a lower risk of monotherapy failure than metformin or glibenclamide. There was a high overall drop-out rate in the study but there was no difference between treatment arms. In terms of secondary endpoints, there was a significant increase in weight gain in the rosiglitazone group (mean increase of 4.8 kg) versus a fall of 2.9 kg in the metformin group over the median 4.4 years of follow-up. These results have been interpreted as demonstrating that rosiglitazone is an effective first-line agent in the treatment of type 2 diabetes, though at a greater cost than metformin and at the expense of weight gain, leaving metformin as the initial treatment of choice in type 2 diabetes (Nathan, 2006).

The RECORD (Rosiglitazone Evaluated for Cardiac Outcomes and Regulation of Glycaemia in Diabetes) (Home *et al.*, 2005) study is looking at just under 4000 patients with established type 2 diabetes to examine cardiac outcomes in patients treated with combination therapy of either metformin plus SU, or rosiglitazone in combination with metformin or SU.

Acarbose

Acarbose, introduced in the early 1990s, is the only α-glucosidase inhibitor currently licensed for use in the UK. A wider range is available in Europe and the USA. They delay the absorption of glucose by inhibiting brush-border enzymes in the small intestine, which act to cleave oligo- and disaccharides. Unfortunately, their clinical use is limited by troublesome gastrointestinal side-effects that result from increased delivery of oligosaccharides to the large intestine, where they undergo fermentation by commensal bacteria leading to flatulence, diarrhoea and abdominal discomfort. These side-effects may be limited to an extent by dose titration and a diet high in complex carbohydrate. Acarbose is unlikely to cause hypoglycaemia as a monotherapy, but if used in combination with other oral anti-diabetic agents it should be noted that if hypoglycaemia occurs then the correcting substrate should initially be glucose and not sucrose (a disaccharide).

STOP-NIDDM (Chiasson *et al.*, 2003) was a large multicentre, double-blind, placebo-controlled trial of acarbose versus placebo of 1429 men and women with impaired glucose tolerance. Mean follow-up was 3.3 years. The primary endpoint was a reduction in the number of patients developing type 2 diabetes as diagnosed by the oral glucose tolerance test, and secondary endpoints looked at cardiovascular risk. Despite 211 and 130 patients discontinuing treatment in the acarbose and placebo groups, respectively, analysis by intention to treat and adjustment for major risk factors led to statistically significant reductions in the risk of cardiovascular disease ($P = 0.02$) and hypertension ($P = 0.004$). Treatment with acarbose led to a 49% relative risk ($P = 0.03$) and 2.5% absolute risk reduction in the development of cardiovascular events. This trial also achieved its primary endpoint of a reduction in the progression to type 2 diabetes in the group receiving acarbose, and this is discussed in greater detail in Chapter 10.

Insulin-sensitising agents and cardiac failure (see also Chapter 5)

There are concerns about the safety of both metformin and the TZDs in patients with type 2 diabetes and heart failure, a group of patients who would seem to benefit from insulin sensitisation due to their established vascular disease and insulin resistance, exacerbated by the neurohumoral activation seen in cardiac failure. Because of the benefits of metformin seen in the UKPDS, the previously accepted contraindications to metformin use have come under scrutiny. The historical concern regarding biguanides and lactic acidosis was based largely upon data from phenformin therapy. Mechanistically, the two drugs have differing effects on lactic acid metabolism, while plasma metformin levels do not correlate with lactate levels. In large observational studies, it is very hard to separate the effects of metformin from the effects of acute illness that may have precipitated lactic acidosis, such as renal failure, cardiac failure and liver failure. Despite this, data from Brown and colleagues are certainly reassuring in that in 41 000 patient-years of therapy with metformin, they found no increase in the incidence of lactic acidosis compared to the period prior to its availability (Brown *et al.*, 1998). A subsequent meta-analysis suggested the incidence of lactic acidosis to be 9.9 per 100 000 patient-years in those not taking metformin and 8.1 per 100 000 patient-years for those receiving metformin (Salpeter *et al.*, 2003). Of the few cases that did develop, increasing age and renal impairment appear to increase the risk. Recent data in fact suggest that there may be a beneficial role of metformin therapy in heart failure (Salpeter *et al.*, 2003; Eurich *et al.*, 2005). Eurich showed that in 1833 patients with type 2 diabetes on oral therapy who developed heart failure, rates were higher in the group receiving SUs alone than metformin alone or metformin and SU in combination. As discussed earlier, since the University Group Diabetes Project there have been unanswered questions concerning the cardiovascular safety of SUs and these data may be confounded by this potential interaction.

As discussed earlier, with the increasing use of the TZD class of oral agents in type 2 diabetes, it has become apparent that they are associated with fluid retention and so may precipitate cardiac failure. Patients with NYHA class III and IV cardiac failure were excluded from pioglitazone and rosiglitazone clinical trials, and so these drugs should not be prescribed in this patient group. More debate has centred upon the use of these drugs in patients with mild cardiac failure, and the identification of asymptomatic patients who may be at risk of developing cardiac failure when prescribed these drugs.

In 2004, the American Heart Association and American Diabetes Association published a consensus statement on the use of TZDs, fluid retention and congestive heart failure. It was suggested that prior to introducing a TZD, consideration is given to previous cardiac history, a history of exertional dyspnoea, presence of oedema and any electrocardiograph changes that may represent undiagnosed cardiac disease. It was suggested that patients are encouraged to report increasing weight, oedema and shortness of breath once therapy is commenced. Although not licensed in Europe, combination therapy of TZDs with insulin may provoke more oedema and weight gain. In patients with cardiac risk factors, asymptomatic abnormalities of cardiac function or NYHA class I/II heart failure, TZDs should be initiated with caution at a low dose. Patients with NYHA grade III/IV heart failure should receive a TZD. Once on therapy, patients should be monitored for weight gain and oedema. If they develop oedema, assessment for other signs of cardiac failure, and investigation if appropriate, should be undertaken. If a new diagnosis of heart failure is established, the use of TZDs in that patient should be reviewed (Nesto *et al.*, 2004).

Since this statement, both the PROactive and ADOPT studies have reported and offered additional information on the relationship between TZDs and cardiac failure. In the ADOPT study, while there was a significant increase in the hazard ratio of investigator-reported heart failure in the rosiglitazone versus the glyburide group, there was no difference between rosiglitazone and metformin. In the PROactive study, while there was an increase in reported heart failure versus placebo, there was no increase in deaths from heart failure, suggesting that the heart failure was relatively easily managed.

When these results are considered in the context of the findings of a large observational study of over 16 000 patients with a principal discharge diagnosis of heart failure, in which there was a reduced mortality (hazard ratio 0.87; 95% CI 0.80–0.94) in those prescribed TZDs, it is clear that large, well-designed, prospective trials are necessary to address this issue properly (Macfarlane and Fisher, 2006).

Novel agents in the treatment of type 2 diabetes

Following many years of having little therapeutic choice in the treatment of type 2 diabetes, it appears that there are an increasing number of agents that will become available to treat hyperglycaemia in the very near future. While the development of PPAR agents that act at the delta and alpha as well as the gamma receptors has faltered, new agents that increase insulin secretion via the incretin system, which is based in the stomach and small intestine, seem to offer safe and efficacious therapy through a novel mechanism of action. The next few years will see these and other agents enter the clinical arena, and it seems likely that careful consideration of the phenotype of an individual with type 2 diabetes will be required in order to select the most effective therapeutic approach.

In addition, drugs that modify the activity of the cannabinoid receptors appear to have beneficial effects on hyperglycaemia and obesity. Rimonabant is a new agent that works as a selective cannabinoid type 1 receptor blocker. Four large studies were performed for registration purposes, and RIO-Diabetes is the last of these to be published (Scheen *et al.*, 2006). As in the other RIO groups, 20 mg of rimonabant caused a reduction in weight of 5.3 kg in patients with type 2 diabetes compared to a reduction of 1.4 kg with placebo, with an associated increase in HDL-cholesterol and reductions in triglycerides and systolic blood pressure. In the placebo group HbA1c increased by 0.1% at the end of 1 year, whereas it fell by 0.6% in the group receiving rimonabant. The authors offer a not particularly convincing statistical analysis that around half of the effect on HbA1c can be explained by weight loss, and suggest that the other half could be explained by other peripheral mechanisms. A worrying side-effect was depression, which was more common in the rimonabant group and may limit its use in clinical practice. It is also noteworthy that compliance with therapy (placebo and rimonabant) was poor and only two-thirds of people were taking therapy at the end of 1 year. Longer term studies of metabolic and cardiovascular outcomes are required.

11.8 Conclusions

With increasing worldwide prevalence of diabetes, obesity and the metabolic syndrome, it seems inevitable that there will be an associated rise in the global burden of cardiovascular disease. Cardiologists need to have a working knowledge of the increasing number of agents that are used to treat diabetes, and an appreciation of the therapeutic regimens that are most likely to achieve metabolic control in these individuals. In the last 10 years, diabetologists have become more aggressive in targeting cardiovascular risk factors rather than focusing entirely on the management of hyperglycaemia, and it seems likely that the most effective way of reducing cardiovascular complications in diabetes will be for both disciplines to work closely together in developing more effective primary and secondary preventive strategies in the management of patients with diabetes.

References

Alberti KG, Zimmet P. Shaw J (2006). Metabolic syndrome – a new world-wide definition. A consensus statement from the International Diabetes Federation. *Diabetic Medicine* **23**: 469–80.

Ashcroft FM, Rorsman P (1989). Electrophysiology of the pancreatic beta-cell *Progress in Biophysics and Molecular Biology* **54**: 87–143.

Bailey CJ, Day C (2003). Antidiabetic drugs. *British Journal of Cardiology* **10**: 128–36.

Bailey CJ, Turner RC (1996). Metformin. *New England Journal of Medicine* **334**: 574–9.

Boden G, Zhang M (2006). Recent findings concerning thiazolidinediones in the treatment of diabetes. *Expert Opinion on Investigational Drugs* **15**: 243–50.

Bolli GB, Di Marchi RD, Park GD, Pramming S, Koivisto VA (1999). Insulin analogues and their potential in the management of diabetes mellitus. *Diabetologia* **42**: 1151–67.

Brown JB, Pedula K, Barzilay J, Herson MK, Latare P (1998). Lactic acidosis rates in type 2 diabetes *Diabetes Care* **21**: 1659–63.

Buse JB, Tan MH, Prince MJ, Erickson PP (2004). The effects of oral anti-hyperglycaemic medications on serum lipid profiles in patients with type 2 diabetes. *Diabetes Obesity and Metabolism* **6**: 133–56.

Cheal KL, Abbasi F, Lamendola C, McLaughlin T, Reaven GM, Ford ES (2004). Relationship to insulin resistance of the adult treatment panel III diagnostic criteria for identification of the metabolic syndrome. *Diabetes* **53**: 1195–200.

Chiasson JL, Josse RG, Gomis R, Hanefeld M, Karasik A, Laakso M (2003). Acarbose treatment and the risk of cardiovascular disease and hypertension in patients with impaired glucose tolerance: the STOP-NIDDM trial *Journal of the American Medical Association* **290**: 486–94.

Chiquette E, Ramirez G, Defronzo R (2004). A meta-analysis comparing the effect of thiazolidinediones on cardiovascular risk factors. *Archives of Internal Medicine* **164**: 2097–104.

Derosa G, Cicero AF, Gaddi A, Ragonesi PD, Fogari E, Bertone G, Ciccarelli L, Piccinni MN (2004). Metabolic effects of pioglitazone and rosiglitazone in patients with diabetes and metabolic syndrome treated with glimepiride: a twelve-month, multicenter, double-blind, randomized, controlled, parallel-group trial *Clinical Therapeutics* **26**: 744–54.

Diabetes Control and Complications Trial Research Group (1993). The effect of intensive treatment of diabetes on the development and progression of long-term complications in insulin-dependent diabetes mellitus. *New England Journal of Medicine* **329**: 977–86.

Diabetes Control and Complications Trial Research Group (1997). Hypoglycemia in the Diabetes Control and Complications Trial. *Diabetes* **46**: 271–86.

Diabetes Control and Complications Trial/Epidemiology of Diabetes Interventions and Complications (DCCT/EDIC) Study Research Group (2005). Intensive Diabetes Treatment and Cardiovascular Disease in patients with type 1 diabetes. *New England Journal of Medicine* **353**: 2643–53.

Dormandy JA, Charbonnel B, Eckland DJ, Erdmann E, Massi-Benedetti M, Moules IK *et al.* (2005). Secondary prevention of macrovascular events in patients with type 2 diabetes in the PROactive Study (PROspective pioglitAzone Clinical Trial In macroVascular Events): a randomised controlled trial *Lancet* **366**: 1279–89.

Dornhorst A (2001). Insulinotropic meglitinide analogues *Lancet* **358**: 1709–16.

Ehtisham S, Barrett TG (2004). The emergence of type 2 diabetes in childhood. *Annals of Clinical Biochemistry* **41**: 10–6.

Eurich DT, Majumdar SR, McAlister FA, Tsuyuki RT, Johnson JA (2005). Improved clinical outcomes associated with metformin in patients with diabetes and heart failure *Diabetes Care* **28**: 2345–51.

Evans JM, Wang J, Morris AD (2002). Comparison of cardiovascular risk between patients with type 2 diabetes and those who had had a myocardial infarction: cross sectional and cohort studies. *British Medical Journal* **324**: 939–42.

Ford ES, Giles WH (2003). A comparison of the prevalence of the metabolic syndrome using two proposed definitions. *Diabetes Care* **26**: 575–81.

Ford ES, Giles WH, Dietz WH (2002). Prevalence of the metabolic syndrome among US adults: findings from the third National Health and Nutrition Examination Survey. *Journal of the American Medical Association* **287**: 356–9.

Ford ES, Giles WH, Mokdad AH (2004). Increasing prevalence of the metabolic syndrome among U.S. Adults. *Diabetes Care* **27**: 2444–9.

Forouhi NG, Merrick D, Goyder E, Ferguson BA, Abbas J, Lachowycz K, Wild SH (2006). Diabetes prevalence in England, 2001 – estimates from an epidemiological model. *Diabetic Medicine* **23**: 189–97.

Gale EA (2005). The myth of the metabolic syndrome *Diabetologia* **48**: 1679–83.

Gerich JE (1989). Oral hypoglycemic agents *New England Journal of Medicine* **321**: 1231–45.

Gerstein HC (2006). Intensive insulin therapy reduced cardiovascular disease in type 1 diabetes *American College of Physicians Journal Club* **144**: 63.

Goldner MG, Knatterud GL, Prout TE (1971). Effects of hypoglycemic agents on vascular complications in patients with adult-onset diabetes. 3. Clinical implications of UGDP results. *Journal of American Medical Association* **218**: 1400–10.

Grant PJ, Stickland MH, Booth NA, Prentice CR (1991). Metformin causes a reduction in basal and post-venous occlusion plasminogen activator inhibitor-1 in type 2 diabetic patients *Diabetic Medicine* **8**: 361–5.

Gross GJ, Auchampach JA (1992). Blockade of ATP-sensitive potassium channels prevents myocardial preconditioning in dogs. *Circulation Research* **70**: 223–33.

Haffner SM, Lehto S, Ronnemaa T, Pyorala K, Laakso M (1998). Mortality from coronary heart disease in subjects with type 2 diabetes and in nondiabetic subjects with and without prior myocardial infarction. *New England Journal of Medicine* **339**: 229–34.

Haines L, Wan KC, Lynn R, Barrett TG, Shield JP (2007). Rising incidence of type 2 diabetes in children in the United Kingdom. *Diabetes Care* **30:** 1097–101.

Hermann LS, Schersten B, Bitzen PO, Kjellstrom T, Lindgarde F, Melander A (1994). Therapeutic comparison of metformin and sulfonylurea, alone and in various combinations. A double-blind controlled study *Diabetes Care* **17**: 1100–9.

Higgs ER, Krentz AJ (2004). ABCD position statement on glitazones. *Practical Diabetes International* **21**: 293–5.

Hills SA, Balkau B, Coppack SW, Dekker JM, Mari A, Natali A, Walker M, Ferrannini E (2004). The EGIR-RISC STUDY (The European group for the study of insulin resistance: relationship between insulin sensitivity and cardiovascular disease risk): I. Methodology and objectives. *Diabetologia* **47**: 566–70.

Home PD, Pocock SJ, Beck-Nielsen H, Gomis R, Hanefeld M, Dargie H, Komajda M, Gubb J, Biswas N, Jones NP (2005). Rosiglitazone Evaluated for Cardiac Outcomes and

Regulation of Glycaemia in Diabetes (RECORD): study design and protocol *Diabetologia* **48**: 1726–35.

Hossain P, Kawar B, El Nahas M (2007). Obesity and diabetes in the developing world – a growing challenge. *New England Journal of Medicine* **356**: 213–5.

Hu G, Qiao Q, Tuomilehto J, Balkau B, Borch-Johnsen K, Pyorala K (2004). Prevalence of the metabolic syndrome and its relation to all-cause and cardiovascular mortality in nondiabetic European men and women. *Archives of Internal Medicine* **164**: 1066–76.

Kahn R, Buse J, Ferrannini E, Stern M (2005). The metabolic syndrome: time for a critical appraisal: joint statement from the American Diabetes Association and the European Association for the Study of Diabetes. *Diabetes Care* **28**: 2289–304.

Kahn SE, Haffner SM, Heise MA, Herman WH, Holman RR, Jones NP, Kravitz BG, Lachin JM, O'Neill MC, Zinman B, Viberti G (2006). Glycemic durability of rosiglitazone, metformin, or glyburide monotherapy *New England Journal of Medicine* **355**: 2427–43.

Kannel WB, McGee DL (1979). Diabetes and cardiovascular risk factors: the Framingham study. *Circulation* **59**: 8–13.

Kennedy DL, Piper JM, Baum C (1988). Trends in use of oral hypoglycemic agents 1964–1986. *Diabetes Care* **11**: 558–62.

Langtry HD, Balfour JA (1998). Glimepiride. A review of its use in the management of type 2 diabetes mellitus. *Drugs* **55**: 563–84.

Macfarlane DP, Fisher M (2006). Thiazolidinediones in patients with diabetes mellitus and heart failure: implications of emerging data *American Journal of Cardiovascular Drugs* **6**: 297–304.

Mather KJ, Verma S, Anderson TJ (2001). Improved endothelial function with metformin in type 2 diabetes mellitus. *Journal of the American College of Cardiology* **37**: 1344–50.

Matthews DR, Cull CA, Stratton IM, Holman RR, Turner RC (1998). UKPDS 26: Sulphonylurea failure in non-insulin-dependent diabetic patients over six years. UK Prospective Diabetes Study (UKPDS) Group. *Diabetic Medicine* **15**: 297–303.

Morris AD, Boyle DI, McMahon AD, Greene SA, MacDonald TM, Newton RW (1997). Adherence to insulin treatment, glycaemic control, and ketoacidosis in insulin-dependent diabetes mellitus. The DARTS/MEMO Collaboration. Diabetes Audit and Research in Tayside Scotland. Medicines Monitoring Unit. *Lancet* **350**: 1505–10.

Murphy EJ, Davern TJ, Shakil AO, Shick L, Masharani U, Chow H, Freise C, Lee WM, Bass NM (2000). Troglitazone-induced fulminant hepatic failure. Acute Liver Failure Study Group. *Digestive Disease Science* **45**: 549–53.

Nathan DM (2006). Thiazolidinediones for initial treatment of type 2 diabetes? *New England Journal of Medicine* **355**: 2477–80.

Nathan DM, Lachin J, Cleary P, Orchard T, Brillon DJ, Backlund JY, O'Leary DH, Genuth S (2003). Intensive diabetes therapy and carotid intima-media thickness in type 1 diabetes mellitus. *New England Journal of Medicine* **348**: 2294–303.

NCEP/ATPIII (2001). Executive summary of the third report of the National Cholesterol Education Program (NCEP) expert panel on detection, evaluation and treatment of high blood cholesterol in adults (Adult Treatment Panel III). *Journal of the American Medical Association* **285**: 2486–97.

Nesto R (2004). C-reactive protein, its role in inflammation, Type 2 diabetes and cardiovascular disease, and the effects of insulin-sensitizing treatment with thiazolidinediones *Diabetic Medicine* **21**: 810–7.

Nesto RW, Bell D, Bonow RO, Fonseca V, Grundy SM, Horton ES, Le Winter M, Porte D, Semenkovich CF, Smith S, Young LH, Kahn R (2004). Thiazolidinedione use, fluid retention, and congestive heart failure: a consensus statement from the American Heart Association and American Diabetes Association *Diabetes Care* **27**: 256–63.

Nichols CG, Ripoll C, Lederer WJ (1991). ATP-sensitive potassium channel modulation of the guinea pig ventricular action potential and contraction. *Circulation Research* **68**: 280–7.

Norhammar A, Tenerz A, Nilsson G, Hamsten A, Efendic S, Ryden L, Malmberg K (2002). Glucose metabolism in patients with acute myocardial infarction and no previous diagnosis of diabetes mellitus: a prospective study. *Lancet* **359**: 2140–4.

Purnell JQ, Hokanson JE, Marcovina SM, Steffes MW, Cleary PA, Brunzell JD (1998). Effect of excessive weight gain with intensive therapy of type 1 diabetes on lipid levels and blood pressure: results from the DCCT. Diabetes Control and Complications Trial. *Journal of the American Medical Association* **280**: 140–6.

Reaven GM (1988). Banting lecture 1988. Role of insulin resistance in human disease. *Diabetes* **37**: 1595–607.

Rendell M (2004). The role of sulphonylureas in the management of type 2 diabetes mellitus. *Drugs* **64**: 1339–58.

Rosenstock J, Hassman DR, Madder RD, Brazinsky SA, Farrell J, Khutoryansky N, Hale PM (2004). Repaglinide versus nateglinide monotherapy: a randomized, multicenter study. *Diabetes Care* **27**: 1265–70.

Ruige JB, Assendelft WJ, Dekker JM, Kostense PJ, Heine RJ, Bouter LM (1998). Insulin and risk of cardiovascular disease: a meta-analysis *Circulation* **97**: 996–1001.

Salpeter SR, Greyber E, Pasternak GA, Salpeter EE (2003). Risk of fatal and nonfatal lactic acidosis with metformin use in type 2 diabetes mellitus: systematic review and meta-analysis *Archives of Internal Medicine* **163**: 2594–602.

Sartor G, Dahlquist G (1995). Short-term mortality in childhood onset insulin-dependent diabetes mellitus: a high frequency of unexpected deaths in bed *Diabetic Medicine* **12**: 607–11.

Scheen AJ, Finer N, Hollander P, Jensen MD, Van Gaal LF (2006). Efficacy and tolerability of rimonabant in overweight or obese patients with type 2 diabetes: a randomised controlled study *Lancet* **368**: 1660–72.

Stamler J, Vaccaro O, Neaton JD, Wentworth D (1993). Diabetes, other risk factors, and 12-yr cardiovascular mortality for men screened in the Multiple Risk Factor Intervention Trial. *Diabetes Care* **16**: 434–44.

Stephens JW, Ambler G, Vallance P, Betteridge DJ, Humphries SE, Hurel SJ (2004). Cardiovascular risk and diabetes. Are the methods of risk prediction satisfactory? *European Journal of Cardiovascular Prevention and Rehabilitation* **11**: 521–8.

Stratton IM, Adler AI, Neil HA, Matthews DR, Manley SE, Cull CA, Hadden D, Turner RC, Holman RR (2000). Association of glycaemia with macrovascular and microvascular complications of type 2 diabetes (UKPDS 35): prospective observational study. *British Medical Journal* **321**: 405–12.

Tattersall RB, Gill GV (1991). Unexplained deaths of type 1 diabetic patients *Diabetic Medicine* **8**: 49–58.

Thordarson H, Sovik O (1995). Dead in bed syndrome in young diabetic patients in Norway *Diabetic Medicine* **12**: 782–787.

Toombs CF, Moore TL, Shebuski RJ (1993) Limitation of infarct size in the rabbit by ischaemic preconditioning is reversible with glibenclamide. *Cardiovascular Research* **27**: 617–22.

Turner RC, Cull CA, Frighi V, Holman RR (1999). Glycemic control with diet, sulfonylurea, metformin, or insulin in patients with type 2 diabetes mellitus: progressive requirement for multiple therapies (UKPDS 49). UK Prospective Diabetes Study (UKPDS) Group. *Journal of the American Medical Association* **281**: 2005–12.

UK Prospective (UKPDS) Diabetes Study Group (1998a). Intensive blood-glucose control with sulphonylureas or insulin compared with conventional treatment and risk of complications in patients with type 2 diabetes (UKPDS 33). *Lancet* **352**: 837–53.

UK Prospective Diabetes Study (UKPDS) Group (1998b). Effect of intensive blood glucose control with metformin on complications in overweight patients with type 2 diabetes (UKPDS 34). *Lancet* **352**: 854–65.

World Health Organization (1999). *Definition, Diagnosis and Classification of Diabetes Mellitus and its Complications: Report of a WHO Consultation.* Geneva: World Health Organization.

Yki-Jarvinen H (2004). Thiazolidinediones. *New England Journal of Medicine* **351**: 1106–18.

Zimmet P (2000). Globalization, coca-colonization and the chronic disease epidemic: can the Doomsday scenario be averted? *Journal of Internal Medicine* **247**: 301–10.

Zimmet P, Alberti KG, Shaw J (2001). Global and societal implications of the diabetes epidemic. *Nature* **414**: 782–7.

Study Acronyms

Chapter 1

DARTS/MEMO	Diabetes Audit and Research in Tayside Scotland/Medicines Monitoring Unit
MRFIT	Multiple Risk Factor Intervention Trial

Chapter 2

ARIC	Atherosclerosis Risk in Communities
WOSCOPS	West of Scotland Coronary Prevention Study

Chapter 3

ARTS	Arterial Revascularisation Therapy Study
ATC	Antiplatelet Trialists' Collaboration / Antithrombotic Trialists' Collaboration
BARI	Bypass Angioplasty Revascularisation Investigation
BARI 2D	Bypass Angioplasty Revascularisation Investigation 2 Diabetes
BIP	Bezafibrate Infarction Prevention
CABRI	Coronary Angioplasty versus Bypass Revascularisation Investigation
CAPRIE	Clopidogrel versus Aspirin in Patients at Risk of Ischaemic Events
CARDIA	Coronary Artery Revascularisation in Diabetes
CASS	Coronary Artery Surgery Study
CHARISMA	Clopidogrel for High Atherothrombotic Risk and Ischaemic Stabilisation, Management and Avoidance
CREDO	Clopidogrel for Reduction of Events During Observation
CURE	Clopidogrel in Unstable Angina to Prevent Recurrent Events
EAST	Emory Angioplasty versus Surgery Trial
ECSS	European Coronary Surgery Study
EPISTENT	Evaluation of Platelet IIb/IIIa Inhibition in Stenting
ESPRIT	Enhanced Suppression of the Platelet IIb/IIIa Receptor with Integrilin Therapy
ETDRS	Early Treatment Diabetic Retinopathy Study

Diabetic Cardiology   Editors Miles Fisher and John J. McMurray
© 2007 John Wiley & Sons, Ltd.

EUROPA	European Trial on Reduction of Cardiac Events with Perindopril in Stable Coronary Artery Disease
FINESSE	Facilitated Intervention with Enhanced Reperfusion Speed to Stop Events
FREEDOM	Future Revascularisation in Patients with Diabetes Mellitus
GABI	German Angioplasty Bypass Investigation
HOPE	Heart Outcomes Prevention Evaluation
HOT	Hypertension Optimal Treatment
IONA	Impact of Nicorandil in Angina
ISAR	Intracoronary Stenting and Antithrombotic Regimen
ISAR-REACT	Intracoronary Stenting and Antithrombotic Regimen – Rapid Early Action for Coronary Treatment
ISAR-SWEET	Intracoronary Stenting and Antithrombotic Regimen – Is Abciximab a Superior Way to Eliminate Elevated Thrombotic Risk in Diabetics
PCI-CURE	Percutaneous Coronary Intervention – Clopidogrel in Unstable Angina to Prevent Recurrent Events
PEACE	Prevention of Events with Angiotensin-converting Enzyme Inhibition
PRAGUE-2	Primary Angioplasty in AMI Patients from General Community Hospitals Transported to PCI Units versus Emergency Thrombolysis 2
PROSPECT	Providing Regional Observations to Study Predictors of Events in the Coronary Tree
RITA	Randomised Intervention Treatment of Angina
SIRIUS	Sirolimus-eluting Balloon Expandable Stent in the Treatment of Patients with De novo Native Coronary Artery Lesions
SIRTAX	Sirolimus-eluting Stent compared with Paclitaxel-eluting Stent for Coronary Revascularisation
TARGET	Do Tirofiban and ReoPro Give Similar Efficacy Outcomes Trial
TAXUS-IV	Paclitaxel-eluting Coronary Stent Implantation IV
VACSS	Veterans Administration Cooperative Study of surgery for Coronary Artery Disease

Chapter 4

ACUITY	Acute Catheterisation and Urgent Intervention Triage Strategy
CLARITY-TIMI 28	Clopidogrel as Adjunctive Reperfusion Therapy – Thrombolysis in Myocardial Infarction 28
COMMIT	Clopidogrel and Metoprolol in Myocardial Infarction Trial
CURE	Clopidogrel in Unstable Angina to Prevent Recurrent Events
DANAMI	Danish Trial in Acute Myocardial Infarction
DANAMI-2	Danish Trial in Acute Myocardial Infarction 2
DIGAMI	Diabetes Mellitus Insulin–Glucose Infusion in Acute Myocardial Infarction
ESPRIT	Enhanced Suppression of the Platelet IIb/IIIa Receptor with Integrilin Therapy
FRISC II	Fragmin and Fast Revascularisation during Instability in Coronary Artery Disease II
GISSI-2	Gruppo Italiano per lo Studio della Sprovvivenza nell'Infarto Micardico 2
GISSI-3	Gruppo Italiano per lo Studio della Sprovvivenza nell'Infarto Micardico 3

GUSTO I	Global Utilisation of Streptokinase and Tissue Plasminogen Activator for Occluded Coronary Arteries I
GUSTO IIb	Global Use of Strategies to Open Occluded Coronary Arteries IIb
GUSTO IV-ACS	Global Utilisation of Strategies to Open Occluded Coronary Arteries Trial IV in Acute Coronary Syndromes
ISIS	International Study of Infarct Survival
OASIS-5	Fifth Organisation to Assess Strategies in Acute Ischaemic Syndromes
OPTIMAAL	Optimal Therapy in Myocardial Infarction with the Angiotensin II Antagonist Losartan
PCI-CURE	Percutaneous Coronary Intervention – Clopidogrel in Unstable Angina to Prevent Recurrent Events
PRISM-PLUS	Platelet Receptor Inhibition in Ischaemic Syndrome Management in Patients Limited by Unstable Signs and Symptoms
PURSUIT	Platelet Glycoprotein IIb/IIIa in Unstable Angina: Receptor Suppression Using Integrilin Therapy
RITA-3	Randomised Intervention Trial of Unstable Angina 3
SAVE	Survival and Ventricular Enlargement
TACTICS	Treat Angina with Aggrastat and Determine Cost of Therapy with an Invasive or Conservative Strategy
TIMI	Thrombolysis in Myocardial Infarction
VALIANT	Valsartan in Acute Myocardial Infarction Trial

Chapter 5

A-HeFT	African American Heart Failure Trial
ARIC	Atherosclerosis Risk in Community
ATLAS	Assessment of Treatment with Lisinopril and Survival
BEST	Beta-blocker Evaluation of Survival Trial
BIP	Bezafibrate Infarction Prevention
CHARM	Candesartan in Heart Failure: Assessment of Reduction in Mortality and Morbidity
CIBIS-II	Cardiac Insufficiency Bisoprolol Study II
COMET	Carvedilol or Metoprolol European Trial
COMPANION	Comparison of Medical Therapy, Pacing and Defibrillation in Heart Failure
CONSENSUS	Cooperative North Scandinavian Enalapril Survival Study
COPERNICUS	Carvediolol Prospective Randomised Cumulative Survival
DCCT/EDIC	Diabetes Control and Complications Trial/Epidemiology of Diabetes Interventions and Complications
DIABHYCAR	Diabetes, Hypertension, Cardiovascular Events and Ramipril
DIAMOND-CHF	Danish Investigations of Arrhythmia and Mortality on Dofetilide in Congestive Heart Failure
DIG	Digitalis Investigation Group
ECHOES	Echocardiographic Heart of England Screening
ELITE-I	Evaluation of Losartan in the Elderly I
ELITE-II	Evaluation of Losartan in the Elderly II
EUROPA	European Trial on Reduction of Cardiac Events with Perindopril in Stable Coronary Artery Disease
HOPE	Heart Outcomes Prevention Evaluation
IDNT	Irbesartan Diabetic Nephropathy Trial

LIFE	Losartan Intervention for Endpoint Reduction in Hypertension
MERIT-HF	Metoprolol CR/XL Randomised Intervention Trial in Heart Failure
MICRO-HOPE	Microalbuminuria, Cardiovascular and Renal Outcomes in the Heart Outcomes Prevention Evaluation
NHANES	National Health and Nutrition Examination Survey
PERSUADE	Perindopril Substudy in Coronary Artery Disease and Diabetes
PROactive	Prospective Pioglitazone Clinical Trial in Macrovascular Events
RALES	Ramdomised Aldactone Evaluation Study
RENAAL	Reduction of Endpoints in NIDDM with the Angiotensin II Antagonist Losartan
RESOLVD	Randomised Evaluation of Strategies for Left Ventricular Dysfunction
SCD-HeFT	Sudden Cardiac Death in Heart Failure Trial
SOLVD	Studies of Left Ventricular Dysfunction
UKPDS	United Kingdom Prospective Diabetes Study
VAL-HeFT	Valsartan Heart Failure Trial
V-HeFT	Vasodilator-Heart Failure Trial
V-HeFT II	Vasodilator-Heart Failure Trial II

Chapter 6

ABCD	Appropriate Blood Pressure Control in Diabetes
ABCD2	Appropriate Blood Pressure Control in Diabetes 2
ALLHAT	Antihypertensive and Lipid-lowering Treatment to Prevent Heart Attack Trial
ALPINE	Antihypertensive Treatment and Lipid Profile in a North of Sweden Efficacy Evaluation
BENEDICT	Bergamo Nephrologic Diabetes Complications Trial
CALM	Candesartan and Lisinopril Microalbuminuria
CAPPP	Captopril Prevention Project
CONVINCE	Controlled Onset Verapamil Investigation of Cardiovascular Endpoints
DCCT	Diabetes Control and Complications Trial
DETAIL	Diabetics Exposed to Telmisartan and Enalapril
DREAM	Diabetes Reduction Assessment with Ramipril and Rosiglitazone Medication
EDIC	Epidemiology of Diabetes Interventions and Complications
EUCLID	EURODIAB Controlled Trial of Lisinopril in Insulin-dependent Diabetes
FACET	Fosinopril versus Amlodipine Cardiovascular Events Trial
HDS	Hypertension in Diabetes Study
HOPE	Heart Outcomes Prevention Evaluation
HOT	Hypertension Optimal Treatment
IDNT	Irbesartan Diabetic Nephropathy Trial
INVEST	International Verapamil SR/Trandolapril
IRMA2	Irbesartan Microalbuminuria Type 2 Diabetes in Hypertensive Patients
LIFE	Losartan Intervention for Endpoint Reduction in Hypertension
LIPID	Long-term Intervention with Pravastatin in Ischaemic Disease
MARVAL	Microalbuminuria Reduction with Valsartan
MRFIT	Multiple Risk Factor Intervention Trial

ONTARGET   Ongoing Temisartan Alone and in Combination with Ramipril Global
             Endpoint Trial
RENAAL   Reduction of Endpoints in NIDDM with the Angiotensin II Antagonist
             Losartan
SCOPE   Study on Cognition and Prognasis in the Elderly
SHEP   Systolic Hypertension in the Elderly Programme
STOP-2   Swedish Trial in Old Patients with Hypertension 2
SYST-EUR   Systolic Hypertension in Europe
UKPDS   United Kingdom Prospective Diabetes Study
VALUE   Valsartan Antihypertensive Long-term Use Evaluation

Chapter 7

DIGAMI   Diabetes Mellitus Insulin–Glucose Infusion in Acute Myocardial Infarction
GIST-UK   Glucose Insulin in Stroke Trial – United Kingdom
HDS   Hypertension in Diabetes Study
HOPE   Heart Outcomes Prevention Evaluation
HOT   Hypertension Optimal Treatment
MATCH   Management of Atherothrombosis with Clopidogrel in High-risk Patients
PROGRESS   Perindopril Protection against Recurrent Stroke Study
UKPDS   United Kingdom Prospective Diabetes Study

Chapter 8

4S   Scandinavian Simvastatin Survival Study
ABCD   Appropriate Blood Pressure Control in Diabetes
CAPRIE   Clopidogrel versus Aspirin in Patients at Risk of Ischaemic Events
CARDS   Collaborative Atorvastatin Diabetes Study
CURE   Clopidogrel in Unstable Angina to Prevent Recurrent Events
DCCT   Diabetes Control and Complications Trial
HOPE   Heart Outcomes Prevention Evaluation
HPS   Heart Protection Study
PROGRESS   Perindopril Protection against Recurrent Stroke Study
UKPDS   United Kingdom Prospective Diabetes Study
VA-HIT   Veterans Affairs High-density Lipoprotein Cholesterol Intervention Trial

Chapter 9

4S   Scandinavian Simvastatin Survival Study
ALLHAT   Antihypertensive and Lipid-Lowering Treatment to Prevent Heart
             Attack Trial
ALLHAT-LLT   Antihypertensive and Lipid-lowering Treatment to Prevent Heart
             Attack Trial – Lipid Lowering Therapy
ASCOT-LLA   Anglo-Scandinavian Cardiac Outcomes Trial – Lipid Lowering Arm
CAPPP   Captopril Prevention Project
CARDS   Collaborative Atorvastatin Diabetes Study
CARE   Cholesterol and Recurrent Events

DAIS   Diabetes Atherosclerosis Intervention Study
DIGAMI   Diabetes Mellitus Insulin – Glucose Infusion in Acute Myocardial
                Infarction
EUCLID   EURODIAB Controlled Trial of Lisinopril in Insulin-dependent Diabetes
FIELD   Fenofibrate Intervention and Event Lowering in Diabetes
HOPE   Heart Outcomes Prevention Evaluation
HPS   Heart Protection Study
INSIGHT   International Nifedipine GITS Study Intervention as a Goal in
                Hypertension Treatment
LIFE   Losartan Intervention for Endpoint Reduction in Hypertension
LIPID   Long-term Intervention with Pravastatin in Ischaemic Disease
LIPS   Lescol Intervention Prevention Study
MICRO-HOPE   Microalbuminuria, Cardiovascular and Renal Outcomes in the Heart
                Outcomes Prevention Evaluation
NORDIL   Nordic Diltiazem
OASIS   Organisation to Assess Strategies for Ischaemic Syndromes
PROactive   Prospective Pioglitazone Clinical Trial in Macrovascular Disease
PROSPER   Prospective Study of Pravastatin in the Elderly at Risk
SHEP   Systolic Hypertension in the Elderly Programme
STOP-2   Swedish Trial in Old Patients with Hypertension 2
SYST-EUR   Systolic Hypertension in Europe
UKPDS   United Kingdom Prospective Diabetes Study
VA-HIT   Veterans Affairs High-density Lipoprotein Cholesterol Intervention Trial

Chapter 10

CAPPP   Captopril Prevention Project
DECODE   Diabetes Epidemiology Collaborative Analysis of Diagnostic
                Criteria in Europe
DPP   Diabetes Prevention Program
DPS   Diabetes Prevention Study
DREAM   Diabetes Reduction Assessment with Ramipril and Rosiglitazone
                Medication
HOPE   Heart Outcomes Prevention Evaluation
LIFE   Losartan Intervention for Endpoint Reduction in Hypertension
NAVIGATOR   Nateglinide and Valsartan in Impaired Glucose Tolerance
                Outcomes Research
PROactive   Prospective Pioglitazone Clinical Trial in Macrovascular Events
STOP-NIDDM   Study to Prevent Non-insulin-dependent Diabetes Mellitus
TRIPOD   Troglitazone in the Prevention of Diabetes
UKPDS   United Kingdom Prospective Diabetes Study
XENDOS   Xenical in the Prevention of Diabetes in Obese Subjects

Chapter 11

ADOPT   A Diabetes Outcome Progression Trial
DCCT   Diabetes Control and Complications Trial

DECODE	Diabetes Epidemiology Collaborative Analysis of Diagnostic Criteria in Europe
EDIC	Epidemiology of Diabetes Interventions and Complications
EGIR/RISC	European Group for the Study of Insulin Resistance Relationship between Insulin Resistance and Cardiovascular Disease
MRFIT	Multiple Risk Factor Intervention Trial
NAVIGATOR	Nateglinide and Valsartan in Impaired Glucose Tolerance Outcomes Research
NCEP	National Cholesterol Education Programme
NHANES	National Health and Nutritional Examination Survey
PROactive	Prospective Pioglitazone Clinical Trial in Macrovascular Events
RECORD	Rosiglitazone Evaluated for Cardiac Outcomes and Regulation of Glyaemia in Diabetes
RIO-Diabetes	Rimonabant in Overweight/Obesity-Diabetes
STOP-NIDDM	Study to Prevent Non-insulin-dependent Diabetes Mellitus
UKPDS	United Kingdom Prospective Diabetes Study

Index

Note: Page references in *italics* refer to Figures; those in **bold** refer to Tables. Studies are entered in the index under their acronyms (see Study Acronyms p. 280).

4S   214

ABCD   146, 215
ABCD2   145
Abciximab   57, 58, 79
Acarbose   249–50, *250*, 253, 272
ACE inhibitors   40–1, 74, 159, 231
  in cardiovascular risk reduction   146
  in diabetic nephropathy   154
  hypoglycaemia and   118
  in microalbuminuria   152
  reducing development of chronic heart
    failure in patients with diabetes   110
  stroke and   186, 188
  treatment of chronic heart failure in
    patients with diabetes   117–18
Activating protein-1 (AP-1)   28, 204
ACUITY   79
Acute coronary syndrome   223
Acute-phase markers   26
Adipokines   16, 26–7
Adiponectin   16, 26–7, 31, 32
Adipose tissue and insulin resistance   104
ADOPT   271, 273
Advanced glycosylation end-products (AGEs)
  29–30, 105–6, 192, 203–4,
  226, 229
Age, mortality and   3–4, 5, 7–8, 7, 10
A-HeFT   **98**
Aldose reductase pathway   204–5
ALLHAT   142, 143, 145, 146, 157,
  158, 160, 230, 231
ALLHAT-LLT   230
ALPINE   158

Alzheimer's dementia   176, 191–2
Amlodipine   110, 145, 146, 152, 156,
  158, 231
Amputation, below knee   12
Amyloid A   25
Angina pectoris   40, 223
Angiotensin   23
Angiotensin II   225
Angiotensin receptor blockers (ARBs)   41,
  74–5, 110, 120, 216
  in cardiovascular risk reduction   146–7
Anisoylated purified streptokinase activator
  complex (anistreplase)   71
Anistreplase   71
Ankle-brachial pressure index (ABPI)
  206–7
Antihypertensive drugs, risk of diabetes
  mellitus with   156–60
Antiplatelet therapy   40, 41–2, 69–71,
  212–13
  in stroke   190
Antithrombin III   28
Antithrombin III inhibitor therapy   79
ANZ   **98**
Apolipoprotein A (ApoB):ApoAI   22
Apolipoprotein E (ApoE)   192
APSAC   71
ARIC   26, 108
Arrhythmia, ischaemia-related   38
Arterial stiffness   107–8
ARTS   52, 53
ASCOT-LLA   230
Aspirin   41, 42, 56, 69, 212, 213
  in cardiovascular risk reduction   141

ATC 41
Atenolol 73, 110, 119, 145, 146,
    231, 251
  diabetes mellitus risk with 157, 158
  in kidney disease 151
  in stroke 186
Atheroma 178
Atherosclerosis 203
  endothelial role in 225
Atherothrombosis, risk factors 227–9
  coagulation defects 229
  dyslipidaemia 227
  elevated blood pressure 227–8
  insulin resistance and hyperglycaemia
    228
  intimal calcification 229
  low-grade inflammation 228–9
  obesity and central obesity 228
  smoking 228
ATLAS **98**, 103, 117
Atorvastatin 230
Atrial fibrillation/flutter 38
Azotaemia 148

BARI 42, 44–50
  BARI 2D 55
  CABG vs PTCA survival benefits
    48–50
  diabetes subgroup analysis 45–6
  registry 46–7
BENEDICT 151
BEST 101, 102, 112, 119
Beta-blockers 73–4
  in chronic heart failure in patients with
    diabetes 118–20
  in coronary heart disease in people with
    diabetes 40
  frequency of hypoglycaemic episodes
    119
  in hypertension 157, 159
  hypoglycaemic awareness 119
  in peripheral artery disease 215
  in pre-diabetes 251
  recovery from hypoglycaemia 120
  in stroke 186
Biguanides 273
BIP 40, 100
Bivalirudin 79
British Regional Heart Study 27
Bx Velocity stent 53

CABRI 51–2
Calcium channel blockers 40
  in cardiovascular risk reduction 145, 151
  in hypertension 159
CALM 155
Candesartan 109, 120, 158
CAPPP 146, 158, 231, 251
CAPRIE 42, 207, 212
Captopril 74, 75, 119, 146, 151, 158,
    186, 251
CARDIA 55
Cardiac autonomic neuropathy 108
Cardiac resynchronisation therapy (CRT)
    120
Cardialysis Core Laboratory 53
Cardiomyopathy 6
Cardiovascular disease (CVD) 1
  dyslipidaemia 229–31
  elevated blood pressure 231–2
  epidemiology in diabetes 2
  hyperglycaemia 232
  mortality from 8–10
  multifactorial intervention 233
  non-pharmacological intervention
    140–1
  pharmacological risk reduction 141–7
  risk reduction 140–9
  treatment effects of cardiovascular risk
    factors 229–31
CARDS 214, 230
CARE 230
Carnitine palmitoyltransferase 107
Carotid disease 177–8
Carvedilol 120
CASS 42
Central obesity 16, 139, 228
Cerebrovascular disease 6
CHARISMA 42
CHARM **98**, 99, 101, 112, 120
CHARM-added **98**, 120
CHARM-alternative 120
Chlorpropamide 268
Chlorthalidone 157, 158, 231
Chronic heart failure
  abnormalities of insulin and glucose
    metabolism 103–5
  complex pacemaker therapies 120
  diagnosis of diabetes in clinical trials 17
  inhibition of RAAS 109
  lifestyle changes 109
  myocardium, effects on 105–7

non-pharmacological measures 110
pharmacological therapies 117–20
reason for patients with diabetes developing 105–9
reducing risk of diabetes in 109
reduction of development in patients with diabetes 109–10
risks of developing 99–100
screening in patients with diabetes 110
treatment of diabetes in patients with, treatment 110–17
treatment of, in patients with 117–21
CIBIS-II **98**, 118
Cilostazol 207
CLARITY-TIMI 28 71
Clopidogrel 42, 58, 70–1, 212
PCI and 56–7
Coagulation defects 229
Coamilozide 232
Cohort studies 2–4
Colestipol 188
COMET **98**
COMMIT 71
COMPANION **98**
CONSENSUS **98**, 117
CONVINCE 145
COPERNICUS **98**, 118
Coronary artery bypass grafting (CABG) 42–3, 47–8
vs PTCA 48–50
vs stents 51–2
Coronary artery disease in type 2 diabetes 223–7
epidemiological and clinical findings 223–4
pathophysiology 224–7, *226*
Coronary heart disease 37–59
mortality from 6–8
nature of 37–8
non-invasive investigation 39
pharmacological treatment 40–2
presentation 38–9
Coronary revascularisation 42–50
Coronary syndrome, acute 27
C-reactive protein (CRP) 25, 26, 27, 32, 225
CREDO study 56–7
CURE study 56, 57, 70–1, 212

DAIS 230
DANAMI 80–1, 85

DANAMI-2 81
DARTS/MEMO Study 12
DCCT 142, 213, 264, 265, 266
DCCT/EDIC 94, 109
'Dead in bed' syndrome 267
DECODE 241, 244, 261, 263
DETAIL 155
Device therapy post-MI 84
Diabetes Epidemiology Research International Study Group 3
Diabetes UK Cohort Study 3, 5, 6, 7, 8, 9, 10, 11
Diabetic autonomic neuropathy 38
Diabetic cardiomyopathy 108–9
Diabetic microangiopathy 108
DIABHYCAR 102
Diacylglycerol (DAG) 205
Diagnostic criteria for diabetes mellitus 260–1
DIAMOND-CHF 101
Diet 245–7
DIG **98**, 101
DIGAMI-1 86
DIGAMI-2 85–6
DIGAMI studies 84–6, 183, 232
Digoxin 117
Dihydropyridine 151
Diuretics 117
DPP 245
DPS 245
DREAM 158, 248, 251
Drug-eluting stents 53–5
Duke Medical Center 47, 48
Duke University registry 50
Dysglycaemia 181
Dyslipidaemia 16, 137, 227, 229–31
correction of 149
peripheral arterial disease and 213–14
stroke and 188–90
type 2 diabetes and 19–22
Dysmetabolic syndrome, *see* Metabolic syndrome
Dysrrhythmias 6

EAST 42
ECHOES **95**
ECSS 42
Ectopy 38
EDIC 142, 264
Edinburgh Artery Study 215
EGIR/RISC 263

Egr-1 28
ELITE-I 120
ELITE-II 120
Emory register 48
Enalapril 109, 152, 155, 231
End-stage renal disease 137, 139
Endothelial dysfunction 24, 107
Endothelial function and type 2 diabetes
    23–5
Endothelin-1 29
Enoxaparin 76
Epidemiological studies 1–12
    appraisal 10–11
    of diabetes mellitus 258–60
    role of 1–2
EPISTENT trial 57, 58
Eptifibitide 57, 77, 78
ESPRIT trial 57–8, 77, 78
ETDRS 41–2
Etomoxir 121
EUCLID 231
EUROPA 40, 110
Exercise 245–7
Exercise ECG testing 39
Express stent 53, 54, 55

FACET 146
Factor VII levels 28
Fatty acid transport protein 270
Fenofibrate 230
Fibrinogen 28
FIELD 230
FINESSE 79
Fondaparinux 76
Fosinopril 146
Framingham studies 2, 98, 99, 259
Free fatty acids (FFAs) 20, 106
FREEDOM 55
FRISC II 82–3

GABI 44
Gangrene 208
Gemfibrozil 230
Gender and cardiovascular disease risk
    11–12
GISSI-2 71–2
GISSI-3 trial 74
GIST-UK 184
Glibenclamide 116, 142, 268, 271
Gliclazide 268
Glimepiride 269

Glipizide 268
Glitazones, see Thiazolidinediones
    (glitazones)
Glucose–potassium–insulin (GKI)-based
    regimen 183
α-glucosidase inhibitors 268
GLUT-1 transporters 204
GLUT 4 270
Glycaemia, management 84–7, 109, 142
    in peripheral arterial disease and 213
Glycoprotein IIb/IIIa inhibitors 76–9
    and PCI 57–8
    in STEMI 78–9
    in unstable angina and non-ST-elevation
        MI (UA-NSTEMI) 76–8
GUSTO I 72–3
GUSTO IIb 79–80
GUSTO IV-ACS 78

Haemostatic changes in type 2 diabetes
    27–8
HDL-cholesteryl ester 20
HDL-cholesteryl ester 20
HDS 135, 136
Health Professionals Study 27
Heparin 76
High-density lipoprotein (HDL) 201, 226
HMG-CoA reductase inhibitors (statins)
    188, 189
HOPE 40, 41, 110, 146, 158, 160, 187, *216*,
    216, 231
HOT 41–2, *144*, 144, 187–8
HPS 189, *190*, 214, 230
Hydralazine 117
Hyperglycaemia 6, 16, 17, 107, 201–5, 225,
    232
    atherothrombosis and 228
    epidemiological studies 240–1
    ischaemic cerebral damage and 181–2
    mechanistic studies 242
    peripheral arterial disease 201–3
    as risk factor for cardiovascular disease
        240–3
    as risk for cardiovascular disease in
        diabetes 242–3
    role of 29–*30*, 30
Hyperinsulinaemia 17, *28–9*, 28, 105,
    137, 225
Hyperkalaemia 148
Hypertension 6, 30, 135–62
    atherosclerosis and 22–3

blood pressure control 142–5
cardiovascular risk reduction 140–9
diabetes mellitus risk with antihypertensive
    drugs 156–60
dietary modification 141
insulin resistance in 136
kidney disease risk reduction 149–56
lifestyle measures 140–1, **141**
multifactorial intervention 149
obesity in 139
peripheral arterial disease and 214–15
physical activity 141
prevalence 135–6
risk stratification 139–40
stroke and 185–6
tobacco cessation 141
weight loss 141
Hypertriglyceridaemia 30
Hypoglycaemia 5, 266–7
  beta-blockers and 40
  cardiovascular effects 267

ICAM-1 28SOS (stent or Surgery) trial 52
IDNT 110, 153, 154
Impaired fasting glucose (IFG) 243–4, 261
Impaired glucose tolerance (IGT) 176,
  243–4
Implantable cardioverter-defibrillator (ICD)
  120
Indapamide 187
Inflammation 25–6
INSIGHT 231
Insulatard 267
Insulin 1, 26, 112–13
  effects in chronic heart failure 113
  incidence of chronic heart failure in
    patients with diabetes 112
  mortality in chronic heart failure 112–13
  role of 17, 19, *20*
Insulin regimes **265**
Insulin resistance 32
  adipose tissue and 104
  atherothrombosis and 228
  definition 17–19, *18*
  in hypertension 136
  parameters associated with 16, *17*
  skeletal muscle and 104
  see also Metabolic syndrome
Insulin resistance syndrome, *see* Metabolic
  syndrome

Insulin-sensitising agents and cardiac failure
  272–4
Interleukins
  IL-1 204
  IL-6 229
Intermittent claudication 12, 205–7
  clinical signs 206
  criteria for surgical referral 207
  investigations 206–7
  management 207
  natural history 206
Intervention trials in pre-diabetes 245–52
  acarbose 249–50
  diet and exercise 245–7
  metformin 247–8
  orlistat 250–1
  renin-angiotensin blockade 251–2
  thiazolidinediones 248–9
Intimal calcification 229
Intracranial haemorrhage 182
INVEST 145
IONA 40
Irbesartan 110, 153, 155, 156
IRMA2 155
ISAR 55
ISAR-REACT 58
ISAR-SWEET study 58
Ischaemic penumbra 181
Ischaemic preconditioning 269
ISIS-1 73
ISIS-2 69, 71
ISIS-3 71
ISIS-4 74

Ketoacidosis 5
Kidney disease risk reduction 149–56
  blood pressure control 150–1
  dyslipidaemia correction 156
  glycaemic control 150
  microalbuminuria and 151–3
  non-pharmacological interventions
    149–50
  pharmacological interventions 150–1
  renin–angiotensin system blockade 154–6

Lacunar infarction (LACI) 178, **179**
Left ventricular hypertrophy 22
Leptin 26
LIFE 110, 146, 158, 231, 251
Lipaemia, postprandial 21
LIPID 149, 230

Lipoprotein lipase 270
LIPS 230
Lisinopril 74, 117, 145
Losartan 75, 110, 146, 147, 158, 231, 251
Lovastatin 230
Low-density lipoprotein (LDL)-cholesterol 203

Macroalbuminuria 148
MARVAL 155
MATCH 190
MCP-1 28
Meglitinide analogues 268
MERIT-HF **98**, 103, 118
Metabolic memory 265
Metabolic syndrome 17, 23, 24, 30–1, *31*, 137, 242
  cardiovascular risk and 263
  clinical management **138**
  C-reactive protein and 25
  definition and classification 261–2, **262**
  prevalence 262–3
Metformin 31, 113, 253
  lactic acidosis and 111
  in obesity 213
  outcomes of patients with diabetes and chronic heart failure on 111–12
  in pre-diabetes 247–8
  in type 2 diabetes 268, 269–70, 271, 272, 273
Metoprolol 119
MICRO-HOPE 110, 231
Microalbuminuria 24–5, 148, 151–3, 271
Mitogen-activated protein kinase (MAPK) pathway 29
Morning (rebound) hyperglycaemia 267
Mortality
  causes 5–6
  clinical trials 101
  in coronary heart disease 6–8, **7**
  gender and 6–7
  gender differences 101–2
  in patients with chronic heart failure and diabetes 100–2
  population studies 100–1
  rates 1
MRFIT study 9, 10, 135, 139, 259
Multicentre Automatic Defibrillator Implantation Trial 84
Myocardial infarction 23, 27, 41–2, 43, 260
Myocardial perfusion imaging 39

Nateglinide 252, 268, 269
NAVIGATOR 252, 269
NCEP 259, 261, 263
NFκB 28, 204
NHANES 98, 99, 262
Niacin 188
Nicorandil 40
Nicotine replacement therapy (NRT) 211, 212
Nifedipine 232
Nisoldipine 145
Nitrates 40, 117
Nitric oxide (NO) 23, 28, 29
Nitric oxide synthase (eNOS) 23, 29
Nocturnal hypoglycaemia 267
Non-ST-elevation MI (NSTEMI) 76, 77
  revascularisation in 82–4
Non-SU secretagogues 269
Non-valvular atrial fibrillation (NVAF) 212–13
NORDIL 231
Nuclear stress testing 39
Nurses Health Study 9

OASIS 224
OASIS-5 76
Obesity 6, 22
  atherothrombosis and 228
  central 16, 139, 228
  hypertension in 139
  parameters associated with 16, *17*
Obstructive peripheral vascular diseases 39
Off-pump revascularisation 43
ONTARGET 156
OPTIMAAL trial 75
Orlistat 250–1, 253

Pacemaker therapies 120
Partial anterior circulation infarcts (PACI) **179**
PCI-CURE trial 56, 57, 70–1
PEACE 41
Percutaneous coronary intervention (PCI) 37, 42, 44
  drug therapy and 56–9
  stenting with 52–3
  vs surgical revascularisation 55
Percutaneous transluminal coronary angioplasty (PTCA) 44, 47–8

Perindopril   40, 187, 216
Peripheral arterial disease (PAD)   5, 6,
    199–218
  acute limb ischaemia   209
  clinical features   205–9
  diabetic vs non-diabetic   **200**, 200
  future therapy   217
  gangrene   208
  hyperglycaemia and   201–3
  intermittent claudication   205–7
  lower extremity revascularisation
      209–10
  medical therapy   210–17
  molecular mechanisms   203–5, *204*
  pathogenesis   200–5
  pathophysiology of glycaemic vascular
      injury   203–5
  rest pain and critical ischaemia   208–9
  risk factors for amputation   199–200
  risk factors in patients with diabetes
      201
  secondary prevention   210
  therapeutic angiogenesis   217
Peroxisome proliferator activated receptor-γ
    (PPAR-γ) agonists   114, 249, 270
Peroxynitrite   29
PERSUADE   110
Phenformin   111, 273
Pioglitazone   59, 114, 115, 270,
    271, 273
Plaque burden   38
Plasminogen activator inhibitor-1 (PAI-1)
    29, 270
Polycystic ovarian syndrome (PCOS)   26
Post Coronary Artery Bypass Graft Trial
    230
Post-stroke hyperglycaemia (PSH)
    180–1
Posterior circulation infarcts (POCI)   **179**
Postprandial glucose regulators   269
PRAGUE-2   81–2
Pravastatin   230
Pre-diabetes
  risk of cardiovascular disease in
      243–4
  screening for   252–3
Presyncope   38
Prevention of diabetes   240–54
  intervention trials   245–52, *246*
PRISM-PLUS   76–7
Pro-inflammatory state   25, 26

PROactive   115, 271, 273
PROGRESS   187, 216
Propanolol   120
PROSPECT   54
PROSPER   230
Prostacyclin   23, 28
Prostaglandins   225
Protein C   28
Protein kinase C   106, 203
PURSUIT   77, 78

Quinapril   41

RALES   117
Ramipril   40, 187, 251
Rancho Bernardo Study   12
Reactive oxygen species (ROS)   29, 106
Reaven's syndrome, *see* Metabolic syndrome
Rebound hyperglycaemia   267
Receptor for AGEs (RAGEs)   29–30
Recombinant tissue plasminogen activator
    (rt-PA)   182
RECORD   272
RENAAL   110, 147, 152, 154
Renin–angiotensin–aldosterone system
    (RAAS)
  effect of abnormalities of glucose and
      insulin on   105
Renin–angiotensin system
  blockade   154–6, 187, 251–2
  in peripheral arterial disease   216–17
  role of   147–8
  stroke and   187
Renal artery stenosis   148, 217
Renal disease as cause of death   6
RESOLVD   **98**, 102, 103, *104*, 117
Reteplase   71
Retinopathy   5, 108, 213
Revascularisation for acute coronary
    syndromes   79–84
  in NSTEMI   82–4
  in STEMI   79–82
  stent thrombosis   84
RIKS-HIA   82
Rimonabant   274
RITA   44
RITA-3   83–4
Rosiglitazone   59, 114, 115, 116, 142, 253,
    270, 271, 272, 273
Ruboxistaurin   205

St Vincent declaration 1
Sarcoplasmic/Endoplasmic-Reticulum
    Ca^{2+}-ATPase 2α (SERCA2α)
    106, 107
SAVE trial 74
Scavenger pathway 22
SCD-HeFT **98**, 120
SCOPE 158
Selectin 226
SHEP 143, 186, 231
Silent ischaemia 38
Simvastatin 189, 230
Single-photon emission computed
    tomography (SPECT) 39
SIRIUS 53, 54
SIRTAX 55
Skeletal muscle and insulin resistance 104
Smoking
    atherothrombosis and 228
    in peripheral artery disease 210–12
Sodium reabsorption, renal 23
SOLVD **98**, 101, 117
Spironolactone 117
ST-elevation MI (STEMI) 71
    revascularisation in 79–82
Standardised mortality ratio (SMR) 4–5, 6,
    7, 8, 9, 11
Steno-2 Study 233, *234*
Stents
    vs CABG 51–2
    for coronary artery disease 50–3
    drug-eluting 53–5
    PCI with 52–3
    restenosis after 53
    revascularisation in thrombosis 84
STOP-2 158, 231
STOP-NIDDM 249, 272
Streptokinase 69, 71
Stress echocardiography 39
Stress hyperglycaemia 84
Stress testing 39
Stroke 39
    burden 176
    cognitive impairment and dementia in
        191–2
    definition 175–6
    diabetes as risk factor for 176–8
    hyperglycaemia and ischaemic cerebral
        damage 181–2
    intensive blood pressure lowering 187–8
    intracranial 10, 11

    ischaemic, non-haemorrhagic 11
    management of diabetes and
        hyperglycaemia following 182–5
    management of hyperglycaemia 183–5
    prevention in diabetic patients 185–90
    prognosis 178–80
    subarachnoid 10, 11
    in type 2 diabetes 9
Sudden death 223
Sulphonylureas 31, 111, 119, 268–9
    incidence of chronic heart failure in
        patients with diabetes 114
    mortality and 113–14
Superoxide ion 29
Surgical revascularisation, complications
    after 43–4
Sympathetic nervous system (SNS)
    effect of abnormalities of glucose and
        insulin on 105
    insulin resistance and 104
Syncope 38
Syndrome X, *see* Metabolic syndrome
SYST-EUR 142, *143*, 231

TACTICS 83
TARGET 58
Target lesion revascularisation (TLR) 51
TAXUS-IV 54
Telmisartan 155
Tetrahydrobiopterin 29
Thiazides 151, 156–7, 159, 251
Thiazolidinediones (glitazones) 31, 59,
    114–17
    cardiac structure and function 116
    cohort studies 115–16
    contraindication 116–17
    in pre-diabetes 248–9
    in type 2 diabetes 268, 270–2,
        273–4
Thienopyridine 58
Thorax Centre, Rotterdam 50
Thrombolysis 71–3
Ticlopidine 212
TIMI 72, 73, 83
Tirofiban 57, 58, 78, 83
Tissue plasminogen activator (tPA) 71
TNF 204
TNF-α 29, 229
Tolbutamide 268
Total anterior circulation infarcts (TACI)
    179

Transient ischaemic attack 175–6
  see also Stroke
Triglyceride intolerance 21
Triglyceride, plasma 20
TRIPOD 248
Troglitazone 59, 116, 270
Type 1 diabetes
  benefits of good glycaemic control in
    264–6
  causes of death from 5–6
  cohort studies 2, 3–4
  microalbuminuria in 152
  mortality from cardiovascular disease
    8–9, **9**
  treatment of 264–6
  weight gain and improved glycaemic
    control 266
Type 2 diabetes
  atherosclerosis and vascular disease in
    16–32
  cohort studies 2–3
  coronary artery disease in 223–7
  microalbuminuria in 152–3
  mortality from cardiovascular disease
    9–10, **10**
  stroke in 9
  treatment of 268–74

UKPDS 22, 99, 100, 109–10, 112–14, 119,
    135, 137, 143, 150, 177, 186, 187,
201–2, 213–15, 232, 242, 261, 268,
    270, 272
Ulcers, ischaemic 208

VA-HIT 214, 230
VACSS 42
VAL-HeFT **98**, 120
VALIANT 74–5, *75*
Valsartan 75, 152, 252, 269
VALUE 158
Vascular cell adhesion molecules (V-CAM)
    204
Vascular dementia 191, 192
Vascular endothelial growth factor (VEGF)
    106–7, 217
Vasocrine signalling 29
Ventricular arrhythmia 38
Verapamil 73, 145, 151
Very-low-density lipoprotein (VLDL) 20,
    21, 226
Von Willebrand factor 28

Warfarin 212–13
White cell count 25
WHO Multinational Study of Vascular
    Disease in Diabetes 3, 4, 11
WOSCOPS 26

XENDOS 250